NATURALLY HEALING AUTISM

The Complete Step-by-Step Resource Guide for Parents Includes Autism Prevention

KAREN THOMAS, C.M.T, C.S.T.-D

Pylorus Press

Dedicated to my son Jacob and my daughter Carly for always being my best teachers and for allowing me their trust.

ISBN: 978-0-9962363-1-7

Cover design by Debbie O'Byrne

www.naturallyhealingautism.com

Where parents go to find the natural resources they need to help heal their children from the symptoms of autism.

CONTENTS

SECTION III: THE HOW—3 STEPS TO WELLNESS

DISCLAIMER

By agreeing to the terms set forth below and using the information from this book or website, www.naturallyhealingautism.com, you release and hold harmless Karen Thomas, Naturally Healing Autism, and all of it's affiliates, agents, members, supporters, and staff from any damages resulting from your subsequent contact with any information or practitioner listed in this work, or thereof.

The information herein is provided for educational purposes only. This information is not intended to be a substitute for informed medical advice or care provided by your own physician or other qualified medical professional.

You should not use this information to diagnose or treat any health problems, disease, or illnesses without consulting your own physician or other qualified medical professional.

The Food and Drug Administration has not evaluated the statements regarding the products and services in this book. These products and services are not intended to diagnose, treat, cure, or prevent any disease.

If you rely on any information provided by Naturally Healing Autism, www.naturallyhealingautism.com, authors, Karen Thomas, Karen Thomas' authors, or other content providers whose information appears on this website or in this book at their request, you do so solely at your own risk.

All the service providers appearing in this book are independent practitioners and are to be used at your own personal discretion and wisdom.

The practitioner and website directory is intended solely to provide basic information concerning practitioners and products to be used at your own discretion. Before selecting any practitioner or product, please make appropriate inquiries and consult with other sources.

ACKNOWLEDGEMENT

I would like to acknowledge all of the great parents who try so hard every day to make their child's life happier and healthier. I personally know the challenge and the perseverance you go through.

PREFACE

The definition of "recovery" is to regain health. Autism is a biological disorder, not a mental illness, and can therefore be healed.

As other moms in my community began to recognize the changes in my son and to hear me talk about treating my daughter's stomach pain and gluten allergies, I began getting approached on a regular basis. With almost 30 years in the holistic health field, I could offer them remedies that they knew were natural and safe.

Even in the grocery store, a mom would come up to me with questions. As I began to answer, she would hurriedly pull out a piece of paper from her purse, usually an old receipt, and write on the back of it while I spewed out information. This type of encounter became so regular that I finally realized I had to write a book. I wanted to have it all written down in an easy-to-follow step-by-step guide specifically for moms.

The number of children diagnosed with autism has more than doubled since 2002. The Center for Disease Control (CDC) now reports that for every group of 68 children, one has autism! This is not a sudden genetic issue, neither has the diagnostic ability of health professionals gotten that much better. We have an epidemic on our hands, and it is time we do something about it—now.

One morning, after I dropped my daughter off at school, I overheard a woman telling a friend that her young daughter was undergoing tests at Stanford Medical Center for stomach problems. After getting tubes pushed down her throat, and many other costly tests, they found nothing. The child was sent home with Maalox. That was it.

I couldn't help wondering about the possibility of food allergies, gluten intolerance, parasites, and liver congestion. All of which could be found without much cost and definitely without bodily invasion or trauma to the child.

I offered her information about how to get testing done at top quality labs that I know of (labs where they don't miss things) and more specific information including possible natural treatments for any illnesses, if found. She was so grateful. I cannot tell you how often I run into this kind of need and how many people are searching for answers.

A mom will do anything to help her child. If there is even a possibility that something will help, it is worth trying. She will keep forging ahead, no matter the cost.

Not everyone can afford all of the expensive therapies that doctors suggest, especially when therapies don't work. Many people do not have health insurance or do not wish to see only the providers on their plan. Some would prefer to save the time and money on tests and diagnostics because they think that they could diagnose themselves from home if they only knew how.

It is crucial that we heal the causes that exist, not mask symptoms. Symptoms help us know what might be wrong. In order to make it right, the body must be built back up on a solid foundation. While no two people are alike and no two people need exactly the same thing, there are certain principles that we all must follow. The natural approach is a way of building the system back up from the core, or the cause, rather than a way to mask a symptom.

I have spent countless hours and dollars weeding through products in order to find the ones that are most helpful and that work the best. Many moms have approached me because they know the success I have had through my research. They are looking for answers and they need guidance. The information I compiled grew to such an extent that it could fill even the longest receipt a mom might pull out of her purse. This reminded me constantly that I needed to put everything into an easy-to-read guide that I could hand to those who needed and wanted it. This, mom, is your handbook.

As we well know, mom is expected to be the main practitioner for the family. No one cares more for your child or spends more time with your child than you do. Mom is up in the middle of the night nursing a fever, a cough, or a panic attack. Mom administers the majority of the vitamins and medications. No one knows better what is truly going on than you. This is why you need to be the most educated.

We're not told before having children that parenthood requires having a sort of medical degree. Even those whose children do not have autism may find themselves in the middle of some very trying times, wishing they knew what to do for their ailing child. Often, too much trust is put into a practitioner who has less of an idea about what is going on with your child than you do. As a result, the practitioner ends up guessing at a prescription that has negative side effects and that only makes things worse.

INTRODUCTION

After seeing so many moms go through the same struggles I did, I knew I had to share the blueprint that healed my own child, so that they could heal theirs. This book is the result of eight years of research and six years of writing. I hope this guide inspires others to take action! I know there will always be more to add, but this book is thorough and timeless.

Autism is the fastest growing developmental disorder in the world. If one in 68 children has autism, that is equivalent to one diagnosis every 20 minutes in the United States. There are many neurodevelopmental conditions, but autism is the fastest growing. The database from the state of California reports that autism rates in the state have increased 1,000% since 1990. More than half of a million people have autism.

It takes time, effort, and money to study, utilize, and figure out the best health balance for your child. It is an art. No two individuals are exactly alike. What works for one person may have to be completely modified to work for another. Many of us have more than one child. We also must take care of ourselves and, often, other family members at the same time. At least, I hope you are taking care of yourself! You may discover that your child's health needs may very well be yours too. Stress can deplete us all, and we have to take very good care not to let it do damage.

A friend of mine who has a child on the Spectrum once said to me, "Unless you have a child like this of your own, you have no idea what it's like." I never forgot that because it is so true.

The majority of information in this book comes from personal experience. All the members of my family have benefited in some way from the bulk of information that is written here. Let me be clear that the information in this book is not just for people with a diagnosis of some kind. I simply wanted to be sure that it got into the hands of those who have been given one. The need to balance the biology of the body, and therefore, the brain (since they are so interconnected), heightens greatly for those who have been diagnosed with an Autism Spectrum Disorder and all that that implies. Many children today who were once diagnosed with autism no longer have any symptoms and are living as typical kids going to mainstream schools with no diagnosis or services needed.

HOW TO USE THIS BOOK

The focus is on natural resources and self-care. When I asked other moms what they wanted from a book they all said simplicity. What they need is a guide to what to do and how to do it. I strove to provide enough information without making it overwhelming. I have most often referred to the term "him" for your child for the sake of simplicity in writing. I want to be clear that this in no way means that I do not understand that there are many girls with autism, as well as boys.

Some people are more linear minded and want to know more scientific information, others just want to know how to do it—now. For this reason, I have divided the book in half: the first half is more scientific and includes the "what and why" information, and the second half includes the "how to". This way you can get going with the stages of healing at the same time as you go back and fill in the rest of the blanks for yourself.

First of all, relax. This information does not have to be overwhelming. I want you to know that you can do this. I have chosen to provide just enough information so that the importance of what you are reading about can be understood. I do not give every minute detail of every study. If I did this, the book would be five times as long as it is. Too much information tends to overwhelm those who are already overwhelmed. Many moms would put the book down and never return to it. The greatest thing you can do for your child is to read the information and put it into action!

As with anything, you must be sure a product is right for you. This is an art. We will go over how to begin and where to go if the results are not what you hoped for. What worked at first for one of my children did not work for the other, but I was able to figure it out in the end. There will be different avenues to take and, as the main caregiver, you will use your instincts, along with the occasional help of a practitioner, to decide where to go next. If it is safe, it cannot hurt to try it. Dosages and frequencies of dosages vary per individual. Keeping a journal is a helpful way to remember what is working and what is not.

The information in this book can be of great benefit to anyone. I emphasize children because I see so many who act out or are made to feel like something is wrong with them. They are being fed Ritalin because their parents don't know what else to do. I am not criticizing those who have gone down this path, but rather, I would like to offer another method of treatment.

Know there is a better way and that you have more choices. It will require patience, especially in the beginning when your child's health has not yet been restored. There are even withdrawal symptoms from foods and the established bacteria in your gut. Sometimes it gets worse before it gets better, but it is worth it.

Even if the information in this book were to help your child just a little bit, ask yourself, "Would it be worth a try?" For the sake of your child, yourself, and the rest of your family, I hope your answer is yes. What I offer here are suggestions to help find and keep the balance. I know your life feels crazy. Wouldn't it be nice if it were a bit more peaceful?

Children today are entering a world filled with more toxins than ever before. The food we eat is not what it used to be, and neither is the air we breathe. We must protect our children so that they can thrive and become the person they were born to be!

It is my heartfelt passion to share the information that has been so valuable to my family and, already to many others, with you. I have provided a lot of information. You will take from it what you need. When people get overwhelmed they just stop listening and they don't do anything. I don't want that to happen to you. *Move forward one step at a time and one issue at a time.*

Moms want to know what to do, but they also need to know how to do it. We're all extremely busy, overwhelmed, and many of us lack the funds to go through all of the costly trial and error. This book is a sum of the most needed information on Autism Spectrum Disorders. How do we know how to truly help someone unless we've walked through it ourselves?

When I asked parents what they wanted in a book, the answer was clear. They replied, "The books that are out there are too hard to read and too overwhelming." It was obvious to me that a book was needed for the layperson, the mom, dad, grandparent, or caregiver who could not only understand the information in a book about holistic health, but who could use the information easily too.

I have done my best to provide scientific information while still keeping it as simple as possible. My real goal is simplicity. I will provide a summary of the information at the end of each chapter, and a quick guide is offered in the final pages. If you feel compelled to jump right to the quick guide, then please do so. The most important factor is that you and your child get the information and that you *use it.* I hope you have as much success as I did and that, someday, you can share it with me. Please let me know. You can email me at info@naturallyhealingautism.com. To assist you with finding the products you need, I have listed many of them on my website and have included a link to them. They are under "healthy home products" at www.naturallyhealingautism.com.

TOO MUCH TESTING

I would like to clearly say that I believe the testing for autistic children has been blown out of proportion, not to mention the expense and the trauma to the child. I like to avoid a blood draw whenever possible, and the added expense. I have offered ways to test that are mostly non-invasive such as muscle testing, saliva, urine, and hair analysis. This is only necessary when and where you feel it would be helpful for you as a parent to know specific information.

We know that all of our kids are low in omega 3 fatty acids, B vitamins, magnesium and their liver enzymes are going to be out of balance. The liver supplement I mention in this book is safe for just about anyone, and can only assist the health of the liver when used in the right dosages. You will learn to muscle test for a product's bioavailability in your child and individual dosage levels for his particular needs. My point is: don't think that every time you see a test you have to do it, especially if your child's symptoms are obvious. There is a strong list of various natural practitioners to help you, so relax. What you do not know right now you will be learning shortly, and all of your family members and friends can benefit from your new found knowledge.

WHAT IS AUTISM AND ASPERGER'S SYNDROME?

In case you are new to all of this, and perhaps reading about autism for a friend or loved one, let's begin with the basics. Generally, the symptoms of autism refer to a difficulty processing emotions and a heightened sensitivity to external stimuli.

Autism is defined as the autism spectrum disorder, or ASD, because the symptoms range in severity from profound disabilities like lack of speech; uncontrollable body movement such as spinning, or head banging; to milder forms like Asperger's syndrome.

Asperger's Syndrome is also known as high functioning autism. Those with Asperger's syndrome commonly have an obsessive interest, high intellectual ability, but lower social awareness. The child may seemingly have a lack of emotion or an inability to love. They do feel emotions and, in fact, are often quite sensitive, but they have an impaired ability to communicate their feelings. Any way you look at it, it is simply a difference in the way the brain is wired.

In 2014, after almost two decades, the American Psychiatric Association decided that the term Asperger's is to be removed from the psychiatrists' Diagnostic and Statistical Manual (DSM) of Mental Disorders. The DSM is regarded as one of the most influential references for the psychiatric profession around the world. The term "Asperger's disorder" will not appear in the DSM-5, the latest revision of the manual. Instead, everyone with symptoms of autism, at any level, will now be put under the newly added umbrella term "autism spectrum disorder." The "spectrum" is quite broad. Each child has his or her own unique symptoms from very severe to very mild. Dropping the term "Asperger's" was quite ill received, especially by moms.

The real problem is in its current epidemic-like rise in numbers. In 2000, the CDC established an Autism and Developmental Disabilities Monitoring program (ADDM). In 2002, one in every

150 children was diagnosed with autism. In 2006 the number rose to one in 110. By 2008, the CDC released the current number: one in every 88 children was now diagnosed on the Autism Spectrum. From 2002 to 2008, the number rose 78%! Currently, in 2014, the most recent number released by the CDC is one in 68. An estimate has been made of one in two by 2025!

Symptoms are most often seen after the age of 3. The earliest known diagnosis is 18 months. It can be hard to tell prior to this age. It is four and a half times more prevalent in boys than in girls. One in 42 boys is diagnosed with an Autism Spectrum Disorder verses one in every 189 girls.

Some children that are diagnosed on the Autism Spectrum are properly treated and no longer exhibit symptoms. Let's look at what's going on and what can be done.

PROLOGUE: HOW I GOT HERE

When I began seeking help for my son, it was easy to see that I had to educate myself on what to do for him. I have been in the holistic health field for over 25 years and have learned enough to know that there are alternatives choices that do work, without the harmful side effects found in so many pharmaceutical drugs.

There is often no need for drugs. Most prescription medications numb the mind and injure the body. The side effects alone are enough to make us say, "There has got to be a better way," and there is.

THE JOURNEY TO THE DIAGNOSIS

My son, Jacob, was born in 1996. From a very young age, he required that we discipline him and we had a lot of trouble doing so. Of course, others would say that we were just not being tough enough when it came to consequences. I always felt that there was more to the picture. Because he was my first child, I didn't have anything else to base his behavior on.

My husband noticed that somewhere, just before the age of three, Jacob's personality changed. Our pediatrician suggested that we give Jacob the Hepatitis B vaccination at the age of two. After receiving this vaccination Jacob went from being a happy boy to a much more serious and introverted one. He was outgoing enough to make friends but being social seemed to be a bit awkward for him. Academically, he was exceptionally bright so we knew he was intelligent enough to understand us. What happened and why was disciplining him such a difficult task? It felt like he was purposely ignoring us. We just could not get through to him.

One day, I asked Jacob a question. He was sitting on the couch watching television so I thought he didn't hear me. I asked again and again, not in anger but in amazement. He was literally not hearing me. I had to walk over, stand in front of him, and get into his line of vision before he knew I was there. I realized that he was not just being ornery, but that there was more going on than I had previously thought. He was so hyper-focused that he could not hear me.

I began experimenting with him. I would ask a question when he was involved in a task and wait for a response. There would be none. We noticed how family members felt like we were just not good enough at disciplining him. Because he was our first child, we thought that maybe it was our fault. Perhaps it was something we were doing.

When he was angry, he would often act out violently. His preschool teacher had the same difficulties with him. When he entered kindergarten and the teacher approached us regarding Jacob's behavior once again, we decided to seek professional help.

We took Jacob to his first therapist when he was five years old. We needed guidance. We didn't know what to do. Over the next several years we would see many different therapists. No one seemed to have an answer for us. All we ever heard was that we should just have stronger disciplinary consequences, and they would give their suggestions, but nothing ever worked. As his tantrums and aggressive behavior grew with his age, we were, at times, exhausted.

We had moved to a new town, but carried the same problems with us. My husband worked out of town during the week and I was acting as a single mom with two kids, one who was most often out of control. I was desperate for help. I sought yet another therapist. In the third session, the counselor asked to speak to me privately and told me that he thought that Jacob had Asperger's syndrome. I said, "What's that?" He replied that he really didn't know much about it but that I should research it for myself.

The year was 2006. At the time, my local bookstores carried no information on the subject. As a Craniosacral therapist, I was continuing my education and was scheduled to be in Berkeley for a class. Berkeley is a large college town that has many bookstores. I walked into a small corner bookstore and asked if they had any books on Asperger's syndrome. The clerk said, "Yes, we have many. The owner's son has it." I do not believe in coincidences.

The first book I bought is still my favorite, even though I now own many on the subject. The title is, *A Parent's Guide to Asperger Syndrome and High Functioning Autism*, and it is written by Sally Ozonoff, Geraldine Dawson, and James McPartland.

As I read this book, I felt a sense of relief. I felt like they knew my son. After all these years I had finally found the answers I had been searching for. I had known all along that there was something more going on with him. I wasn't looking for a label; I was looking for answers so that I would know how to help him. If I didn't know how his mind worked and what he had been trying to deal with inside then how could I know what I could do for him?

Jacob didn't have all of the characteristics I read about, but he had some. I needed to know exactly what I could do for him. By knowing what characteristics of Asperger's he had, I would be able to help him more effectively as his parent.

Although labels may sometimes be necessary, we must also deviate from using them on a regular basis. People are simply wired differently. These types of children born today are gifted. They are ultrasensitive, multifaceted, multidimensional people. Perhaps we are watching evolution move faster than we ever imagined possible right before our very eyes. No one should be looked at as weird just because they're not like you. All they need is some acceptance of who they are and the way they are. After all, we want to be accepted the way we are, don't we?

All of the other therapists we had seen over the years had missed it completely. Asperger's can be missed and difficult to diagnose due to high functioning abilities unless you really know what you are looking for. Even PhDs in psychology miss it.

It is vital to seek a psychologist who is a *specialist* in the field of Asperger's and autism. I called a friend whose son I knew was on the Autism Spectrum and asked her which specialist I should take Jacob to. We soon had an appointment and a diagnosis. Jacob did indeed have Asperger's syndrome. The shock and the relief came all at once. We learned all of this only two months before his 11th birthday. Now, what to do?

Our therapist was leaving on maternity leave that day. We were given no guidance about what we should do except see a social therapist. The social therapist ended up telling me that we should put him on medication! There was no way I was going to do that. I have always believed in treating the causes, not masking symptoms with drugs and their potentially harmful side effects. We felt completely lost.

Our son also had other health issues concerning his stomach and his immune system. No one seemed to have answers for me about those problems either.

Throughout his life, Jacob had suffered from stomach pain. We once found parasites and treated him for it, but there seemed to be more to it. When he was upset, he would experience so much stomach pain that he often ended up on the floor, doubled up in pain.

As we drove to a swimming lesson one day, he complained of his stomach hurting him. I didn't want him to go to the lesson but he really wanted to go. I had him run up and down the parking lot to prove to me that he was ok. He did and he seemed to be all right so we went into the lesson. In his first lap, he grabbed hold of the side of the pool and started screaming. I took him to the emergency room thinking maybe it was appendicitis. They took a blood sample that came up with a somewhat elevated white blood cell count. This indicates that the body is fighting some kind of infection. His symptoms had subsided, so they told me that we should just go home. I was still concerned but didn't seem to have much choice. They wouldn't do anything more for us, so we left.

That night Jacob woke at 2:00 a.m. screaming from stomach pain. Remembering how unhelpful they had been in the emergency room, I stayed and observed Jacob all night waiting until it was late enough in the morning for his doctor to be in. We went in that morning and, after pushing and prodding him for a few minutes, I was told it probably wasn't appendicitis but to observe him that day. I begged for at least a blood test but they refused because the doctor did not feel it was necessary! I thought, "What can it hurt to do a blood test?!"

Later that same day Jacob was still having stomach pain. I couldn't just wait around anymore to see what was going to happen. I called the doctor again pleading for a blood test at least. The reply was, "If you don't trust your doctor, then you should find a new one," and she hung up on me.

I wasn't interested in treating the ego of the doctor. I needed help from someone. We got into the car and drove once again to the emergency room. I told them of the events of the past 24 hours. They put Jacob into a gown and a nurse took his temperature and blood pressure. When the doctor came in, I explained what had happened again: his doctor would not give a blood test, so I had come here for one. That was my biggest mistake. The doctor left the room for a few minutes. When he came back, he refused to do any tests. I don't know if he made any calls or just decided on his own not to go against what another doctor had said to me previously. I learned later that a doctor will never go against another doctor's recommendation. Be careful what you say.

I thought to myself, "What am I doing here? This is so not my world. I am much more holistically oriented than this." I needed to know the cause of his pain so I could do something to heal it. Fear had gotten hold of me and I had reacted.

As the doctor continued to talk *at* me saying nothing of value, I stood up, pulled the gown off of Jacob, helped him get dressed, and we walked out of the hospital. I was furious. However, I am grateful for that experience. What it did was fuel my fire. I was determined to find out what was the matter with my son *and to fix it naturally.* It was clear to me that I was on my own. Being more interested in holistic health, I headed straight to the health food store and that's where my research for this journey began.

I will now begin to tell you my reasoning behind the purpose of writing this book. I feel compelled to share what I have learned regarding a holistic approach to creating healthier, happier children today.

How I wish I knew before I ever became pregnant what I know now. This is what I wish to share with you in hopes that you and your children will benefit from it in any way that you can.

There will be bits and pieces to pull from the information I am about to give you. Please always go with your own gut instinct when deciding what to do. If you have a strong feeling that a piece of this information can benefit your child or yourself, then please follow that. If you ask your doctor about it and find that they are against it and your own gut says, "But this feels right", then go with that!

I am not telling you that you should not listen to your doctor. What I am telling you is that if someone is closed off to a new piece of information or is clinging to *one* study in particular, yet there are people getting better who are trying the new technique, then it may be time for a second opinion. I am a strong believer in second opinions and of people following their own instincts instead of being led by someone else or bullied. Seek out the name of someone who has a good reputation and who your friends and relatives have gone to successfully. Find someone you feel you can trust, and who will listen to you. It is OK to doubt what I say and do more research on your own to verify any information you feel compelled to do so on.

I have been through what you are going through. A mother will do anything for her child. She is the one who cares for the child the most and who knows best what is going on with her child day and night, seven days a week. We will do anything necessary, like dipping into the college fund so that you can continue getting the remedies needed to help your child get better. We will stop at nothing, knowing that we can make a difference and help our child to get better. The financial pressure and the frustrations thicken, but we still forge ahead. Moms also seem to hold the weight of responsibility when it comes to the outcome for their child.

I have weeded out many products and treatments that I found were not of value and I have been able to find the ones that are. It was worth every minute of my time and every penny. It is my hope that the information in this book will save you both.

Autism will fool you. The opposite of what you think might happen, will happen. It can take time, but your child can get better. The sooner your child is treated, the better. A one year old is 100 times easier to treat than a ten year old. However, as I just mentioned, my own son was almost 11 when he was diagnosed. It's never too late. Autism is a biological disorder, it is not a mental illness, and therefore, it can be healed. There's no time to waste. Let's go.

By the way, Jacob currently has no special needs, runs his own life away at college, is social, happy, healthy, and is doing great now!

SECTION I:

WHERE TO FIND HELP

CHAPTER 1

MUSCLE TEST RESPONSE

The first person to look to for help is you. You know your child best and you are his or her best advocate. No one else, not even a doctor, is with your child seven days a week, 24 hours a day. Others do not see the changes you do. Do not be afraid to take charge. One of the first tools to learn is muscle test response or muscle testing.

Muscle test response, or muscle testing, is not testing the muscle, but the energy flowing through the reflexes of the body and the response associated with it. It is also referred to as Autonomic Response Testing. Autonomic Response Testing is the more appropriate term, as it does not imply testing of any kind, but only a response instead. For the sake of clarity, I will use the term muscle testing here.

Muscle testing uses the body's own electrical currents. If the circuitry along a pathway has too much energy or too little, the body acts as though a fuse has been blown. This tells us there is an energy imbalance, which can, or already has, caused a health problem in the body. Here we find the root cause and protocol necessary to help the patient, not just something to treat the symptoms.

The body can be tested to see if an issue is chemical, emotional, neurological, structural, or circulatory. It can be used for assessments in personal protocol. As no two people are the same, it may help to determine what the body still needs in supplementation. Be mindful of the suggested dosages of medication as the body's needs change over time. Proper vitamin ratios are important. Too much of one vitamin can cause a deficiency in another.

The body will instantly turn weak in response to negative emotional attitudes and stress, just as it does in reaction to physical properties.

LEARNING TO TEST

First, be sure that the person being tested is well hydrated by a pure water source. Choose which muscle you are going to test. The most common way to perform a muscle test is to have a person hold his or her arm straight out in front of them at about eye level. Be sure that the arm is completely straight and that the elbow is not bent at all. When a substance is beneficial to the system, it will test strong. If the substance is negative for the health of the system, then the muscles will test weak. Any muscle can be tested and surrogates can even be used to do this (see surrogate testing below).

Using only a few fingers on the person's wrist say "resist," and test his or her strength by gently pushing down. Test for strength of the muscle alone before adding any substance so that you know your base point. Also, remember that this is not a competition. A couple of your fingers will do the job. Lightly press downward on the back of the person's wrist and pay attention to the amount of strength the muscle shows you. Then stop. There is no need to keep pressing or to push harder. The person's initial strength is what you are looking for. This is your baseline strength point to use. If they are weakened by a product or object, the body won't lie.

Once you have your baseline strength point, put the substance (i.e. a vitamin, a piece of bread), into either of the person's hands, on his or her body anywhere, even in the person's pocket or sock. It works the same way. This is good when someone cannot hold an item. Be sure to retest the same muscle (in this case, the arm). If their muscle is weak where it once was strong, you know that the substance you are testing for is not good for them right now. I say "right now" because our bodies can change over time. Examples are after gut cleansing or heavy metal detoxification the body is much stronger. Muscle testing is a great tool for testing allergy related items such as various foods. Retest as often as you feel necessary.

There is a lot of good information about muscle testing in a question and answer forum found at www.curezone.com/forums/am.asp?i=1749436.

SURROGATE MUSCLE TESTING

Surrogate testing is great for babies, young children, the very weak, someone who is completely passive, or who is even asleep. Two test people are needed for this. One acts as the surrogate and is muscle tested first. Find out the person's strength so that you will have your baseline. He or she will then touch the person to be tested with one of his or her hands anywhere on the patient's body.

Direct contact is best but not necessary. It is important that the person being tested is touched over an area of natural clothing, such as cotton. Polyester and some synthetic fabrics can interfere with testing.

Next, the person who is the tester will place a substance into the hand of the surrogate while he or she is touching the child. Then the surrogate is tested again. If he or she is weak now where he or she was strong before then the substance is not good for the child. This can also be used to help find appropriate dosages.

ONE EXAMPLE STUDY

Here is an example of a study where the unknowing mind does not play a part in the outcome of the response to muscle testing. In an audience of 1,000 people, 500 envelopes were passed out holding artificial sweetener in them and another 500 contained organic vitamin C. The audience alternated the envelopes among themselves and muscle tested each other. When the envelopes were opened they saw that those containing the artificial sweetener were the ones that made everyone go weak. The envelopes with the organic vitamin C proved to test strong for all.

The prevalence of muscle testing has grown tremendously since the early 1960's when it was introduced by Dr. George Goodheart, a well-known Applied Kinesiologist (AK). Originally, muscle testing was referred to as AK. AK doctors are licensed healthcare professionals.

In the late 1960's, Dr. John Thie wrote the book, *Touch For Health*, www.touch4health.com. This book advocated a drug-free approach and began a movement to use the same general principals and reflex stimulation methods as AK. Dr. Thie's book was so influential because it was written for the layperson. This meant anyone, licensed or not, could learn how to use AK at their own discretion. Today, over 80 forms of muscle testing are used. It is important to find someone you trust, but also to know that you can learn the simple principles and general uses yourself. It can easily be done by anyone.

Muscle testing can be very helpful when deciding which supplements to purchase. There may be several different brands, strengths, and dosages of the same supplement from which to choose. Ask an employee at the store to muscle test you for a supplement. It is easy to teach muscle testing quickly, right there in the store. Have an employee muscle test you for a baseline strength with a particular muscle such as the arm straight out in front of you (as described above). Next, have the employee muscle test you again, using the same muscle tested the first time, while you are holding the supplement of choice in your hand. If you remain strong the supplement shows to be beneficial for your system. If your muscle goes weak it is not good for you right now. I say "right now" because as our bodies strengthen over time with detoxification and gut cleansing we can ingest various foods, and supplements, or use materials that we once could not.

To find the right dosage amount, first find the product that tests strong. As the employee holds the product, ask and muscle test with each question: "Is the dosage one per day?" Test the muscle and stop. "Two per day?" Test again and stop. "Three per day?" Continue until the muscle goes from strong to weak. The last one that answered strong is the answer to your question.

OCCASIONAL UNDEFINED RESULTS

There can be undefined results. This can be due to factors such as an imbalance in the cerebral hemispheres in the brain, or cause and effect by a practitioner who has the same ailment or toxic load as the patient. The clinician must be healthier than the client.

If you suspect that you or your doctor have any of the same issues as your child, the responses may be affected. In return, the patient can have the same effect on the examiner. This is why no two examiners may find the same results on the same patient, unless the patient is healthy and toxin free. If the results vary with your doctor you may want to seek another for a second assessment.

This is not meant to leave you concerned regarding its use. It is very effective. If you find that your results vary I would suggest finding a practitioner who is well educated and experienced in muscle testing. I find that I get clear results when I test my daughter, but when I test my son the results are sometimes unclear. This is likely the result of a cause and effect relationship between the two of us. I may carry in my tissues some of the same issues as he does.

Holistic practitioners, such as chiropractors and acupuncturists, commonly use muscle testing as a reliable and important assessment tool, and they become proficient at it. Some doctors in mainstream medicine are beginning to take advantage of this method due to the growing knowledge of its usefulness and accuracy.

There are those who try to disclaim it, but I, and millions of others, have found it to be immensely helpful for many years. Throughout this book, I urge you not to let others tell you what you should believe or not believe.

TESTING POINTS AND ORGANS ON THE BODY

Always place the *back* of your hand over the area to be tested. The back of the hand is non-confrontational and therefore, non-threatening to the system. This can be helpful to remember when your child is having a tantrum or when you initially approach anyone or anything, including animals. There are several different points on the body that can be checked for various issues.

Remember that it is a good idea to be specific and ask pointed questions. Many points are close to each other. For example, ask, "Is this a parasite issue? Is this the flu virus?" Place the back of your hand over the point and test the child using only one or two of your fingers on the wrist of his outstretched arm (elbow straight), or using a surrogate for testing, you may check some of the most commonly needed points. When you are testing, think and ask about what you are testing for:

- Candida: directly over your child's belly button
- viruses (general): one inch below the belly button
- viruses (flu): one inch to the left of the belly button (ask and think about the flu)

- parasites: one and a half inches left of the child's belly button (ask and think about the parasite)
- bacteria (for colds): the area just below the angle of the jawbone (close to where it meets the ear lobe), on the patient's right side
- lymph: place the back of your hand in front of the left pectoral region. It is the upper soft spot there just medial to the armpit.
- allergies: point the index and middle fingers toward the medial portion of each eye, one on each side of the bridge of the nose
- If the left cheek tests weak it is because of an issue with the body's organs. The organs must be tested individually if this comes up. Seek the help of a qualified practitioner when necessary.
- liver: since the liver and gallbladder are so close to one another ask, "liver?" as you place the back of your hand over the area just under the lowest rib on the patient's right side.
- gallbladder: just medial to the space tested for the liver ask, "gallbladder?"
- stomach: directly center, below the sternum, or center of the stomach
- small intestine: right side of abdomen
- large intestine: left side of abdomen (think about the colon)
- adrenals: cup your hand and place your fingers inside of the left armpit with your thumb reaching just in front of it.
- kidneys: Place the back of your hand on the back just below the last rib, (think kidneys).
- thyroid: back of hand over the lower portion of the throat

To see my example video of muscle testing for bacterial colds, viruses, and allergies go to http://youtu.be/1krEhJ4dzJM.

FUN WITH LEARNING

Keep practicing on everyone in your family. Have fun learning how to do it. One test that I enjoy doing to disbelievers, or anyone for that matter, is asking the patient to say, "My name is (their own name)," and then I test his or her strength. The person's strength will be strong. Then I ask them to say, "My name is (using a name other than their own)," and the person will test weak.

You can practice on family members and on your child. Learn to test your child before going to see your practitioner and see if the answers the practitioner gets are the same as the ones you got. This is a good way to build self-confidence as a tester. This also helps you to prevent reading any information you get incorrectly when you are a novice. Practitioners are usually happy to help you learn.

Three sources to help you find a practitioner who uses muscle testing or autonomic response testing are:

- www.crawellness.com;
- www.appliedkinesiology.com; and
- www.naet.com.

SUMMARY

Muscle testing, or muscle test response is an easy and effective way to test the body for substance tolerance, dosages, assimilation, and more. Anyone can learn how to do it, even you. Surrogate testing is even useful with infants, or people who are unable to be directly tested. Many practitioners such as chiropractors, acupuncturists, and even some medical doctors use muscle testing.

The products found in this chapter can be found at http://naturallyhealingautism.com/a-healthy-home/

CHAPTER 2

ALTERNATIVE THERAPIES AND PRACTITIONERS

To find a good holistic practitioner, look for referrals. Ask friends and family if they know anyone or have heard of anyone who is good. Going into a local health food store is a great way to find one too. Ask the employees or the owner if they have people in different fields that they recommend. I have given you some good resources to look into as well.

NATURAL ALLERGY ELIMINATION

One of the most important alternative techniques I have found for my children and myself has been natural allergy elimination or desensitization. It is a natural way to stop the immune system from over reacting to substances in both its internal environment and in the external environment. Millions of people suffer from environmental allergies and food allergies, but do not realize all of the culprits that cause them harm. The reaction to an allergen may not appear for up to 72 hours (three full days) after exposure. This can make it nearly impossible to determine what has triggered the response.

Common symptoms of allergens are:

- frequent abdominal cramps, gas, bloating, diarrhea, or constipation
- acid reflux or Gastroesophageal Reflex Disease (GERD), ulcerative colitis, or Crohn's disease
- joint pain, muscle aches, fibromyalgia, or chronic fatigue

- asthma, eczema, psoriasis, unexplained skin rashes, or swollen limbs
- extreme fatigue after meals
- depression
- brain fog, forgetfulness, lack of focus, short attention span, ADD or ADHD
- headaches or irregular heart beats
- itchy eyes, nasal congestion, sinus headaches, or sneezing
- frequent colds, flu, and respiratory infections

We know that allergies are just an overreaction of the immune system. When the immune system is battling imaginary issues, it is weak in its defense against common bacteria and viruses. It is the immune system's defense that gives us our symptoms.

Through muscle testing by our natural allergy desensitization practitioner I was shocked to find that at the age of 11 my son's body was having a constant immune reaction to measles. He had never had the measles except when he was vaccinated for it. What irony. The very action we took that we thought would immunize him for the potential virus put it into his body and was causing him harm. Prior to his vaccinations I did not have the knowledge about them that I do now. This book will help you on that journey. Thankfully, I had found this treatment, and could help undo the damage, and regain his health.

We also found that although my son was taking the highest quality, most bioavailable form of essential fatty acids, Captain's krill oil, his body was not processing or absorbing them. Essential fatty acids are a critical piece of healing and maintaining health for a child on the autism spectrum. Once he was treated, his body could assimilate the nutrients from the very same supplement and gain its benefits. Afterward, we all noticed how much calmer Jacob was on a regular basis. The brain requires essential fatty acids in order to function properly and stabilize mood, among other things. I will provide more detailed information about essential fatty acids later.

HOW DOES IT WORK?

Natural allergy elimination treatment combines kinesiology, homeopathy, and acupressure to determine which allergens you are sensitive to. This technique can be done on an individual of any age. The first appointment is about an hour and is used for assessment. The skilled practitioner will test your body's immune response by muscle testing or performing computerized testing while the patient contacts vials of homeopathic tinctures corresponding to serums that contain potential allergens.

Sensitivity levels are gauged from one to ten. These serums cover every base from foods, chemicals, various toxins, pollens, barometric pressure, electromagnetic fields, to your own animals' hair, supplements, medications, and much more. Supplements, medications, dust, or animal samples from your own home can be brought in for assessment and treatment too.

Once the allergens are found, future 30-minute sessions are scheduled. During treatment, the patient holds onto or touches the vial with the homeopathic allergen in it. The vial can also be laid on top of a person or put into the person's sock to hold it against the body. While the patient is in contact with the vial, the practitioner gently stimulates specific acupressure points along the spine in order to stimulate the central nervous system. Then acupressure points are stimulated on the arms and legs to open the rest of the meridians throughout the body. This opens the energy flow and allows the energy from the vials to flow through the body so that the body now recognizes that energy as safe.

Once this is complete the patient rests for fifteen minutes while in contact with the homeopathic vial containing the allergen. After the treatment is over the patient must stay out of contact with the allergen for a specific amount of time (see below). Once complete the body sees the energy of the molecule, but now knows it is safe and stays calm. It changes the old patterns of defense.

It is always a good idea to go in for a quick retest, via muscle testing, to be sure that the allergen has been cleared. This can be done the next day or the next week, but it is wise to be sure that the treatment worked properly on your body.

Afterwards, highly restricted diets are often no longer necessary. Once you are desensitized, you can eat or use the products, but do so with some discretion. My own daughter could not eat gluten without severe stomachaches prior to being desensitized. She now eats gluten without having any problems, unless she really overindulges. Even then, the reactions are mild compared to what they used to be. Remember that wheat, or gluten, is not a healthy foods as it once may have been. Through bioengineering of our crops they are no longer good for anyone, especially in large amounts.

The body will let you know if you have had too much of something through showing symptoms. Do not worry. This will rarely undo the treatment; it just lets you know your level of tolerance. Treatment is very individualized.

The allergy elimination technique has gone through three generations. All are generations are still available today. I will explain some of the important differences between the generations.

The first generation allergy elimination technique was developed by Dr. Devi S. Nambudripad. It is commonly known as Nambudripad's Allergy Elimination Technique or NAET.

NAET can only desensitize an individual for one allergen per appointment. If only one, two, or three allergens show up, then this is fine. The downside of this is/that commonly ten, twenty, or more allergens show up so it can take many more appointments, which mean more time and more money. The patient also needs to stay out of contact with the allergen for 24 hours after the treatment. That being said, NAET does work well, and my family has had great success with it but additional options do exist. Practitioners are easy to find as many have been trained over the years. To find one near you go to www.naet.com.

The second generation allergy elimination technique was developed by one of Dr. Nambudripad's students, Ellen Cutler. Dr. Cutler developed a refined program she calls BioSET. It is a combination of organ detoxification, enzyme therapy, and allergy desensitization. Muscle testing and homeopathic vials are not commonly used to identify allergens in BioSET. Instead, computer software is used to detect potential allergens to the system.

As the patient holds onto a small metal rod, his or her energies become connected with the computer program. Thousands of allergens have been programmed into the system. The practitioner uses a small probe on the palm of the hand to connect with the computer software system.

Once the allergens are found, the same acupressure points along the spine are stimulated. An additional benefit to this method is that multiple allergens can be desensitized in one treatment, taking less time and costing less money. The amount of time one stays away from the allergen after treatment varies per individual. For some, it may be a few hours, but for others it may need to be closer to 24 hours. For a BioSET practitioner near you go to www.drellencutler.com, and look under "BioSET system," or call (415) 384-0200.

The third generation allergy elimination technique is called Sensitivity Reduction Technique (SRT). This method was developed by Dr. Shari Tenpenny. Dr. Tenpenny is one of the country's most knowledgeable and outspoken physicians regarding vaccines and the right to refuse them. She has developed additional attributes to allergy desensitization. For more information please visit www.tenpennyimc.com.

SRT uses muscle testing and homeopathic vials, but has the additional benefit of using Chinese energy medicine balancing vials. It gives the body a new template. After the immune system has been told to stop doing what it has been doing incorrectly, it needs to be redirected to do something it is supposed to do instead. It is like telling a child not to do something. The child needs to be given an action that he or she can do or the child may begin doing something else that he or she is not supposed to do.

SRT is capable of desensitizing multiple allergen groups in one treatment. Usually a total of only one to six treatments are needed. Allergens can be done in groups and are done in a specific order called foundations. Foundations of the body build upon one another, so they must be done in order.

1. **Foundation one** is the immune system. It includes things in our internal environment that are always with us and that we cannot get rid of. These things include blood, lymph, urine,

saliva, glandular secretions, the immune system, and the central nervous system.

2. **Foundation two** is phenol compounds. These include things we are surrounded by and cannot permanently get away from. The main compounds we are exposed come from petroleum products, mostly plastics.
3. **Foundation three** is the molecules that make up our nutrition, such as proteins, fats, amino acids, vitamins, and minerals. Once these are addressed, we will see more digestion of more beneficial nutrients.

A three-hour wait time is all that is needed after a treatment. During this three-hour period, the patient must stay away from all foods and potential allergens. In comparison to the other treatments, this is a very short wait time. Due to deprogramming old cellular memory, after three hours the system knows the proper way to handle the energy from any of the treated allergens.

Many years before his SRT treatments, my son had been desensitized from gluten by our NAET practitioner. When retested, he was still clear, but tested positive, or allergic, to white flour. They seem so similar but have a different molecular makeup. Although green food coloring had come up years before, now red food coloring tested positive. It was the SRT treatment that picked up that my son's body was not processing essential fatty acids (EFA's), and she was able to balance his body so that it could now assimilate them. EFA's are crucial for optimum physical and mental health.

In studies of patients treated through SRT, 87% were still completely allergy-free five years later.

INTEGRATIVE/ALTERNATIVE MEDICAL DOCTORS

Integrative medical doctors are western medical doctors. The difference between western medical doctors and integrative medical doctors is that they integrative medical doctors have been trained in multiple proven therapies of both conventional medical applications and alternative medical treatments. The combination of integrative medicine and western medicine allows the doctor to have a broader perspective. A doctor who excels in both types of medicine can treat the individual as a whole with knowledge of natural, drug-free treatment sources. The philosophy is to heal the causes, not the symptoms.

Types of medicine employed by integrative medical physicians include:

- Western medicine
- Allopathic medicine
- Osteopathic medicine
- Regenerative medicine
- Holistic medicine
- Naturopathic medicine
- Functional medicine

For a medical doctor that focuses on the complimentary, alternative, and integrative body as a whole see the websites below.

How do I find another practitioner that offers alternative resources?

Integrative medicine practitioners are scattered across the country. You can find doctors in your area through the websites of the following professional organizations:

- American Academy of Osteopathy (AAO)
- The Cranial Academy
- American Academy of Environmental Medicine (AAEM)
- American Academy for the Advancement of Medicine (ACAM)
- International College of Integrative Medicine (ICIM)
- Institute for Functional Medicine (IFM)
- American Holistic Medical Association (AHMA)
- American Board of Holistic Integrative Medicine (www.abihm.org)
- Academy of Integrative Health and Medicine (www.aihm.org)

ORTHOMOLECULAR MEDICINE

First theorized by double Nobel laureate Linus Paling, orthomolecular medicine is based on restoring the entire biochemical make-up specific to an individual using natural sources such as vitamins, minerals, amino acids, trace elements and fatty acids to restore optimum health. The distinctive differences of molecular medicine lie in its focus on genetic factors and how they affect all biochemical aspects specific to the individual.

For more information on orthomolecular societies internationally go to, www.orthomed.org.

MERIDIAN STRESS ASSESSMENT (MSA)

Meridian stress assessment (MSA) is a non-invasive tool that assists practitioners in learning what energy patterns are weak in the body. This is a computerized program similar to Dr. Cutler's approach described above. The practitioner tests the body using gentle probing of acupressure points on the feet and hands. The test will allow for assessment of organ weaknesses, allergens, chemical and heavy metal toxicity.

The MSA by Biomeridian is the only FDA approved class II system which assures both safety and effectiveness. It does not replace the need for blood or urine tests, but it does access meridians quickly and accurately to help with patient protocol during homeopathic, nutritional, or herbal supplementation. It assists with dosages including those of medications to ensure effectiveness, accuracy, and safety. For more information and studies go to www.biomeridian.com/meridian-stress-assessment.htm.

CHIROPRACTIC WITH MUSCLE RESPONSE TESTING

Many chiropractors who are proficient in muscle testing are also known as Contact Reflex Analysis (CRA) doctors. Other types of chiropractors who also use muscle testing are Applied Kinesiology (AK) doctors. I would suggest finding one who is skilled with this technique as it offers a far more comprehensive approach. It gives the ability to see the body as a whole rather than to just see the places that hurt on the body.

Assessment determines if an issue is caused by a chemical, structural, emotional, nutritional, or neurological imbalance.

Once this is determined, the practitioner will be able to assist in the protocol necessary to heal the body. Doctors are often well educated in nutritional analysis and can be of great assistance when this is indicated during the assessment. To find a practitioner skilled in CRA near you call (616) 669-5534, or go to www.crawellness.com. CRA Wellness also has a phenomenal line of nutritional supplements available at www.vervita.com. For an AK doctor see www.appliedkinesiology.com.

NATUROPATHIC DOCTORS

Naturopathic doctors are not medical doctors; they are primary care doctors. They combine modern science with nature. These doctors' protocols work to assist the body back into a natural state of health through its own innate abilities by treating the whole person and not just the symptoms. These physicians work in hospitals, clinics, and private practices. They combine modern science with nature. Their protocols work to assist the body back into a natural state of health through its own innate abilities to heal.

A licensed naturopathic physician attends a four-year, graduate-level medical school studying all of the same basic sciences as an M.D, but has additional training in holistic and non-toxic therapies focusing on prevention. Training includes study in homeopathy, botanical medicine, nutrition, and psychology. For more on naturopathic doctors go to, www.natuopathic.org. For the directory of The Pediatric Association of Natural Physicians go to, www.pedanp.org/find_nd.html. For a rating of naturopaths in your area go to, www.healthgrades.com.

HOMEOPATHY

Although used commonly in Europe and India, homeopathy is not quite as accepted in America mostly because it is not well understood. Although many studies have been done, those in who do not understand how it works disclaim it. This is just like anything else, so you need to be informed.

Homeopathy is a very different concept to grasp. It is based on the Law of Similars. This law states that "a disease can be cured by a substance if that substance can cause, in a healthy person, symptoms similar to those of the disease." The word *homeopathy* comes from homeo meaning similar and pathy meaning suffering.

This excerpt was taken from the book, *The Impossible Cure* by Amy Lansky. It is my favorite book about homeopathy for two reasons: firstly, it is written for the layperson and is very easy to understand; secondly, the author, Amy Lansky, also has a child who "was" on the autism spectrum. After her son's 18-month measles, mumps, rubella shot he began exhibiting symptoms of autism. Homeopathic remedies have since cured him. For the whole story you can read all about it in her book.

The rise in cases of autism coincides with the increase in vaccinations. Another benefit homeopathy offers is to remedy illnesses or damage that the body has been affected by from vaccinations. This is what happened with Amy Lansky's son. Homeopathy can repair the damage done by vaccinations including the body's response to allergies, asthma, and behavioral problems that are a result of vaccinations. A homeopathic remedy should help the body do what it needs to do. It is used to inspire the vital force. Homeopathy works on susceptibility. It comes from recognizing the weakness in the body that has already occurred and the symptoms that are already present.

A "constitutional" remedy takes in both mental and physical components. The homeopathic doctor will take into account every aspect. The emotional and physical components are accounted for in order to help understand the larger picture of a person's distress. Treatment is determined, generally, by matching symptoms. There is a common factor in that homeopaths take into account what is unusual about an individual's pattern. Remedies are specific to each individual. Be patient, it can take some time for a good homeopath to find the proper remedy.

With the assistance of homeopathic practitioners my children and I have received constitutional remedies. Separately, the constitutional remedy Thuja was also prescribed for Jacob by a homeopathic doctor. Thuja assists with nervousness around strangers, is helpful for extra sensitive people, and addresses any residual susceptibility or symptoms from vaccines that his body carries, has adapted to or compensates for. The remedy inspires the vital force to restore that back to health. See the chapter on "Healing the Brain" for the explanation of homeopathy using products from the company Seroyal. I used this to heal my son's neurological ailments along with the help of a natural practitioner.

I too am a true believer in homeopathy. Every member of my family has benefitted from its use. We have all used the over-the-counter, commercial flu remedy Oscillococinum by Boiron for years with great success. When a bacterial cold is present we often use Bacteriotox from Apex Energetics, available at www.pureformulas.com.

Amy Lansky's book is filled with homeopathic remedy studies on all kinds of illnesses. Homeopathy is a proven medical method with hundreds of double blind, placebo-controlled studies done over decades. A man by the name of Wayne Jonas, MD, who was the former director of the Office of Alternative Medicine at the National Institute of Health, has coauthored another great book on homeopathy and homeopathic research studies called, *Healing With Homeopathy: The Complete Guide* (Jonas and Jacobs).

It may be helpful to know that homeopathic doctors can work long distance on the phone or by Skype. This can be great news if you live in a tiny town far away from any homeopaths. I will pass on a name to you from an interview I heard on Autism One radio. The mother of a child diagnosed with autism spoke only long distance with homeopathic Doctor Robert Ullman in Edmonds, Washington. Dr. Ullman provided the mother with a homeopathic remedy that cured her son of his symptoms. Dr. Ullman can be found at http://healthyhomeopathy.com.

The main homeopathic doctor directory is, www.homeopathicdirectory.com, or www.homeopathy-cures.com. See the chapter on vaccinations to learn more about healing genetic defects from vaccinations with homeopathy.

DIETRICHT KLINGHARDT

Dr. Klinghardt is one of the foremost doctors in the natural treatment of autism. He has successfully treated individuals who experience dysfunctions within the autonomic nervous system and who have brain disorders. He is a wealth of information and the mothers of those who are on the autism spectrum should know about him. He has also successfully treated Lyme Disease for many years. Lyme Disease is common among those who are on the autism spectrum.

Dr. Klinghardt looks into and treats not only the outcome of toxic damage, but also the causes. He works with everything from the biomagnetic field to biotoxins and molds. He demonstrates how the release of toxins from molds increases up to 600 times in the presence of an electromagnetic field. He also shows how a woman can be treated safely during pregnancy for these illnesses.

He is not taking patients any longer but suggests those looking for treatment see one of his certified practitioners he has trained, with names located on the website at www.klinghardtacademy.com.

He teaches exclusively with the Klinghardt Academy. Anyone may attend one of their lectures or purchase one of the training DVD's for Healing the Brain or Autism for the latest protocols. They have a full protocol DVD for Autism that you can purchase. It is called, "What's working Today?"

HOLISTIC OR BIOLOGICAL DENTISTRY

Remember that when you go to any doctor, you are hiring him or her. Do not be afraid to ask questions. Call ahead and ask to speak to an office manager or someone who knows the procedures of the office. In dentistry, it is important to be assured that doctors do not use mercury in their practice. The removal of mercury amalgam fillings must be done correctly so that your body is not made additionally toxic as a result of the vapors from the mercury and the mercury's residue. You also need to know if doctor's have proper waste procedures for this toxic metal so that it does not end up in our rivers and oceans. See the chapter on heavy metals for more on mercury and mercury amalgam fillings.

The dangers that mercury presents are significant, especially to the neurological system. Biological dentists should also have certain protective barriers in place such as:

- eye protection for both patient and staff
- dental dams for the reduction of inhalation during removal of mercury amalgam fillings or other materials
- air suction devices
- cooling of mercury during removal (usually done with cool water)

Biological dentists generally follow certain criteria:

- they are mercury free
- they use no fluoride
- they do not use latex
- they do not perform root canal treatments
- they do not offer metal or titanium implants
- they either use homeopathy or are open to using homeopathy

How do biological dentists test to see if certain materials are compatible with your body? Ideally, they have biofeedback machines or they perform Meridian Stress Assessments (MSA). This enables them to check for problems in a particular area of your body and also allows them to see if materials they will use or materials already in your mouth are compatible with your body. Some dentists may use Applied Kinesiology or muscle response testing for this purpose.

Teeth are connected to energy meridians in your body. Distal pain or systemic illness can be a result of problems associated with your teeth. The heart is directly connected to your teeth. A panoramic x-ray may also be needed for further examination. If a cavitation (bacterial pocket under the gums), has formed, it will compromise the blood supply to the affected bones and teeth. The blood vessels here are very small and can get squeezed off. This will inhibit healing. Most traditional dentists are not trained in how to find a cavitation on an x-ray.

Doctors should *only* use digital x-rays because digital x-rays emit 90% less radiation than analog x-rays.

Upon waking in the morning, palpate the masseter muscle. This muscle is located in the side of your cheek and begins around your temporomandibular (jaw) joint, and moves downward. If the area is sore then you have likely been grinding your teeth while sleeping. Grinding will cause micro trauma and will not allow the bone to heal.

As I am not a big fan of night guards due to their inhibition of cranial bones, I also know there are times when they are necessary. Grinding your teeth at night has two common causes: The first common cause is emotional stress, and the second is parasites. If grinding is damaging the teeth and preventing healing, then using a night guard for a short time while sleeping may be necessary. During this time, it is crucial that you also receive Craniosacral therapy to keep the cranial bones mobile and in balance. The Craniosacral work will also help to release the emotional trauma that is contributing to the grinding. This is the same case with orthodontia.

When the cranial bones are inhibited from their original micro-movements, it can create a domino effect of cranial faulting. This means that the cranial bones are unable to fluctuate in their normal pattern. This can have a direct effect on the brain and its ability to function properly. It can also affect the spinal cord, its nerves, and any of its organ connections. The sacrum at the base of the spine is also affected, and therefore the lower back and pelvic region are affected too.

EARLY CAVITY PREVENTION TIPS

The teeth can tell us a lot about what is going on inside of a person's body, especially the gut. The mouth and the digestive tract are the greatest areas to cause inflammation in the body. If your child is prone to cavities or any other oral issues be sure to look further into his health. The first place to go is the gut. When the digestive tract is not functioning properly there will commonly be weakness in the teeth. There is a bacteria called Streptococcus Mutans that is *the* cavity causing bacteria. Pathogenic bacteria in the gut, such as candida, also lives in the mouth. The information in this book will assist with all of that, as will a good bio-dentist.

Do not exchange saliva with your child. As odd as this may sound, when we exchange saliva it is quite possible that we exchange other hosts. The bacterium that enables cavities to grow is called Streptococcus Mutans and it lives and colonizes in the mouth of anyone who has cavities. We can even pass this along to our infants, who do not yet have teeth. Compromised microflora in the gut allows for Strep. Mutans to breed. This bacteria live in the pockets and pits of gums and teeth. It is also passed on to other individuals via saliva. When we test the temperature or the taste of our child's food and we hand them that spoon or bottle without properly cleaning it first, we can spread infections and this bacteria.

XYLITOL

Xylitol, pronounced (zy-li-tall), is an all-natural sweetener extracted from hardwood trees. It was approved by the FDA in 1963. It has been sited in the *Journal of The American Dental Association*, *The international Dental Journal*, *The Journal of Dental Research*, and many others.

Xylitol has the ability to destroy the dental cavity bacteria Strep. Mutans by 90% with regular usage. It also helps to maintain an alkaline environment, inhibits plaque formation, and causes an inability to metabolize oral bacteria.

When my son began getting cavities, my dentist recommended that I purchase lollipops made with xylitol to help prevent the growth of the Strep. Mutans bacteria and future cavities. After Jacob began eating several of these lollipops per day. Now, several years later, he has not had a cavity since.

I occasionally buy the gum or the candies, but I feel the greatest benefit for cavity prevention comes from the lollipops. I purchase them in large quantities. When we eat a xylitol lollipop it is in our mouth for an extended period of time, therefore increasing its benefits. Your teeth feel like you have just brushed them after eating a xylitol lollipop. The benefits of xylitol also go deeper into your system than just your mouth. By ingesting xylitol, we can reduce the Strep. Mutans in our bodies. This is helpful for pregnant women and their growing fetus too.

Xylitol ranks a low seven on the glycemic index (white sugar gets a 68), does not cause a spike in blood sugar, and will not contribute to Candida overgrowth. Xylitol is an excellent sugar replacement anytime and is great for baking. There are no known toxic levels in xylitol, although many people do have difficulty digesting it, so watch your child for reactions. Always start with small amounts. Always start with small amounts and watch for any signs of digestive disturbance such as stomach ache. Xylitol is safe from humans, (but not for dogs).

Although xylitol is sold in health food stores there are also some good websites you can purchase it from. One is www.drjohns.com (888) 375-6462. The other is www.xylitolusa.com. This company, once called Emerald Forest, uses pharmaceutical grade xylitol that is 99.4% pure xylitol crystals. Additional filtering is used to remove any possibility of impurities, such as corn fiber, and it has a sweeter taste. This process also makes it allergen-free. Make sure you purchase the lollipops that are naturally flavored and not the ones that have food coloring in them.

We use xylitol toothpaste in our family. It gives us all of the benefits of xylitol listed above without the fluoride. See the chapter on heavy metals for information regarding fluoride.

The company NOW makes great toothpaste called Xyliwhite in fruit flavor for kids and in cinnamon flavor for everyone else. Both can be purchased at www.swansonvitamins.com and www.pureformulas.com. My teeth feel so much cleaner using this toothpaste than they do with any other toothpaste I have used. Xylitol is amazing.

The following organizations can help you to find a mercury-free, biological dentist:

- www.holisticdental.org
- www.toxicteeth.org/dentistsdoctorsproducts.aspx
- International Academy of Oral Medical Toxicology, www.iaomt.org

For additional information:

- International Academy of Biological Dentistry & Medicine (IABDM) (http://internationalacademyofbiologicaldentistryandmedicine.org/find-a-biological-practitioner/)
- Dental Amalgam Mercury Solutions (DAMS) (http://www.dams.cc/) E-mail them at: dams@usfamily.net (mailto:dams@usfamily.net) or call (651) 644-4572 for an information packet

- Huggins Applied Healing (http://www.hugginsappliedhealing.com/find-dentist.php) You'll need to fill out a form and they will connect with you to find a suitable dentist in your area

CRANIOSACRAL THERAPY

I became certified as a massage practitioner in 1988. For about the first five years I practiced basic massage, sports, deep tissue, etc. Through these years I noticed how much of the physical issues that people were experiencing were due to emotional issues. I began looking for a way to alleviate the symptoms from the cause. In 1993, I took my first craniosacral class. Once I took this class forward all I wanted to do was craniosacral work, and now, this is all I do in my practice (I also research and write).

The affects that I have seen with cranial work far surpass anything I have seen in other forms of bodywork. Many individuals that I work with have symptoms from an emotional or physical trauma that happened many years prior. Birth is the first place to look. As a child grows up with cranial imbalance, he or she also grows up with the symptoms related to that imbalance. These symptoms do not go away until the problem is taken care of with proper cranial balancing.

What is the most important organ in your body? You're right! It's the brain. It runs everything: all of our cells, tissues, and organs. It makes sense that this delicate organ must be structurally protected by bones. The word *craniosacral* comes from "cranium", the bones of the skull, and "sacrum", the bone at the lower end of the spinal cord. The two are joined by a tube (the Dural tube) that runs along the spinal cord.

Craniosacral therapy is a very gentle, yet effective, form of bodywork. Using the most noninvasive touch possible, about the weight of a nickel, the educated practitioner is able to gain knowledge regarding the health of the cranial system (the skeletal system responsible for protecting and influencing your brain and spinal cord). With this gentle touch, a craniosacral therapist is able to assist the bones back into balance and alleviate the symptoms. Some chiropractors will adjust cranial bones such as the atlas (where the occipital bone of the skull meets the first cervical vertebrae of the spine), but many do not have extensive education in cranial imbalances with the other bones in the head.

There are 22 bones in the head. All of these bones move independently with their own subtle micro-movements called the cranial wave. This cranial wave is critical to the function of the bone and its impact on the brain. The bones are separated by sutures. These are the places where the bones come together. The sutures allow the bones to move and they also create shock absorption to protect the brain in case of head trauma.

Each bone affects another and its specific movement. Due to physical and/or emotional trauma the bones in our head can become faulted out of balance. Bones, nerves, and neurotransmitters are all affected. Neurotransmitters are chemicals that transport messages in the central nervous system. These chemicals can be disrupted by cranial imbalances. When these things happen the ability of the brain to function properly has been impaired. We are then left with physical and/or emotional symptoms.

As an example, the most common subluxation (bone imbalance), created during birth is of the occiput. The occiput is the bone on the back of the head that meets with the soft tissue of the neck. It is also where the spinal cord meets with the brainstem. It is quite easy to see that if this bone were out of balance it could cause a lot of problems. Along with its disruption to other cranial bones and their function, the occiput also affects the bones in the neck, the spinal cord, and cranial nerves.

The spinal cord has 32 billion cells and many nerves. One of the nerves disrupted by an imbalance of the occiput is the vagus nerve. The vagus nerve has branches that control areas such as digestion and respiration. It also allows for an immediate response to the environment via the hypothalamus, pituitary, and adrenal axis. When it is compromised, it can cause anxiety in any individual. Babies with colic and children with asthma should be checked for a cervical and occipital imbalance. Colic can also be due to lactose intolerance, stressed thoracic vertebrae, or an inhibited diaphragm.

Some common physical symptoms of cranial bone imbalance are:

- headaches
- migraines

- jaw problems (TMJ)
- neck pain
- earaches and infections
- dizziness
- problems with balance
- low back trouble
- auditory or balance issues
- nausea
- digestive imbalances/colic/spitting up more food than you keep down
- breathing trouble/asthma
- sleep disturbances
- hormonal dysfunction
- sinus issues
- anxiety
- hyperactivity
- anger
- depression
- obsessive/compulsive behavior
- low energy
- lack of mental clarity
- socially withdrawn or disconnected
- learning disabilities
- dyslexia

OCCIPITAL EIGHT-FINGER HOLD
(freeing the occiput)

Cranial work is best done when the patient is lying still. If this is difficult to do when your child is awake then wait until he or she is sleeping. I spent many evenings contorted between the headboard of the bed and my children's pillows to properly reach their heads for cranial work.

As your child is lying down, you will sit at the top of his or her head. Place both of your hands in a supportive, gentle hold with your eight fingers resting along the bottom ridge of the occiput. This is where the soft tissue meets the bone at the back of the neck. Your fingers only need to rest here. You may feel a slight swaying motion or their head may begin to turn from side to side. This is called unwinding in cranial work and it is very beneficial. Be sure that you are only supporting where the head wants to go and not leading it. Stay here as long as you are comfortable. This releases the occiput, the neck, and calms the brain.

When the occiput gets pushed upward in birth it can jam up the bones next to it. Two of the bones that become jammed are the temporal bones. These are the bones around each of the ears. I find this in just about all people with autism, ADHD, and aggressive behavior. When the temporal bones are out of balance there can also be such symptoms as headaches, ear infections, dizziness, nausea, anger, speech and language trouble, and problems with social engagement.

Social engagement comes from cranial nerves 5, 7, 9, 10, and 11. If we can upregulate or balance one, we automatically can upregulate all of them.

TIP: By stimulating the lower part of the earlobe (such as rubbing it between two fingers) it relaxes the vagus nerve and can be very calming for those who are over stimulated or nauseous. The entire ear lobe has many different acupressure points known to calm the system. You can teach your children to gently massage their outer ear when they feel stressed. Some children are seen tugging at their ears. I believe this to be a natural, innate response to self-calming and self-correction. The temporal bones are often imbalanced in children who have an autism spectrum disorder and those with learning and behavioral disabilities.

PICTURE OF 8 FINGER OCCIPITAL HOLD

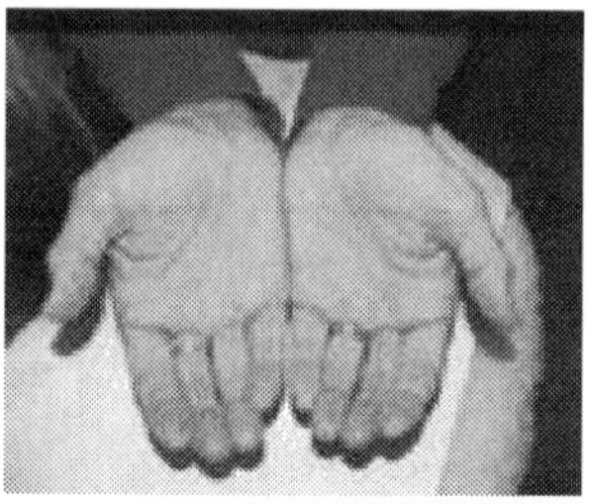

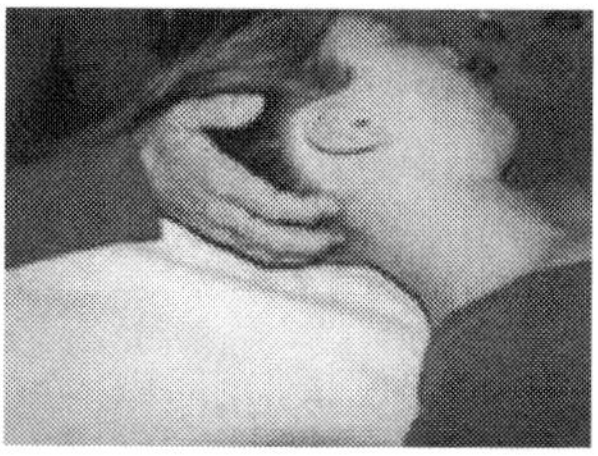

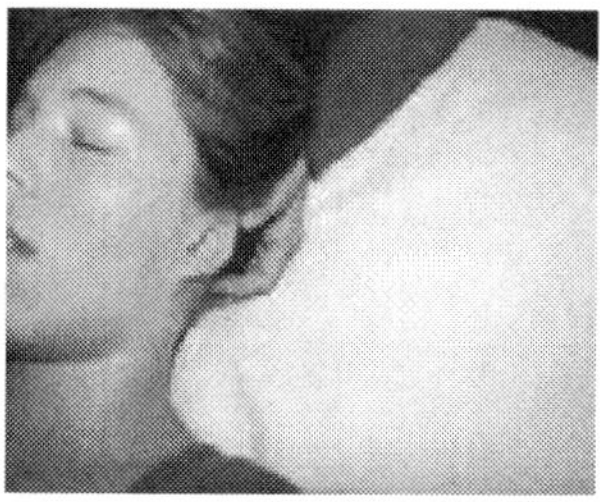

TEMPORAL EAR PULL RELEASE

By gently pulling down and out on the ears (in a 45 degree angle) toward the shoulders it can help free the temporal bones and bring about relaxation. It can also assist in alleviating symptoms of temporal faulting noted above.

Mom can do this hold on her child. However, if the child will not hold still there is a risk of causing additional trauma to the temporal bones. In this case, your best bet is to do it while your child is sleeping.

While he or she is laying face up, reach down and grip the lower portion of the ears with your index finger on the underside of the ear as close to the head as possible. Your thumb should be placed inside the lower portion of the ear (front side) just below the ear canal. Never put your finger into the ear canal itself. Lightly pinch the ear lobe between your fingers to keep your grip as you *gently* pull downward and outward in a 45-degree angle toward the shoulders. Keep this gentle hold for several minutes (as long as you can). When you are done, do not just let go. It is important that you slowly release the downward tension and bring the ears back to a neutral position before letting go.

PICTURE OF TEMPORAL EAR PULL

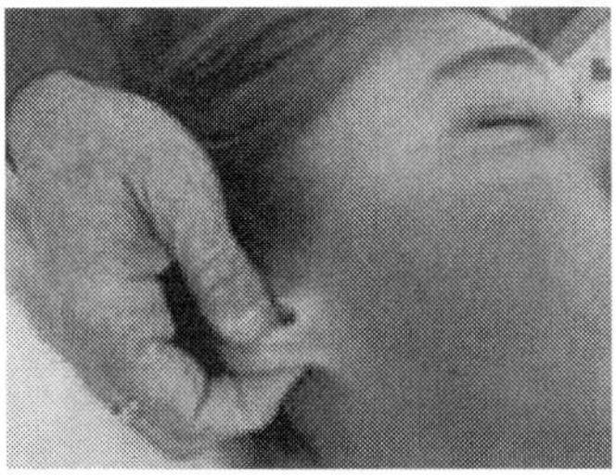

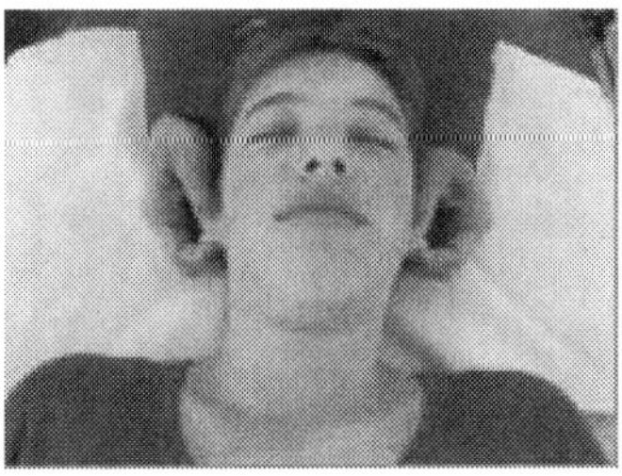

A bone behind the eyes, the sphenoid, touches the optic nerves. It also holds the pituitary gland, which is responsible for keeping the endocrine or hormonal system in balance. When this bone is faulted it can affect more than vision and hormones. The symptoms of a faulted sphenoid can range anywhere from mild headaches to schizophrenic behavior.

When we see a children banging their head it is very possible that they are acting in a self-correcting manner. Their head hurts and they are trying to fix it. When one bone is faulted out of balance others are adversely affected and this can lead to many symptoms.

For a demonstration of these temporal and occipital craniosacral holds please see my Youtube videos at http://youtu.be/1krEhJ4dzJM.

CORE LINK HOLD

TIP: In cases of general hyperactivity or a general need for calming, grounding and balancing, place one hand transversely over your child's sacrum while he or she lies on his or her back (awake or asleep) and simply let your hand rest there. You may pick up a gentle swaying motion. This alone is helpful in balancing the sacrum, which can cause hyperactivity when faulted. For additional assistance with this, place your other hand transversely under the occiput at the same time. This places your hands over both cranial and sacral attachment points. Sometimes the neck will begin to move around or unwind. This is very beneficial. Try to allow the freedom of its movement under your hand and simply act as a support. Nothing more.

Migraines are caused by an inflamed or excessively dilated blood vessels. This commonly comes from two areas: the trigeminal nerve branch in the back of the neck where the spine meets the skull, and the palate (or roof of the mouth). Craniosacral work is extremely effective for migraines. Until you get to a craniosacral therapist you can put a cold compress on the back of your neck, and suck on ice chips to help alleviate the pain. The supplement 5-HTP is also known to be helpful for migraines because it promotes an increase in serotonin, which can also be a cause for the migraine. See the chapter "Natural Supplementation for the Brain" for more information on 5HTP.

PICTURE OF CORE LINK HOLD

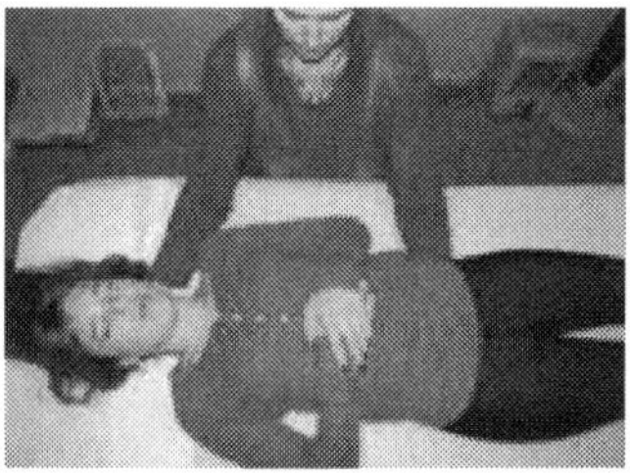

PROTECT YOUR CHILD'S HEAD

Bicycle helmets should be worn anytime your children are on *anything* with wheels or when they do activities, such as ice-skating, where they can hit their head. Advocates of the brain caution against any activity that is a potential danger to the brain.

Dentistry is also very hard on the craniosacral system. It is ideal to seek treatment before and after dental or orthodontic work.

HOW TO FIND A CRANIOSACRAL THERAPIST

The easiest way to find an educated practitioner would be to contact either of the two schools most commonly known for craniosacral instruction. The one I graduated from is The Milne Institute, www.milneinstitute.com. To find a craniosacral therapist who has graduated from this program go to the site and click on "practitioners." The second school is The Upledger Institute, www.upledger.com. On this site, click on "find a therapist."

Both sites will be able to locate the practitioner nearest to you. If, through your screening process, you find a person that you have the best gut feeling about or you find someone who is the most experienced, but this person is far away, I highly recommend driving the extra distance to see that practitioner.

It is important to interview the practitioner on the phone before you make an appointment. Ask where the practitioner received his or her training, how long he or she has been practicing, and how much experience, if any, the practitioner has working with children, babies, or your child's specific issue (i.e. autism, language problems, asthma, etc).

The best time for your children to receive a treatment is when they are their calmest. It is even best if they are sleeping, although this is usually more typical with toddlers and infants. For infants who are still nursing, I find it best to work on them while they are nursing because they are occupied, safe, and relatively still. For older children who are unable to stop moving, you may ask if your practitioner can come to your home when your child is sleeping. I remember climbing into my children's bed at night to do some cranial work on them. Be creative and do whatever works.

HYPERBARIC CHAMBERS AND OXYGEN

A hyperbaric chamber is a safe, effective way to increase the oxygen in the body. When we breathe, we take in limited amounts of this essential gas. Once inhaled, the lungs help transport oxygen to the hemoglobin, or red blood cells. If we are lucky, the oxygen reaches our brain with enough concentration to feed its cells. Most of us do not breathe deeply enough as it is. Today, we have the added issue of less oxygen on the planet.

Oxygen is needed for cellular life. It detoxifies the cells and helps with fatigue. It assists in proper digestion and better absorption of nutrients from the foods we eat. Additionally, most fungi, bacteria, viruses, and parasites are anaerobic. This means they die in an environment filled with oxygen. Oxygen helps balance and maintain the body's pH (acid/alkaline) levels.

The brain consumes more than 20% of the total oxygen used by your body. When concentrating, the brain uses even more. Low levels of oxygen mean lowered brain functioning, including a decrease in memory and concentration. The part of the brain commonly affected by decreased oxygen is the hippocampus. The hippocampus is involved in memory and spatial awareness. It is also the primary part of the brain that is affected in Alzheimer's.

Hyperbaric chambers are commonly used for treating brain injuries, genetic disorders, muscle fatigue, traumatized or burned skin, and issues of the gut. After just ten treatments, brain scans show marked differences in activity.

Some of the benefits of hyperbaric chambers are:

- improved cognition
- improved focus/attention
- reduced stress and heightened affection
- reduced sensory disturbance
- improved motor skills
- improved social skills
- increased linguistic abilities

Hyperbaric chambers have an incredibly high effectiveness rate with autism. The study by Dr. Daniel Rossignol out of the University of Virginia showed marked improvements ranging from 50 percent improvement up to 93 percent improvement in symptoms such as verbal skills, non-provoked outbursts, aloof and withdrawn behavior, tantrums, eye contact, poor response to usual teaching methods, sustained odd play, hyperactivity, hearing impairment, aggressive/self-injurious behavior, imitative or repetitive behavior, apparent over-sensitivity or under-sensitivity to sounds, tastes, smells, fear or pain. Read the full study at www.hyperbaricmedicalassociation.org.

Hyperbaric chambers are not at all the same. There is hyperbaric oxygen therapy (HBOT) which is used in hard-sided chambers. They use 100% oxygen. Hyperbaric air therapy (HBAT) uses air. Soft sided models use HBAT, and cannot reach the necessary pressures above 1.3 ATA (normal atmospheric pressure) needed to produce enough therapeutic oxygen. Also, when used ineffectively hyperbaric chambers can make symptoms worse. Read the details in the article; HBAT vs. HBOT-What's The Difference, by Laura Betts at hyperbaricsrx.blogspot.com.

The short story here is to never use soft-sided models. When you call any hyperbaric treatment facility be sure they use the hard-sided models and do not push the soft sided ones. The soft sided ones are a scam to get parents to spend a lot of money.

For additional information please visit:
www.hyperbaricmedicalassociation.org. The IHMA is a non-profit that has been directly responsible for the clearance of additional insurance reimbursable conditions. (They do not push HBAT.)

Additionally, to improve oxygen levels eat raw, uncooked vegetables. Exercise increases our breathing, forcing us to take in more oxygen. There are also oxygen supplements that can be helpful such as Cellfood, which is sold in most health food stores and at www.swansonvitamins.com or www.brainchildnutritionals.com. Another liquid product called Oxygen Supreme II is sold at www.pureformulas.com.

NEUROFEEDBACK

Neurofeedback is a gentle, noninvasive way to improve brain regulation. It treats supposed life-long problems such as migraines, epilepsy, and autism. It does this without the use of drugs or negative side effects.

The patient sits in front of a computer screen. An educated practitioner chooses the software depending on the patient's symptoms. The computer screen looks like a game. It is very similar to the old Pac-Man game in which a little creature goes up and down the screen eating things. Changing your breath, or even your thoughts, changes brain waves. The more the patient tries to relax, or pays more attention to the object on the screen, the more the brain is regulated. The software program is just a guide. The brain does the work. The brain learns to function on its own in areas it had difficulty functioning before. For example, brainwaves increase where they were underactive before and decrease where they were overactive.

A thin wire with a dime-sized cup on the end is fastened to the scalp with conducting paste. These sensors pick up the brain waves and transmit them to the computer. The computer picks up your brain's activity and gives instant feedback.

Noticeable changes commonly occur between the first and the tenth session. Generally, between 20 and 45 sessions are needed. Training time is between 20 and 50 minutes. A minimum of two to three sessions per week is necessary. More sessions are better. It is like going to the gym for your brain. It needs to learn and remember its new training to stay fit. Once there has been enough consistent training, the benefits last for years. Occasional "tune ups" may be helpful over time. Needs may slightly increase again over time due to a change in nutrition, an increase in allergies, or an unstable home environment.

NEUROFEEDBACK CAN HELP WITH:

- autism
- anxiety
- depression
- addictions
- ADD/ADHD
- sleep problems
- stress reduction
- learning disabilities

- emotional instabilities
- low self-esteem
- migraines
- seizures
- Tourette's
- chronic pain
- symptoms of multiple sclerosis and Parkinson's

Some educated and experienced practitioners estimate a success rate of up to 90% with autism. In cases of autism, look out for a decrease or disappearance in anxiety, sensory overload, frustration, aggression, shyness, and an increase or improvement in emotional awareness, social skills, sleeping habits, and handling stress.

When on medications, the treatment may be so effective that changes need to be made in dosage levels. Work with your medical doctor during treatments.

Many parents have found such profound results that they have purchased a neurofeedback unit for their home. Families can join together to purchase a neurofeedback unit and to help cover the expense. There are online webcast trainings available to learn about the programs. I know of parents who had such great results with their own children that they purchased a unit and now provide sessions for others. There are also practitioners who rent out units.

My own practitioner was injured in an accident and was living with chronic pain. She was told that there was nothing more they could do for her. She found neurofeedback and returned to a healthy, happy life, so she purchased a machine and went to school to share the benefits with others.

Both of my children benefitted greatly from neurofeedback. I highly recommend it.

For more information on Neurofeedback and to find a practitioner near you visit these websites:

- www.eegspectrum.com
- www.isnr.org/nfbarch/nbiblio.htm.

INDIGO BIOFEEDBACK

Indigo is a unique form of biofeedback. Clinical studies show that Indigo's proprietary algorithmic formulas improve the body's ability to adapt to stressors. It retrains both physiological and emotional aspects and shifts the body's energetic response.

Indigo biofeedback measures over 11,000 frequencies through electrical-impulse-skin-response via straps attached to the wrists, ankles, and forehead. Within five minutes it can detect and record the electrical activity of the body, show where there are weaknesses, and provide overall information about the client's health. Resonant frequencies are used on the system as homeopathic, nutritional, and other natural health remedies would be. Biofeedback is used for everything from pain, anxiety, depression, asthma, digestive disorders, and parasitic infections.

These machines can be purchased for your own use, but they are expensive. Most people seek a qualified practitioner. Be sure to ask practitioners where or how they were trained and how long they have been practicing so you know what their level of experience is. For a worldwide listing of Indigo biofeedback practitioners go to www.practitioners.thequantumalliance.com.

HELP FOR SIBLINGS, FAMILY MEMBERS, AND YOU

Siblings of children on the autism spectrum often experience feelings of guilt or anxiety regarding their brother or sister's condition. They are also inflicted by the intensity of their parent's feelings. Luckily, homeopathy and neurofeedback can help them with these issues. Another technique that is tremendously helpful for every family member and can be learned at home by anyone at no cost, is something called Tapping or Emotional Freedom Technique.

TAPPING OR EMOTIONAL FREEDOM TECHNIQUE

Tapping or Emotional Freedom Technique (EFT) is based on a combination of Chinese medicine (acupressure or meridian points), and Western psychotherapy. Meridian points are connected to the body's energy flow. They are like the body's freeway network for energy. Sometimes this freeway has emotional traffic jams. When this energy flow is disrupted, physical and emotional issues arise.

When stimulated, these acupressure points send signals to the stress centers of the brain. These signals bypass the thinking portion of the brain. The thinking portion of the brain is commonly only accessed during talk therapy. In this situation, the body's emotional energy pathways are not shifted. This is the key component to why EFT works. This is treating the causes, rather than just the symptoms.

Multiple studies have been done on the effects of EFT, some even by the prominent Harvard Medical School. The Medical School's analysis described how stimulating the acupressure points reduced the brain's stress and fear response. EFT balances the sympathetic and the parasympathetic nervous systems. One study by Dr. Dawson Church showed that average levels of Cortisol, the body's stress hormone, were reduced by 24% in some 83 subjects, and up to 50% in others. Comparatively, those who underwent an hour of talk therapy showed no significant reduction in Cortisol.

EFT is simple and painless. Anyone can learn to do it. While tapping on specific meridian points, you are to think of an emotional incident in your life that may be the trigger for current feelings and actions like anxiety, distraction, insomnia, relationships, financial pressure, pain, depression, and most disease. Measure this feeling now on a scale from one to ten, ten being the worst.

Think of either the first or the worst incident you can remember. While thinking about, this talk through how you are feeling now. If you cannot think of a specific memory, then just talk about how you feel when certain things happen to you that cause you to feel those emotions. While talking about the issues, concentrate on resolving the negative emotion. This shifts your body's energy and restores balance. Begin tapping with your fingertips on the points shown below. Go through several rounds of it until you notice the negative feelings subsiding. When you are finished, measure the emotions from one to ten again. You will likely feel a difference already.

If you are doing this for children who are unable to express themselves, you can teach them to tap on the points or do it for them. They do not even have to tap in the specific order listed. It will still work. By tapping on any of the points listed below, the energy will shift in the body and bring calmness.

Author Nick Ortner has written a book called, *The Tapping Solution*. For more information and free downloads go to www.thetappingsolution.com.

To find an EFT practitioner go to:
www.thetappingsolution.com/eft-practitioners

WHERE TO TAP

The following advice can be found at www.thetappingsolution.com. Tap five to seven times each on the remaining eight points in the following sequence:

Head (TH): Tap the crown, center, and top of the head with all four fingers on both hands.

Eyebrow (EB): Tap the inner edges of the eyebrows, closest to the bridge of the nose with two fingers.

Side of eye (SE): Tap the hard area between the eye and the temple with two fingers. Feel out this area gently so you don't poke yourself in the eye!

Under eye (UE): Tap the hard area under the eye that merges with the cheekbone with two fingers in a line beneath the pupil.

Under nose (UN): Tap the point centered between the bottom of the nose and the upper lip with two fingers.

Chin (CP): This point is right beneath the previous one, and is centered between the bottom of the lower lip and the chin.

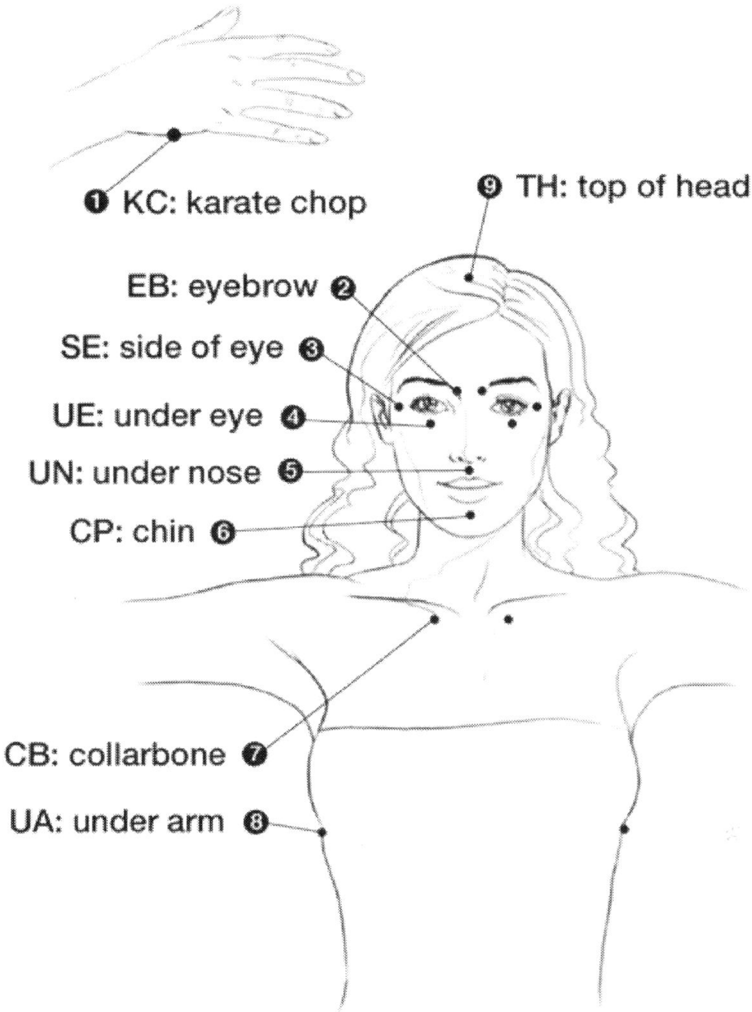

Collarbone (CB): Tap just below the hard ridge of your collarbone with four fingers.

Underarm (UA): Tap your side, about four inches beneath the armpit with four fingers.

Head (TH): And now you're back where you started. You've completed the sequence.

As you tap on each point, repeat a simple reminder phrase, such as "my anxiety" or "my interview" or "my financial situation."

Now take another deep breath!

DONNA EDEN AND ENERGY MEDICINE

Donna Eden is one of the most sought after healers in energy medicine. She has taught over 5,0000 people, both professionals and laypersons. Her book, *Energy Medicine*, is a thorough explanation of how simple body movements can calm the brain and the body. She has also written a condensed version of this book, *The Little Book of Energy Medicine*, which is simple and easy to follow, with pictures of body movements that will calm or energize you in minutes. Both you and your child can learn the simple exercises. They can be very helpful.

EYE MOVEMENT DESENSITIZATION AND REPROCESSING (EMDR)

Children who are on the autism spectrum, have ADHD, or have learning difficulties often have low self-esteem. Their childhood has been plagued with criticism surrounding their behavior. They have had difficulties reading, writing, or just comprehending. Multiple negative experiences reinforce their feelings of failure and they continue to have even more trouble concentrating. This therapy may be helpful for the issues associated with these past experiences. Siblings and parents of these children can benefit from this therapy as well.

Eye movement desensitization and reprocessing (EMDR) is a highly effective form of therapy that allows for the removal of negative emotions. Feelings, thoughts, and physical sensations relating to a negative behavior are addressed. EMDR uses eye movements and other rhythm-based stimulation such as hand tapping. This shifts the brain's information-processing system. EMDR disrupts an old memory and reduces, or removes, the emotion behind it. This therapy has a reputation for working quickly. One trauma can be disabled in one to three sessions. More than one million people have been helped by EMDR.

This is not for those who have a purely biological issue. It is helpful for people whose behavior, such as low self-esteem, depression, anxiety, or nightmares, has been caused by past experiences. There must be a willingness to experience ones feelings.

It is how the psyche feels about an experience that creates the emotion. One person may not be affected by the same incident that traumatizes another. The experience may be seemingly harmless, yet can have a life changing impact.

EMDR therapists must be certified by the EMDR International Association or the EMDR Europe Association.

1. Find a therapist who is professionally trained in EMDR.
2. Be sure it is the right therapist for the individual receiving the therapy. The interaction between the two should be a positive one.

For information on training or for a referral, contact the Institute at this website www.EMDR.com, email address inst@emdr.com, or phone number (831) 372-3900.

SUMMARY

There are many alternative therapies available ranging from natural allergy elimination, and craniosacral therapists to homeopathy an alternative medical doctors. Multiple resources are available to help you find what you are looking for depending on your child's needs.

The products found in this chapter can be found at http://naturallyhealingautism.com/a-healthy-home/

CHAPTER 3

SENSORY PROCESSING DISORDERS

My greatest concern is that parents will be unable to understand that it is not that their children will not act appropriately or do what they are asked, but that their children cannot. Children with sensory processing issues, or unregulated neurological functioning, are often seen as defiant. They are actually incapable of changing their behavior due to a disorganized brain. Our society has programmed us to believe it is just about behavior. These children are thought of as lazy or disrespectful. Professionals and family members told my husband and I for several years that we needed to be firmer with discipline as parents. They were wrong!

Many of the ordinary, daily tasks or responses we take for granted are extremely challenging for those with sensory processing disorders. A toxic body and brain may prevent a child from doing the tasks asked of him, regardless of how hard he tries. Children with this disorder may or may not be on the autism spectrum. There is often a *misdiagnosis* due to these behaviors. Learn about sensory processing disorders (SPD) and exercise patience with your children. It is as hard for them not to be able to act appropriately as it is for you to watch it. Their self-esteem is often damaged due to these issues. We will discuss this on a more neurological level in the chapter on supporting the brain.

Apraxia is an inability to perform a motor task. Epraxia is a difficulty performing any task at all. Children who suffer from these conditions are intelligent, but their brain is consumed by their own processing inabilities. These children can be in a hyper- or hypo-neurological state. The same person can be constantly changing from one state to another. They do not imitate well, so the pressure you put on them makes it worse. Food allergies and environmental factors play a constant role.

Confused neurological states start in the womb when the central nervous system becomes disorganized. The symptoms of sensory processing disorder range greatly.

The four sensory systems are:

1. Tactile problems create the refusal to eat due to issues of both tastes and textures of various foods. Using a fork can be quite difficult. This is the same for holding a pencil and for writing. Proper tactile sense is necessary for language development. Children who face this difficulty need proper awareness of their mouth, lips, and tongue.
2. Vestibular issues come from the inner ear. They create problems with balance and movement. A lack in proprioception, or the ability to know where your body is in space, is very common. Sometimes people just think that their children are clumsy because they do not pay attention to what they are doing. They unconsciously tiptoe because it lessens the touch of the floor on the bottom of their feet with each step. These children may desire a lot of stimulation or prefer none at all. Symptoms of over-responsive vestibular issues can be extreme nausea when riding in a car or playing on a swing. They become dizzy easily. If these children are vestibular seeking, they crave intense movement. They like to hang upside down and enjoy rocking. They may play on the swing for hours. Those with vestibular under-responsiveness may have trouble getting going but have a hard time stopping once they're moving.
3. Visual over-responsiveness creates many fears. Children may over-respond or under-respond to fast moving, shiny objects. They have poor visual discrimination.
4. Auditory issues create fear and anxiety in relation to noise. An auditory-sensory-craver loves loud noise and action.

Children with auditory problems may have difficulty putting their thoughts into words. The cause for auditory problems may have been ear infections. The temporal lobes of the brain are also associated with speech. During Craniosacral therapy, I work with the temporal lobes for this issue (see craniosacral work in the chapter on alternative therapies).

Some common symptoms of SPD are:

- "Sensory Modulating Problems", or children's inability to regulate themselves. This can be overreacting or underreacting to any stimuli.
- "Sensory Discrimination Problems", which create difficulty in distinguishing one stimulus from another.
- "Sensory-Based Motor Problems", which have to do with motor control and their ability or inability to move in the way they consciously choose to.
- "Associated Regulatory and Behavior Problems", which can be a combination of developmental problems and simply, poor biological sensory processing. This may or may not be actual SPD.

Know that no two people are the same. We are born with our very own biological and neurological system. Each symptom can range from mild to severe. It is common to witness both consistent and inconsistent behaviors.

More information for help with auditory and vestibular issues can be found at www.tomatis.com. There is help for visual issues at autisticvision.com. The right occupational therapist can be very helpful too. See below.

THE FIRST STEP

Now that you understand that your child is not just being defiant or lazy, you should also recognize that until his biology is healed, he might not be able to complete the tasks asked of him. I would suggest working with the health information in this book prior to seeking your occupational or social therapist. I am telling you this from my own personal experience. We wasted a lot of our money and time sending our son to work with different types of people before his brain was healed and before he was capable or compliant.

Most of us are told to talk to our pediatrician. After an expensive appointment, they will usually dismiss your feelings and your child's behavior. To save time and money get an initial evaluation by a *specialist* in sensory processing disorders. They will let you know what exactly is going on and what you have to work with. I, and many others, have found occupational therapists to be the best place for your initial evaluation (see below).

You are looking for a therapist within their specialized field who has a background, and hopefully training, with children on the autism spectrum. Many therapists will come to your home. Either way, the therapist will fully engage parents in "homework" with their child. Children must have a strong family structure where they start to learn strong social connections with their parents.

As you follow the processes in this book, your child's system will become healthier. It is important to note that if their body is cleared of many of the underlying chemicals and physiological and anatomical issues, their needs for therapy will often decrease. Once their system is clean, they can be who they truly are. Then you will know what still needs to be worked with.

This is a therapist's, occupational or otherwise, dream. They can come in and get to the core work with the child without having to battle against all of the other factors that prevent the child from fully engaging and learning what he or she has to offer.

Development goes from large to small motor skills. Individuals must be taught in accordance with their needs. Biology should be addressed first so that they are more capable of understanding and carrying out the tasks asked of them.

THE PARENTS' JOB

When it is too much for the child, they will break down behaviorally. It is important that your therapist knows when enough time has been spent with your child for one day. Sometimes very small amounts of time are enough. The therapist should train parents to work with their children when they are most calm. Use play whenever possible and do not push them. If your children know that it is stressful when you ask them to do things, they may develop anxiety every time you approach them with a task. In a hyper state the brain is consumed and cannot learn. Most importantly, maintain their self-esteem so they will continue to work with you. Any constructive attempt your children make should be given positive reinforcement. They understand this from your body language, facial expressions, and words. Your children must trust you. If your children do not trust the therapist, find a new one!

They are unable to regulate themselves, so you need to become tuned into their behavioral responses. A good therapist will be your best guide in the beginning, but you must also be well aware of your children's reactions to stress. In turn, you will teach this to the therapist. You are ultimately working to mature their neurological systems.

Time Timers are visual timers that help show your children the time, and they can be purchased on www.amazon.com. The time remaining for any future event or for the end of a lesson, or whatever else, is in red. When time is up, the red disappears. This can help children relax and feel some sense of control. This way, they are more present for what is going on now.

A helpful book on sensory processing issues and their remedies is *The Out-of-Sync Child* by Carol Stock Kranowitz, M.A.

The book, *More Than Words*, by Fern Sussman helps teach parents how to build social interaction and language skills with their children.

Michelle Garcia developed a program entitled *Social Thinking* fifteen years ago. She has won awards for her social curriculum that targets those with high functioning autism and Asperger's syndrome. Her program teaches parents how to learn social skills and cues and how to tell their children that their behavior affects others and the way others respond to them. It also teaches parents about their own emotions and how to adapt. Professionals, parents, and caregivers all use her program. To receive her newsletter and to learn much more, see her website www.socialthinking.com.

Another good website for more information is www.sensoryprocessing.net. Also, autism apps are now available on your smart phone. These can be very helpful. A learning center that helps those with any difficulty, but has a strong reputation for working successfully with those on the autism spectrum, is www.lindamoodbell.com.

OCCUPATIONAL THERAPY

The first thing to do is get an evaluation from an occupational therapist that is trained in sensory processing disorders. It is an added benefit if they have experience with people on the autism spectrum. If you need to travel a far distance to get this evaluation from the proper person, then do so. The evaluation you get from the proper person can be used by an occupational therapist closer to where you live for ongoing sessions.

Ask for a sensory integration processing disorders (SIPD, dubbed "sipped") certified occupational therapist, if possible. They have additional training in diagnosis and treatment of sensory processing disorders. For a directory of occupational therapists see www.healthgrades.com/occupational-therapy-directory. Another good resource site that has a directory to help you find an occupational therapist near you is www.sensory-processing-disorder.com.

TOOLS TO HELP CALM ANXIETY

In order to calm anxiety, you must calm the nervous system. Using your muscles is one way to do this. Lifting a heavy object actually has a calming effect on the system. Ask your children to carry fairly heavy objects, within their capabilities, like a box with some papers or books in it, out to the garage for you.

One of the best tools for calming anxiety is the doorjamb bar. Easily installed in any doorway, this indoor support bar is strong enough to support pull-ups and has an attachment for a swing or trapeze bar. This is especially helpful on rainy days.

There are many doorjamb bars available, but not all are safe. The bar our occupational therapist recommended, and the one that we have had great success with, is sold by Playaway Toy Company Incorporated. Properly installed, the weight limit is 175 pounds. For more information see www.playawaytoy.com or call (715) 752-4565.

An additional resource is www.sensorygoods.com. This website carries swings, floor products, and weighted blankets. Weighted blankets can help those with over stimulation problems become calm.

A rock-climbing wall of any size enables children to have a great physical and mental exercise that also calms them. Rock climbing increases motor skills and mental focus. It also has a calming effect on the nervous system. There are kits you can buy that will help you build a rock-climbing wall yourself or you can have someone build one for you. More towns now have rock-climbing gyms too.

TRIPLE WARMER POINT

There is an acupressure meridian just behind the ear that helps to calm the entire system in times of stress, anxiety, and overwhelm. Place your index finger on the bone right behind your earlobe and then draw your finger straight back, (not down), about half an inch it will fall into the little dip that is in the soft tissue just below the bone. This is your triple warmer point and it can come in very useful when you or your child are stressed.

NEUROLOGICAL SWITCHING

We all become neurologically "switched" on a semi-regular basis. Simple actions can cause our neurological system to become confused and the hemispheres of the brain to disconnect. This is when we become clumsy and confused.

Two ways to regulate neurological switching and balance the hemispheres of the brain are to:

STIMULATE THE NEURO-BALANCING POINTS: Place the fingers of one hand one inch to the right of your belly button. Place the fingers of the other hand over the area just below the inner portion of your collarbone. These are the same collarbone pressure points as illustrated by number seven in the tapping solutions diagram shown in the chapter on alternative therapies. Rub both of these areas simultaneously for 15 to 30 seconds, or more. Then place your fingers over the same areas on the left side of your body and repeat the stimulation.

1. CROSS CRAWL: While sitting or standing, place your right elbow on your left knee. Then place your left elbow on your right knee. Continue this "cross crawl" patterning, moving back and forth and quickly repeating it several times.
2. A video by Donna Eden shows a great example of how easily the hemispheres of the brain can become disorganized. Donna Eden has taught over 5,0000 professionals and laypersons in the technique of energy medicine. See Donna Eden's cross crawl with kinesiology, www.happiness.com/brain-gym-exercises.html#cross-crawl).

Donna Eden has an excellent explanation of the four types of human characteristics that take in information and deal with stress. The four sensory systems are tonal, visual, kinesthetic, and digital. For a proper explanation see www.energymedicine.com.

AT SCHOOL

Children may be unable to verbally explain what it is that is troubling them. When they can no longer focus or hold still, or when they need stimulation, the following can be helpful if performed discreetly:

- Have the teacher ask your child to carry a box of books over to the next classroom. The box should already be packed with enough weight so that he or she really uses his or her muscle strength, but not too much weight, of course.
- Allow your child to quietly go out and do some pull-ups on the pull-up bar or go on the swings.
- Never allow him or her to miss physical education opportunities. Any movement, even stretching, is helpful.
- Teach the child the temporal-ear-pull hold from the Craniosacral therapy section in the chapter on alternative therapies.
- Gently rub the ear lobes or the entire outer ridge of the ear between his index fingers and his or her thumbs.

- Allow him of her to sit closer to the teacher so there are fewer distractions in between them.
- The act of chewing is very helpful. Chewing gum, if allowed, stimulates cranial nerves that help to engage both wakefulness and social engagement.
- Tell the child what he or she *can* do. The child needs an appropriate action to replace a poor one with.

Healthy food choices are critical. Poor food choices loaded with processed foods, chemicals, and sugars will distract and prevent focus. Vitamin B supplements help too. There is plenty of information on diet and supplementation throughout this book.

See the chapter on supporting the brain for supplements that can help various neurological needs.

Two booklets that can be helpful for parents and school faculty are:

What Every Child with ASD Wishes You Knew
What Every Student with ASD Wishes You Knew

SPEECH THERAPY

Most sensory and motor speech issues are caused by anxiety and stress. Get help sorting these negative feelings out. One speech therapist I saw advised that children who stutter should be made to stutter on purpose. This shows them that they can control it to some degree. I thought this was brilliant. It was so simple. Although this was a simple explanation, it is not always a simple task. Finding someone you trust and, more importantly, that your child trusts is crucial.

Speech is more difficult than we realize. It involves motor planning from breathing in air, getting your vocal chords to do what you want, and your jaw to move just right. Then your mind must be able to put the thoughts you have into words.

Speech therapy has many interactive approaches. One method is The Hanen method, www.hanen.org. This is a software program that also has an interactive bubbles feature to assist those who are on the autism spectrum in their learning process.

Integrated Listening Systems is a program that improves brain function through multiple sensory awareness (www.integratedlisteningsystems.com). This system is customized for emotional regulation during sensory input while learning. You can use it while sleeping or during your daily routine while wearing headphones.

Fast Forward Learning is a self-paced software program focused on strengthening the brain. It helps build essential skills in three to six months. See their website at www.gemmlearning.com/fast-forward-software-program/. It is backed by over 240 research studies including those at Johns Hopkins, Stanford, and Cornell Universities.

APPLIED BEHAVIORAL ANALYSIS (ABA)

Children on the autism spectrum do not learn as easily from their environment. Applied Behavioral Analysis (ABA) is a hands-on training tool that teaches individuals how to interact with their environment properly. The approach of this program is to change brain pathways through early intervention.

Overall, I would suggest that you monitor results and make sure these programs are working. Your children must be treated in accordance with their learning capabilities. Find a therapist that you trust, and still pay attention to your children's outcome. At times, ABA can be too stressful. If you find this to be the case with your children, go with occupational therapy, and remember that they may need more detoxification and brain support to be able to da what is asked of them.

A book that may be helpful for you on ABA is *Let Me Hear Your Voice* by Katherine Maurice.

For additional information and resources a good site is www.rsaffran.tripod.com/aba.html.

SUMMARY

A disorganized brain can prevent a child with sensory processing disorders from performing the tasks asked of him, regardless of how hard he tries. Society has trained us to believe otherwise. A proper diagnosis by a specialist in the field of sensory processing disorders and those on the autism spectrum is essential. There are four different sensory processing disorders: visual, auditory, vestibular, and tactile, so symptoms vary greatly.

Never rule out the strong possibility that your child may still be toxic. If his body and brain are filled with toxins he will not be able to behave or do as he is asked. In order to have success, his biology must be healed and he must have strong support from his teachers and family.

There are ways to support him along the way with calming techniques, various therapeutic options and multiple resources available. It is beneficial to work with his health as much as possible to balance his system and support his brain so that he can have the optimum outcome.

The products found in this chapter can be found at http://naturallyhealingautism.com/a-healthy-home/

CHAPTER 4

GENETIC SUSCEPTIBILITY

Of all factors, genetics play the most important role. Genes are basically just DNA blueprints. They are a pre-set program, but can be effected by the environment. What changes or mutates a gene is the signal it receives. Three reasons for signaling defects are:

1. Trauma: via the nervous system. It impairs brain signals to proteins.
2. Toxins: chemicals interfere with signals to proteins.
3. Mind: wrong signals are sent at the wrong times and create dysfunction and disease.

Less than five percent of humans have genetic defects at birth. Ninety-five percent of defects are from incorrect signals. The outer coating of the cell is the "brain" of the cell, or the cell membrane. Genes are controlled by proteins within the cell. Protein is engaged by signals. The cell membrane can be permeated by one of the three signaling defects noted above and the protein portion of the cell can be disrupted. When the protein is disrupted it creates dysfunction or disease.

The brain contains a protein that excretes toxins, and this protein has three different structural make-ups: APO-E2, APO-E3, and APO-E4. They each have a different capability to remove mercury from the brain. The APO-E2 protein is capable of carrying two atoms of mercury away from the brain, while APO-E3 can only carry one. The APO-E4 protein, however, is not capable of removing any atoms of mercury from the brain.

We get one of these proteins from each of our parents. The two genes we inherit determine our brain's ability to detoxify this neurotoxin. If both of our parents have the APO-E4 protein, we have an 80% chance of getting Alzheimer's disease. One study showed that autistic children commonly have large amounts of APO-E4 protein in their brains.

When there is a mutation in this gene, there may be no symptoms or it can cause many health disorders such as autism, Down's syndrome, heart defects, pulmonary problems, irritable bowel syndrome, chemical sensitivities, chronic fatigue, and hypothyroid. The mutation commonly causes mental and neurological disorders such as depression, anxiety, irritability, epilepsy, and bipolar disorders.

The proteins in cells collect their blueprints from DNA. Genes serve no other function than to store and pass on blueprints. It is now known that the genes we get from our parents can be altered by our environment, a phenomenon known as epigenetics. Even more interesting is that these alterations can be passed on to the next generation. (Reprogramming of Genome Function Through Epigenetic Inheritance; Surani, M. Azim; Nature, Volume 414, Issue 6859, Pp.122-128 92001); 11/2001; Nature; 2001 natur.414.122s.)

Genes lie dormant until a trigger signals its protein receptor and engages it causing either a positive or a negative reaction. If autism, ADHD, pervasive developmental disorder, seizures, juvenile rheumatoid arthritis, Type 1 diabetes, asthma, and bowel disorders were not occurring in epidemic proportions 50 years ago, then what has changed? There appears to be a correlation with an increased number of vaccinations.

For religious reasons, the Amish choose not to vaccinate, and their children have virtually none of the developmental or behavioral issues that the children of our modern society do. Is this merely coincidence? If it were environmental, as in electromagnetic field pollution and toxins in the air we breathe, it would be intelligent to believe that some of their children would be affected, but why none? One separating factor is that they do not vaccinate.

MTHFr GENETIC MUTATION

There is a gene called methylenetetrahydofolate (MTHF). The enzyme in this gene is known as methylenetetrahydofolate reductase, or MTHFr. More than forty mutations in this gene have been detected. This enzyme is responsible for processing amino acids which are the building blocks of protein, synthesizing and utilizing B vitamins (especially folic acid and vitamin B12 to its active form of methylcobalamin). The enzyme is also needed to assist the body in the making of glutathione. A mutation in this gene also causes a disruption in the methylation pathway allowing for multiple detoxifying issues at the cellular level. A mutation in this gene is very common among those with the mold biotoxin genetic disorder discussed in the chapter on underlying issues.

When there is a mutation in this gene there may be no symptoms or it can cause many health disorders such as autism, Down's syndrome, heart defects, pulmonary problems, irritable bowel syndrome, chemical sensitivities, chronic fatigue, and hypothyroid. The mutation commonly causes mental and neurological disorders such as depression, anxiety, irritability, epilepsy, and bipolar disorders.

Treatment for those with this disorder is supplementation with liposomal glutathione or a glutathione transdermal patch, and active forms of B vitamins.

Genetic testing for MTHFr can be tested for through an oral swab, saliva tests, or blood testing. The oral and saliva tests are great for children. Both parents can be tested for this prior to conception to see if either one carries it. It can be tested for during any stage of life. Lab tests run about $150.00. Dr. Ben Lynch is the foremost authority on MTHFr and its findings. For more information or to order a test go to, www.mthfr.net.

Additional genetic mutations to be aware of are:

- MTR/MTRR(Methionine synthase reductase): The combination of these two mutations can deplete methyl B12, (contributing to methylcobalamin deficiency), and they work together to convert homocysteine to Methionine. Treat with B12 and folate.

- MAO-A R297R(monoamine oxidase A): An enzyme necessary for breaking down neurotransmitters for the brain such as serotonin, norepinephrine, and dopamine. This tends to be common in children with autism. Individuals with this mutation may experience neuropsychiatric conditions or symptoms such as obsessive compulsive disorder (OCD), mood swings and/or violent behavior.
- COMT (catechol-O-methyltransferase): This enzyme also breaks down neurotransmitters such as dopamine, epinephrine, and norepinephrine. The enzyme is needed by the area of the brain known as the pre-frontal cortex which is responsible for executive functioning, planning, and the knowledge of consequences per actions, short-term memory, emotion and inhibition of behavior. Common symptoms are irritability, hyperactivity, and abnormal behavior. COMT also assists with the metabolism of estrogens. COMT can be measured through a twenty four hour urine test.
- VDR (vitamin D receptor): Vitamin D receptors are necessary to allow the body to assimilate vitamin D. Vitamin D is necessary in fighting both bacteria and viruses. It is also an essential part of brain health assisting enzymes to build dopamine. Dopamine is essential in attention, focus, and impulse control.
- BHMT(betaine homocysteine methyltransferase): This enzyme assists the methylation cycle in converting homocysteine to Methionine. This enzyme can be greatly affected by stress. A mutation in this enzyme may lead to a breakdown in dopamine. This is the neurotransmitter responsible for attention, focus and impulse control.

For more information go to www.geneticgenie.org/methylation-results-23and me/. Also read the book, Autism: Pathways to Recovery, by Amy Yasko.

GENETIC TESTING

There are a couple of tests that can be done prior to conception or after birth to detect possible genetic abnormalities. We have previously discussed the testing for the gene called methylenetetrahydofolate (MTHF), and the defect to the important enzyme in this gene known as methylenetetrahydofolate reductase, or MTHFr.

An additional test that can be done to test some genetic susceptibilities is called the Buccal test. The Buccal test is by Genova Laboratories. Buccal basically means saliva or inner cheek. This test is done by swabbing the inside of the cheek with a cotton swab provided in the test kit. This is very easy to do for a child of any age. It is then sent to the lab.

Testing collects DNA cells and evaluates genetic variations called single nucleotide polymorphins (SNP's). These genes modulate blood pressure, lipid balance, nutrient metabolism, inflammation, oxidative stress, and possible defects in the immune system. It also tests for susceptibilities in metabolism of liver phases one, two, and three. Your liver enzymes are also tested to detect how they affect your metabolism. Often glutathione is not made properly or at all by people with this issue so supplementation with liposomal glutathione is essential.

Having a gene with a SNP mutation does not necessarily mean that the gene is not functioning properly. What testing does provide is an explanation as to why certain diseases or specific traits such as autism tend to be symptomatic in multiple family members. This can be helpful prior to conception and birth to determine if your child may be more susceptible to the dangers of environmental triggers such as vaccinations.

These tests are available from many health practitioners and can be purchased online at sites such as www.integrativepsychiatry.net, (800)385-7863. The test results can be emailed to you.

HEALING THE GENETIC DEFECT

Genetic defects may be triggered by trauma, injury, or viruses such as those induced by vaccination. These defects caused by vaccines are known to continue for four generations! Energy signals are one hundred percent more effective than physical ones. Genetic mutations are reversible with the use of homeopathic remedies. For more information on this subject please listen to the audio at www.klinghardtacademy.com.

My son was given the constitutional homeopathic remedy Thuja by our homeopathic doctor. This assists with nervousness around strangers, is intended to help over-sensitive people and addresses any residual susceptibility or symptoms that he carries or his body has adapted to or compensates for related to vaccinations. The remedy inspires the vital force to restore that back to health.

A "constitutional" remedy addresses the needs of the entire person including the physical, mental, and emotional. A good homeopathic doctor is essential. Please see chapter two for information on how to find one.

A very informative explanation on genes is given by Bruce Lipton in his CD audio book, *The Wisdom of Your Cells.*

SUMMARY

Genes are DNA blueprints, but they can be effected by the environment. Only five percent of genetic defects happen in utero, from the time of birth. Ninety five percent come from three factors. These three factors are trauma via the nervous system, toxic chemicals and emotional trauma.

Proteins within the cells control them. They receive signals from the environment. We all carry genetics but it is within the signals that the blueprint of the gene is expressed. This can be a positive outcome or a negative one.

Testing is available if you would like to see if any genes are carried by either parent that may make your child susceptible to various issues. Healthy parents and clean environment make the biggest difference. If problems do arise, homeopathy has shown to be very beneficial in healing the genetic defects.

The products found in this chapter can be found at http://naturallyhealingautism.com/a-healthy-home/

SECTION II:

THE WHAT AND WHY BASICS

CHAPTER 5

DETOXIFICATION AND ORGAN SUPPORT

FIRST: SUPPORT THE LIVER

It is more than likely that your child's liver is congested. It is the first organ to support in the healing process. The liver has many diverse functions. It is our main organ of detoxification, it builds and supplies nutrients, enzymes, and hormones to cells, and directly affects growth and functioning of all cells in the body. If the liver cannot supply these nutrients to the cells, the cells cannot perform the activities necessary to keep your body healthy. If the liver is congested, it cannot effectively remove toxins from the body. The liver, among its many duties, also produces hormones, amino acids, and protein. The body can become deprived of these important compounds if the is liver congested. Amino acids are the building blocks of protein. They also build neurotransmitters needed by the brain for its proper functioning.

Imbalanced gut flora, environmental toxins, and poor diet all contribute to liver congestion from the formation of gallstones. High acid foods and beverages begin to thicken the blood. This includes excessive intake of protein rich foods including animal fats. Gallstones block the blood flow through the liver, the bile duct, and the gallbladder. Without proper functioning of the liver's processes disease will form.

The liver can be congested as early as birth. By cutting or clamping the umbilical cord too soon (less than about an hour after birth), it leaves the baby with a reduced volume of nutrient filled blood, and an increased toxic load that was not filtered out via the placenta. A fetus is susceptible to the toxins in the mother's body. The average woman puts about 515 synthetic chemicals on her body every day. These are absorbed through the skin and eventually must be filtered by the liver. When the liver becomes congested it is unable to filter toxins. Many of these toxins are the same ones that congested it in the first place. The liver filters toxic chemicals from food, water, air pollutants, pesticides, medications, plastics, soaps, lotions, vaccinations, and more. This sets up the liver to develop early childhood gallstones.

Children on the autism spectrum almost always, if not always, have an imbalance in gut flora, or gut bacteria. One of the biggest problems is candida or yeast. The toxins released by the yeast organisms are very harmful to the liver. We will discuss candida in great detail in chapter seven.

Sugars, especially high fructose corn syrup, are a big part of the problem for the liver also. Blood sugars and metabolic syndrome must be put under control. Non-alcoho;ic fatty liver is an accumulation of triglycerides and fat in the liver that cause it to start poisoning itself. The skin often tells us if these fats are not being properly broken down. Rashes, hives, very dry or flaky skin are all common indicators.

Blood tests can detect fatty liver too. If the test determines that the enzyme alanine transaminase (ALT) levels are high, then it is positive for fatty liver. ALT is the most important enzyme indicator in fatty liver detection.

Liver enzymes can tell us about inflammation in the body. These enzymes can give a good baseline level to track progress of treatment if done both before and after cleansing. If affordability is an issue, then after treatment is complete would be best.

To avoid trauma to a child via blood tests there is a great alternative. The laboratory Diagnos-Techs offer a panel used with your child's stool that can give their inflammation markers along with a lot of other valuable information. It does not specifically test liver enzymes but inflammation markers tell us a lot about what is going on in the liver. This test can also check for IgA antibodies (gluten allergens), parasites, fungus, and more. Most alternative practitioners use this laboratory and have these tests on hand, or they can order them at Diagnos-Techs, 425-251-0596.

Liver gallstones are basically hardened clusters of cholesterol and organic material such as fatty acids. Due to their structure, they cannot be seen on x-rays, ultrasounds, or computer tomography scans

(CT scans). For this reason, they often go undetected. They will disrupt food digestion, waste elimination, and overall detoxification.

Liver bile is an alkaline fluid that is necessary for the proper digestion of fats and protein, calcium absorption, elimination of toxins from the liver, maintaining the correct pH or acid/alkaline balance in the intestines, and preventing harmful bacteria from growing in the large intestine. For adequate health, the liver must produce one to one and a half quarts of bile per day. It is not uncommon for people to produce less than a cupful per day. The liver filters more than a liter of blood every minute. Although the liver bile may be too low for proper digestion, liver enzymes in blood may still show normal in tests.

A poor working liver and gallbladder will lead to nutrient deficiencies. When the supply of bile, pancreatic lipase (fat enzymes), and pancreatic fat are too low, due to a congested liver and gallbladder, the body cannot absorb the fat-soluble vitamins A, D, E, and K, or the all-important essential fatty acids. These vitamins cannot be properly digested or absorbed from food or supplements. The digestive tract does not have the enzymes it needs and the nutrients necessary for proper digestion are not absorbed from food. The fat soluble vitamins and good fats such as olive oil, coconut oil, and avocado oil are crucial for a number of organ functions including brain protection, healthy vision, viral and bacterial combat, and protection of the intestinal lining.

The nutrition in the blood feeds the brain. When the brain does not receive what it needs, it is starved of its essential nutrients. The brain, therefore, cannot manufacture the chemicals necessary to carry out its vital functions. This can result in fatigue, depression, inability to concentrate, insomnia, irritability, illness, and more.

If we begin to detoxify the system without first supporting the liver, the toxins will back up into the bloodstream. These toxins affect multiple systems of the body, including the brain, and we can become quite ill. Viruses, bacteria, and fungi use the undigested food and waste as food. The liver must be able to remove toxins, damaged cells, and other waste material from the body. Excess toxins congest the lymph glands, which remove cellular waste and keep the immune system healthy. The liver and lymphatic system must be able to feed nutrients to the cells and remove their debris.

Dandelion and milk thistle help to increase the body's production of bile along with increasing the health of the liver.

PHASE I AND PHASE II OF LIVER DETOXIFICATION

There are two different phases in liver detoxification. They are known and referred to as Phase I and Phase II.

Phase I burns toxins with oxygen and enzymes. Phase I breaks down the raw materials. After this takes place the extremely toxic compound benzene is formed. In order to detoxify benzene, and complete full detoxification process, the Phase II enzymes are needed. Phase II can become disrupted if there is a poor diet, especially one containing too many bad fats such as corn, safflower, sunflower, peanut, canola or soybean oils, a deficiency in the body's master antioxidant glutathione, toxins such as medications and pesticides, and heavy metals which are particularly damaging to liver enzymes. High fructose corn syrup and sugars create an imbalance in blood sugar which can also be harmful to the liver. It is important to keep your blood sugar under control.

In Phase II the oxidized chemicals are combined with sulfur, organic acids, and amino acids. Protein builds the necessary amino acids cysteine and methionine which build sulfur for Phase II of liver detoxification. Cysteine and methionine build the additional necessary amino acid taurine. N-Acetyl Cysteine (NAC) carries a sulfhydryl group (thiol) which binds to toxins. The master antioxidant glutathione is made in the liver from NAC. Along with these necessary steps healthy methylation and sulfation pathways are all crucial for proper Phase II detoxification. If this does not carry out correctly the liver can become congested and the oxidized chemicals cannot be excreted via the bile or the urine. If these toxins are not released the entire body, bloodstream, immune system, lymphatic system, digestive system, skin and respiratory system may all become toxic causing a myriad of health and behavioral problems.

Excretion takes place via urine or feces. It is crucial that the bowel is in good health so that these toxins do not get reabsorbed into the body. Roughage from green leafy vegetables, and fruit, especially berries, along with plenty of pure water will assist this. Vitamin C and magnesium will both get the bowel moving. Also minimize foods that bind and may cause constipation if this is an issue. Some examples of binding foods are gluten, cheese, and red meat.

SULFATION AND METHYLATION

Sulfation or sulfur metabolism and methylation are important in detoxification and each are affected by a weak liver.

Sulfation or Sulfate Metabolism

Proteins contain sulfites which turn to sulfates in the body. We need sulfates to assist detoxification, reduce inflammation, and help make stomach acid and digestive enzymes. A lack of ability to properly digest proteins causes the body to become low in sulfates. This combined with a weakened liver make it difficult for the body to properly digest and eliminate many chemicals, including those in foods. Genetically modified foods are known to effect sulfur metabolism.

The enzyme sulfite oxidase converts sulfites to sulfates in our body. Too many sulfites can be dangerous to your health. Too little sulfates also lead to damage to the nervous system, vision, and chronic illness. Due to genetic abnormalities in this enzyme or an improperly working digestive system it is very common to be low in sulfates. The sulfite oxidase enzyme needs molybdenum and vitamin B2, (riboflavin). Both are commonly deficient in children with autism. They can be taken in supplemental form, but foods which build molybdenum are red cabbage and buckwheat.

An additional way to increase sulfates in the body is through Epsom salts baths. Epsom salts are chemically magnesium sulfate. The sulfates pass through the pours of the skin and get into the bloodstream. Very warm water opens the pours and allows this to be most efficient. One cup of water dissolved in bath water one to three times per day can be helpful.

The Methylation Cycle

Methylation is a type of gene expression (see chapter four for more on genes). There are hundreds of different methylation reactions in the body. Most commonly noted is its role in the body's ability to detoxify. Eighty five to ninety percent of people with autism are known to have reduced methylation. Methylation is required to produce glutathione.

When there is heavy toxic burden on the liver it has a strong demand for the body's master antioxidant glutathione. When glutathione level drops low enough, the sulfur metabolism becomes disrupted. The methylation cycle (part of the sulfur metabolism, or detoxification) can become partially blocked and deplete some or all of several important sulfur containing metabolites including S-Adenosyl Methionine (SAMe), cysteine, glutathione, taurine, and sulfate. This can create such a weakening in the system that it allows disease to develop.

Supplements that assist methylation are calcium, DMG, folic acid, vitamin B6, vitamin B12, magnesium, zinc, and SAMe. Glutathione can also be taken in supplemental form. See the chapter on "common nutritional deficiencies" for more information on these supplements and where to buy them.

Individuals on the autism spectrum tend to have difficulty with protein synthesis, low levels of taurine, sulfur and glutathione, thus interrupting the detoxification pathways. Sulfuric molecules are involved in metabolic and methylation processes. Glutathione is especially needed to remove heavy metal toxicity such as those from vaccines. As you can see many of the originating issues for those on the autism spectrum start with liver congestion. It is crucial to get this organ of detoxification working properly.

Some symptoms and illnesses associated with liver congestion are:

- chronic infection
- digestive difficulty
- poor assimilation of nutrients
- obesity
- loss of weight
- loss of appetite
- diabetes
- anemia
- mineral deficiency
- reduced protein synthesis

- kidney problems
- upper respiratory weakness including difficulty breathing, and respiratory infections including pneumonia
- lowered immunity
- hearing trouble and ear infections
- headaches
- depression
- irritability
- fatigue
- ADHD
- skin problems (itching, acne, hives, rashes)
- sinus and tonsil issues
- arthritis
- high blood pressure
- heart trouble, including heart attack
- stroke
- urinary tract issues
- hormonal imbalances
- bone
- allergies
- back pain
- gout
- vision problems
- circulation problems
- tooth decay and gum disease
- viral infections
- parasites
- Hemorrhoids
- thyroid imbalance

RESTORING THE HEALTH OF THE LIVER

The good news is that with proper cleansing, the liver can be restored to health in most cases. When this happens, allergies and other illnesses often disappear. Decongesting and supporting the liver can reduce or eliminate most diseases.

There is an excellent liver flush book that explains everything in great detail. The book, *The Amazing Liver and Gallbladder Flush*, by Andreas Moritz is an easy, do-it-yourself liver cleanse (for adults). There is one drawback for children with this particular flush. It must be followed by colonic irrigation. This liver cleanse can be done by most people over the age of ten, however, without this crucial step, toxic gallstones released from the liver can get lodged in the intestinal tract on their way out and create greater health problems. Most children and teens may not want to try this process. That's OK, but if they do, it is one of the best ways possible to flush the stones from their body and regain health. Professional colonic irrigation is best, but enemas done at home can be very helpful with any liver detoxification program.

COFFEE AND CHLOROPHYLL ENEMAS

For older children, adults, and those who are willing, coffee and chlorophyll enemas are a healthy way to stimulate the cells of the liver and assist it in detoxification. They are also a great idea when doing any type of cleanse or when you feel like you may be catching a cold or flu. They are great for boosting the immune system.

The fluid absorbs into the bowel wall and hemorrhoidal veins, then flows directly into the portal veins and into the liver. Lie on your right side with your knees pulled up against your chest. Hold and allow the fluid to absorb for about ten minutes, if possible.

FORMULA:

1. Add three heaping tablespoons of organic ground coffee (not instant) to two and a half cups of water.
2. Let the solution boil three minutes and then simmer five to ten more minutes.

3. Put two cups of filtered water at room temperature into an enema bag. Add filtered coffee.

It is best to do an enema about two hours after a bowel movement.

Free radicals are released during this process so drink a green drink just after.

Do the coffee enema three days in a row, take three days off, then take four days off from them. Repeat this process three times.

Check with you practitioner regarding the age of your child.

If your child will not agree to colonics or enemas, (as mine did not), then the following supplementation or homeopathic remedies are the next best option. Although, the following supplements are still necessary.

CHLOROPHYLL ENEMA

Follow each coffee enema with a chlorophyll enema using three tablespoons of chlorophyll to two cups of warm filtered water.

FOODS TO ASSIST LIVER HEALTH

Eat organic foods whenever possible. Foods that help create healthy liver enzymes are organic vegetables, fruit, beans, nuts, seeds, whole grains, organically grown meats, poultry, eggs, and fish that has not been farmed or has not come from polluted waters. Protein is necessary to build the amino acids necessary for proper Phase II liver detoxification, but do not eat animal fats in excess because the higher protein content and acidity can be hard on the liver and end up affecting the entire body. Methionine and cysteine build glutathione. Foods that help build methionine and cysteine are cruciferous vegetables such as broccoli, cauliflower, cabbage, and kale. Juicing with fresh organic fruits and vegetables can help the body build bile.

SUPPLEMENTS TO ASSIST RESTORING LIVER HEALTH

There are a few good liver support products to choose from. *You will only need one program from the list below*, but I like to offer choices. For assistance with your decision muscle test prior to purchase and ask the question, "Which one will be best utilized by my child's body?" The cost of each product varies greatly, as does the type of supplement (i.e. liquid, or capsule).

The first liver product I used was Liver Life by Bioray. It is a daily liver and kidney decongestant. It facilitates detoxification and has been shown in laboratory tests to normalize liver enzymes. It also helps to restore pH levels in the body, improve digestion and absorption of nutrients, and help with bowel function. This is a liquid, so it can be added to any beverage easily. The best price for it can be found on www.amazon.com. With any purchase over twenty-five dollars shipping is free if you choose super-saver shipping on Amazon. There is also a good price at www.pureformulas.com, and free shipping.

The company Integrative Therapeutics makes a product that supports both Phase I and Phase II of liver detoxification. The two supplements are Detoxification Factor and Blue Heron. These are professional grade formulas and should be used with the assistance of a healthcare practitioner. Both are available at www.pureformulas.com. It is in capsule form that can be opened up and put into food or beverage.

An additional product, which supports phases I and II of liver detoxification, is the product Liver Support and Detoxification by the company Pharmax. It is sold in most health food stores and online at sites such as www.pureformulas.com. It comes in capsule form.

There are homeopathic remedies that can be very helpful and may be easier to offer children. There is a simple three part Antitox program, by the company Apex Energetics, www.apexenergetics.com (800) 736-4381. They are a twenty-five-year-old, research-based company with the highest quality formulas available. Their products are very easy-to-take liquids that come with a dropper for sublingual use. My family has had great success with many of their products over the past decade for various needs. This liver detoxification program is as follows:

1. The product "Gentle Drainage" is used. Commonly three to five drops under the tongue, one to three times per day, or as directed by your healthcare practitioner until the bottle is gone.

2. The product Lymph Terrain (T2), by Apexenergetics is used the same way as step one.
3. The product Liver Max (H-2), by Apexenergetics is used the same way as the preceding two products.

Additionally, the liver regularly excretes neurotoxins that make their way into the small intestine. These toxins can reabsorb into the nerve endings there and travel up the spinal cord to the brain. The binding agent Beta Sitosterol has been known to stop reabsorption. The company Pharmax makes Beta Sitosterol. Dosages of one to two capsules, four times per day between meals with two doses at bedtime have been known to be helpful. Take this medication for three weeks on, then three weeks off, for six to twelve weeks. Check with your healthcare practitioner for your child's dosage and needs. Beta Sitosterol by Pharmax can be found at most health food stores and online at many sites such as www.pureformulas.com, and www.amazon.com.

ADDITIONAL ASSISTANCE

A few drops of lemon in water a few times a day helps to alkalize the system and, because of its astringency, also assist the liver in detoxifying. The best time of day to do this is first thing in the morning because it stimulates the activity of liver cells and gets them going for the day. The liver of a child on the autism spectrum is usually very congested and it is always a good idea to strengthen it.

The below supplements help to assist the liver processes. In depth information on each can be found in the chapter, "common nutritional deficiencies."

- Silymarin (the active form of milk thistle) carries the necessary bioflavonoids to assist liver detoxification. Generally, 70-210 mg three times per day is helpful.
- N-Acetyl Cysteine (noted above) makes glutathione and binds to toxins.
- Glutathione

- Phosphotidyl choline helps to protect the liver and all other cells of the body. It also assists with brain building, brain chemistry, and cognitive learning. Phosphotidyl choline is contained in krill oil so if you are already giving your children krill oil they will be getting some of this nutrient, as long as fat digestion is working properly. Dosages of 1200-1500mg per day have been known to be helpful.
- Zinc increases the liver's ability to detoxify heavy metals through increased production of metallothioneins. These are proteins and polypeptides that contain large amounts of metal and sulfur. They are found throughout the body. When mercury, lead, or cadmium enters the liver, its cells begin producing large quantities of metallothioneins. Zinc should not be used in excess as it can increase the amount of toxicity from heavy metals. Usually ten to fifteen miligrams per day is plenty, depending on age and weight. Zinc should be balanced with a small amount of copper. See the chapter on common nutritional deficiencies for more on this.

Check with your healthcare practitioner regarding your child's age and size for any supplement. Muscle testing is very helpful also.

Generally, it is a good idea never to overeat as it can reduce blood flow to the liver, which inhibits bile and produces gallstones. Except for those with medical conditions such as diabetes or hypoglycemia, allow your stomach to empty between meals, and do not eat after 6:00 P.M. The liver produces less bile after this time and this hinders digestion.

Healthy water sources are crucial. Fluoride and other heavy metals are often found in tap water along with chlorine and other chemical contaminants. See the chapter on environmental toxins for information on healthy water.

Genova Laboratories makes a liver detoxification profile test done from a buccal (cheek) swab. Your health care practitioner can order one or they can be found at many online sites such as www.completehealthinstitute.com.

For more information, and a resource guide to consultations with experts in liver disease, see the resource section of Andreas Moritz' website, www.ener-chi.com.

GALLBLADDER

The gallbladder is a small organ that protrudes from the bile duct at the back of the liver. It stores liver bile. Before moving down the bile duct into the digestive tract, liver bile must pass through the gallbladder. The walls of the gallbladder release bile for the digestion of foods that contain proteins, acids, or fats. When the amount of bile is too low due to intestinal congestion it leaves fats undigested creating trouble in the GI tract.

Liver gallstones also grow in the gallbladder. These stones will obstruct the movement of bile and disrupt digestion. Stones in the gallbladder are often more calcified and can be seen with an ultrasound. The frightening part is that a stone may grow for up to eight years before it causes any discomfort or problems.

When there is not enough bile to help with the breakdown of foods, especially fats, we often feel nauseous. Nausea is a common symptom of gallbladder weakness. The best supplement I have found to assist the gallbladder is A-F Betafood by Standard Process. Standard Process supplements are food-based. This means that they come from real foods. Most natural practitioners carry them in their offices. A-F Betafood can also be found for a good price at www.amazon.com. Individual needs vary, so muscle test your child or talk to your healthcare practitioner to determine the number of supplements needed per meal. The Standard Process product Phosphood Liquid is an even deeper cleanse for the gallbladder. It helps to remove the buildup of "sludge" in the gallbladder. I have found that it gives almost immediate relief.

When my gallbladder acts up, I muscle test and usually find that I need to take four or five A-F Betafood with each meal. My daughter needs three pills three times per day. If pills are a problem, you can mash them up and add them to food or beverage. A one-third dropper full of Phosfood also does the trick, and it is liquid. Phosfood has a bitter taste, so add it to a small amount of beverage to mask the taste.

The liver flush by Andreas Moritz previously discussed under the chapter heading "Liver" will remove the gallstones from the gallbladder as well as the liver. Do not think that because your gallbladder is clear in diagnostic tests that liver gallstones do not exist. They usually do, but are not detectable. The liver support supplements will assist gallbladder help as well. There is also a specific gallbladder flush program that works very well from Standard Process. Ask your alternative healthcare practitioner for assistance with this, but remember that the liver must be cleansed too.

THE COLON

The health of the colon, or the large intestine, is critical to overall health. Daily bowel movements must release toxic material or it can be reabsorbed into the walls of the large intestine. Constipation allows for toxic reabsorption due to the extended amount of time the waste stays in the bowels. Proper amounts of water are needed to allow for the removal of waste including pesticides, hormones, and antibiotics in animal feed, and carcinogenic agents in the air we breathe. Dehydration and lack of proper fiber can cause constipation.

The bowels effect behavior through toxic reabsorption, but they are also very sensitive to the neurotransmitters in the digestive tract. These brain signaling chemicals include adrenaline, norepinephrine, and serotonin.

Fiber is essential when feces are moving well to keep digestion on track, but contrary to popular belief, if the bowel is constipated and lodged with waste, taking fiber often makes it worse. Fiber acts to further bind what is not moving. If you are constipated, aloe leaf is an excellent choice for getting things moving. More options are listed below. Be sure to avoid binding foods such as gluten, cheese and red meat.

The large intestine also absorbs minerals necessary for our health. An improperly working colon causes nutrient deficiencies. Enemas are helpful to release fecal matter from the lower portion of the large intestine. Coffee enemas will stimulate the nerves in the liver and assist its detoxification processes. Colonic irrigation or colonics are an essential part of health. They gently remove old debris from the entire colon and its walls by cleansing it with distilled or purified water.

Colonics can be done as early as age six, although many children may not agree to this. If they do, be sure to see an Advanced Certified Colon Hydrotherapist. To find and I-ACT certified professional go to, www.i-act.org, or call (210) 366-2888.

The acronym H.O.P.E. is sometimes used to help remember what to do to assist the health of the colon.

H.O.P.E stands for:

- **H**igh fiber
- **Omega-3** oils
- **P**robiotics
- **E**nzymes.

Supplement and food choices to assist bowel regulation:

- Probiotics are the best choice. They naturally help regulate the bowels, increasing movement or slowing it down when needed. Probiotics are discussed in detail in the chapter on Reducing Inflammation.
- Aloe (aloe leaf is best for constipation). Aloe Complete Whole Leaf Concentrate is sold at www.crohns.net.
- No-phenol enzymes from www.houston-enzymes.com help to loosen stool.
- Zyme-Prime enzymes from www.houston-enzymes.com help to firm stool when it is too loose.
- The product Colonmax is helpful for constipation. It contains many beneficial herbs such as slippery elm, marshmallow, magnesium, rhubarb, cape aloe, and triphala, www.advancednaturals.com (866) 594-5468.
- Magnesium pulls water into the bowel and relaxes the smooth muscle to assist excretion. The product Natural Calm/Natural Vitality is best. It is sold at most healthfood stores and at www.pureformulas.com.
- Vitamin C gets the bowels moving
- Curcumin is an antioxidant and can be helpful in colon health.
- N-butyrate is in oat bran or supplemental form. When taken with vitamin E it has been shown to reduce colon cancer and improve colon function.

- Colosan is a magnesium-based product combined with oxides, which release oxygen into the colon. It also assists in the removal of parasites and old fecal matter, www.colosan.com (800) 416-7114.
- Green leafy vegetables
- Fruit, especially berries
- Omega-3 oils
- Drink six to eight glasses of water a day.

Some high fiber foods are:

- Flax
- Chia seeds
- Fruit, especially berries, prunes, avocados, and apples with the skin on.
- Vegetables, especially green leafy ones such as broccoli, kale, and artichokes
- Nuts
- Beans
- Oat bran
- Brown rice

For more information and a resource guide to consultations with experts in colon disease see the resource section of Andreas Moritz' website, www.ener-chi.com.

KIDNEYS

Kidneys filter the blood, and they have the job of keeping the proper balance of pH between alkaline mineral sodium and acidic potassium. The right balance in the blood and other fluids of the body is essential for bodily functions to take place properly. Disease is present when the body is too acidic or too alkaline. Additionally, when toxins are reabsorbed into the blood, they circulate to the brain.

Cell communication and fluid exchange is altered when the kidneys become congested and cannot do their job. Vitamin D cannot be converted into its active form if the kidneys are not working properly.

Kidney congestion is often due to an acidic diet, poor digestion, dehydration, and stress. Our bodies need water to flush out the toxins, not drinks filled with sugar and chemicals that cause them to work harder. Fluid retention begins and bloating and weight gain may be noticeable.

If kidney stones grow large enough, they will block the flow of fluid from the kidneys and create a build up of more toxic waste. Because they are crystalline in nature, kidney stones cannot be detected by x-rays nor do they usually cause pain. If they go unnoticed, these stones can wreak havoc. Aside from toxic build up in the body, the kidneys may become diseased and urinary discharge can become obstructed.

SYMPTOMS OF WEAK KIDNEYS AND ADRENALS:

- dry eyes
- chronic dry cough
- excessive thirst
- low grade fever
- excessive perspiration
- sore back, knees, or legs

Always be sure to drink a lot of pure water to assist the health of your kidneys. The mineral phosphorus also assists kidney function.

There is a simple way to detect sand and stones in the kidneys. Pull the skin under your eyes sideways toward the cheekbones. Any strange bumps, red or white pimples, or discolored skin indicates that sand or stones are present in the kidneys.

Specific herbs are recommended by Andreas Moritz to cleanse the kidneys. These herbs should be taken as directed in his book, The Amazing Liver and Gallbladder Flush, and are sold in an already prepared mixture at www.presentmoment.com.

For more information and a resource guide to consultations with experts in kidney disease, see the resource section of Andreas Moritz' website www.ener-chi.com.

THE ADRENAL GLANDS

The adrenal glands are located just above the kidneys. They are the glands that handle the body's stress. The main way the adrenals react to stress is by releasing the hormone Cortisol. When the adrenal glands sense stress they release the stress hormone Cortisol. Cortisol is a natural anti-inflammatory, but it requires the adrenals to work even harder. Whenever the body endures ongoing stress, whether physical or emotional, the adrenal glands become fatigued. When the liver is congested it will cause an imbalance in hormones and affect the adrenal cortex.

Many children are born today with weak adrenals. The adrenals can become weak in utero due to stress on the mothers' system and pathogenic bacteria stressing both the mother and the fetus. If the immune system is fighting any weakness, the adrenal glands are put to work. When the gut is imbalanced, the body is toxic. Food allergies are created and the ongoing inflammation is a trigger for the adrenal glands, along with the immune system, to fight for the body's health and wellbeing. A drop in blood sugar or hypoglycemia can be created by a lack of absorption of nutrients due to pathogenic bacteria in the gut. Hypoglycemia is another strong trigger for the adrenal glands to release Cortisol.

Hypoglycemia is very hard on the adrenal glands. It is a challenge during the day, but also very hard on your system at night. During sleep, Candida feeds on your blood sugar. This stresses the body and the brain and your glucose levels are lowered significantly. Your brain relies on the right amount of glucose to function properly. Therefore, this stress during sleep overworks the adrenal glands due to this imbalance in blood sugar. When the adrenals become fatigued it creates an imbalance in your thyroid gland.

When cortisol release becomes deregulated by the adrenal glands, it can result in adrenal fatigue. The adrenals will often release too much Cortisol. A common symptom is waking in the night, usually around 3:00 a.m. One supplement that helps this Cortisol regulation, and may help regain sleep balance, is Seriphos by Interplexus available at www.pureformulas.com. I have had personal success with this product. After using it for about three months, the system regains balance and the product should no longer be used. It simply assists the body for a short time to help it get back on track.

When blood sugar drops, it causes low glucose levels in the brain. Thus, the brain's energy supply is low. This causes the brain to secrete toxins such as glutamate. The result is negative behavior and mis-wiring in the brain. This is especially disruptive when the brain is developing and also causes adrenal problems. Hyperactivity, an inability to handle emotions, and aggressive behavior are common symptoms.

An imbalance of adrenal hormones can impair the body's ability to grow and to recover from illness and injury. This imbalance also disrupts the body's ability to build and utilize protein, or to perform what is known as protein synthesis. Proteins are needed for the health of cells and other necessary hormones in the body.

Some medications can be especially hard on the adrenal glands such as corticosteroids, opiates, and insulin. The heavy metal, mercury, can weaken the adrenals and suppress the immune system via injury to the hypothalamus, which has no blood-brain barrier. In turn, an injured hypothalamus can cause lifelong suppression of the immune system and weaken the adrenals and the thyroid.

Symptoms of adrenal fatigue include:

- Insomnia, or awakening in the night with anxiety (commonly between 1:00 a.m. and 3:00 a.m.)
- Cravings for salt or salty foods
- Daily fatigue
- Hormonal imbalance
- Blood sugar imbalance and cravings for sugary foods or carbohydrates
- Lowered immune system
- Gaining weight and trouble losing weight
- Difficulty getting up in the morning
- Dizziness when getting up quickly

- Mild depression
- Lack of motivation even to do fun things
- Memory loss
- Headaches
- Mental fogginess
- Easily agitated or angered
- Feeling better after dinner
- Joint pain
- Water retention
- Extreme loss of energy between 3:00 and 4:00 P.M.

TESTING FOR ADRENAL FATIGUE

Cortisol cannot be tested properly in one urine or blood sample. This is how most conventional doctors will test. False readings are common. Testing should be done on saliva in four different time increments throughout the day because Cortisol levels fluctuate. Natural practitioners carry this test in their offices. They are easy take-home tests that can be done in one day.

This saliva test measures your levels of different hormones including the stress hormone Cortisol, which tells us about the health of the adrenals, and levels of dehydroepiandrosterone (DHEA). DHEA is a hormone produced by the adrenal glands. It helps maintain the sex hormones estrogen and testosterone. Low levels of DHEA often give symptoms of headache, insomnia, and water retention. Balancing DHEA helps to restore adrenal health, the immune system, increases energy, assists mood, and helps build muscle strength.

HOW TO IMPROVE THE HEALTH OF YOUR ADRENALS

Along with rest and deep belly breathing exercises there are exercise and dietary changes that can help. Daily exercise reduces Cortisol levels and increases neurotransmitters in your brain that help you to relax. This lowers Cortisol levels and supports adrenal health. Decongesting the liver will assist in hormonal balance affecting the adrenal cortex. Eat Salt: Himalayan or natural salt only. Adults add ½ to one teaspoon of mineral or Himalayan salt to your water first thing in the morning and add small amounts (1/4 to ½ tsp.) a few times per day, especially when you feel fatigued, children get half to one quarter and adult dosage. Always muscle test first. Phosphorylated serine is helpful to calm adaptive responses in the body to Cortisol. See the chapter, "A Short Lesson in the Brain" under "Sleep" for more information.

Blood sugar balance: eat more protein and less sugars and starches. Combine your fats, carbohydrates, and proteins at each meal. Eat plenty of vegetables, but avoid fried foods, cow's milk (because of the high sugar content), and caffeine. Remember, it is essential to drink pure, non-chlorinated, non-toxic water.

To protect the brain and help keep its energy supply up, eat foods that are high in antioxidants such as deep colored fruits and vegetables. Green leafy vegetables and blueberries are a couple of examples.

In addition there are some supplements that are known to be very helpful for the health and balance of the adrenals.

SUPPLEMENTS THAT CAN ASSIST THE ADRENALS:

- Drenamin from Standard Process (small pill form can be crushed up). Sold by many natural health care practitioners and can be found at www.pureformulas.com. My son, daughter, and I take Drenamin daily. Adults in need take one, three times per day.
- Ribes Nigrum Gemmo homeopathic liquid by Seroyal is a good choice for non-pill takers. It is available at www.pureformulas.com.
- Rhodiola is a natural herbal adaptogen. This means it helps the body adapt to stressful situations, and can be very beneficial in assisting the balance of the adrenals.

ADDITIONAL SUPPLEMENTS FOR CALMING:

- Ashwaganda root: this has been used for centuries to calm the body, and it is a great antioxidant.

- Licorice root extract: an eighth of a teaspoon one to two times per day can be helpful. This is very concentrated so it is recommended to muscle test and ask your healthcare practitioner for dosage levels. Wise Women Herbals makes a quality product. It is sold in healthfood stores and online at www.pureformulas.com.
- Essential fatty acids help to regulate Cortisol.
- Holy Basil
- DHEA: I like the product BioSome liquid liposomal DHEA from Metagenics. It is available in healthfood stores and at most online websites such as www.pureformulas.com, and www.amazon.com. DHEA should be regulated by a practitioner to avoid exceeding dosages.
- Pantothenic acid (vitamin B5)
- Vitamins C, E, B6, B5
- Seriphos by Interplexus
- GABA

A flood-lamp from a true green spectrum light has been shown to lower Cortisol levels. It is available from GE for about $35.00. Turn on the lamp for about twenty to forty five minutes a day, although more is fine, too.

Tip for mom: The simple saliva test can be very accurate. If your hormone levels are off and you need a supplement, a compounding pharmacy can make you sublingual drops. This has been shown to be the best way to receive supplements without overloading the body and potentially creating toxic levels of fatty deposits, as many hormone creams will do. The above-mentioned supplements (just one or two in the right combination) have been known to help balance the system too. Rhodiola and licorice root extract balanced my own adrenals.

It is vital to have your child's liver, thyroid, pancreas, and gallbladder cleared of all health issues to maintain the body's own ability to produce and distribute the proper hormones as needed. This way the body can do what it needs to naturally, without supplements. N.E.A.T. practitioners and naturopaths can be very helpful in giving your child the support he or she needs to do so.

THE LYMPHATIC SYSTEM

We know that 80% of the immune system comes from the gut. The reason for this is largely due to the lymphatic system's association with the intestines. Lymph removes cellular and metabolic waste or toxins from the body. When the blood flow in the liver is congested because of gallstones, the lymphatic system backs up and cause toxic build up in the body. This stresses the immune system further as its waste removal is inefficient. The health of the lymphatic system is crucial for a healthy immune system, and a healthy circulatory system. When the liver cannot filter toxins properly, the blood and lymphatic fluid become toxic.

Mononucleosis and measles are two of the many infections that reoccur with a poor lymphatic system. These diseases are also seen in children. The measles virus was living in my son's system because of vaccinations. He had never been exposed to the measles otherwise. In his research, Dr. Andrew Wakefield found the same measles virus that children had been inoculated with in the intestinal tract of children with autism.

It stands to reason that it is important to keep the lymphatic system, and therefore the liver, healthy in order to have a healthy immune system and assist proper detoxification to fight disease. The endocrine or hormonal system is often weakened. These include the thyroid, parathyroid, adrenal glands, ovaries, and testes. The tonsils, spleen, and thymus gland are also commonly affected.

Common initial symptoms of an improperly working lymphatic system are:

- middle and low back pain
- a swollen abdomen
- swollen hands, arms, feet, and ankles
- a puffy face

Multiple chronic illnesses are associated with lymph congestion such as:

- irritable bowel syndrome
- brain disorders

- memory loss
- asthma, bronchial, and lung problems
- back pain
- vision/ eye trouble
- kidney problems
- circulatory problems
- heart disease
- breast cancer
- ovarian cysts
- sinusitis
- allergies
- thyroid trouble
- stiff neck and shoulders
- headaches
- migraines
- earaches and hearing problems
- vertigo
- dizziness

Lymph nodes (nodules) are positioned throughout the body. Massaging these areas can assist in breaking up and moving out debris. They are located in several places.

- the upper side portion front of the neck just under the angle of the mandible (jaw bone), especially important on the left side as it drains to the heart.
- the creases in the groin where the leg bends
- the front of the armpits
- the area over and just above the belly button

Trampolines or rebounders assist the lymphatic system via the gentle motion of gravity on the internal organs. Although massage in these regions can assist in the removal of lymphatic waste, the body must be able to complete excretion. This comes from overall liver detoxification and cleansing. See "liver" above for more information on liver cleansing and support.

When my daughter's lymph backs up, she will feel like she's getting sick, or just says she feels bad. Several times we have successfully used the homeopathic product Lymphotox by apexenergetics, www.apexenergetics.com, which I purchase from my chiropractor. When she says she's feeling bad I will muscle test her over each of the viral, bacterial, Candida, and lymph points to find the culprit. It is often her lymph point, which is located just in front of her left armpit. After I give her the Lymphotox, she feels better often within thirty minutes. This also lets me know that her liver is in need of support.

To view an example of muscle testing please refer to my YouTube video at http://youtu.be/1krEhJ4dzJM.

THYROID

Women are often familiar with the issues the thyroid can create. The most commonly known symptoms are fatigue and weight gain, but the thyroid can affect many systems of the body, including those in children. Adrenal fatigue can disrupt the thyroid so it is important to assess the health of the adrenals before and during treatment of the thyroid.

The thyroid is a small gland the shape of a butterfly on your throat in the area just below the Adam's apple. It produces several hormones. Thyroid hormones effect the development and functioning of the kidneys and the liver in utero. These are two of our primary detoxifying organs. Kidney disease in turn can cause thyroid dysfunction. These organs are also commonly weak or congested in children on the autism spectrum. Thyroid conditions are known to cause behavioral disorders and dementia. The health of the thyroid is also critical in the early stages of brain development.

The thyroid gland is involved in:

- hormone balancing
- protein synthesis

- determining oxidation in tissues and organs
- energy metabolism
- proper growth, including the growth of the brain
- digestive fluid secretion
- calcium absorption

Many children are being born today with hypothyroidism or low thyroid function. Some symptoms of hypothyroid are an inability to regulate body temperature often having cold hands and feet, swelling under the eyes, fatigue, a lowered metabolism causing abnormal weight gain, GI problems, a lowered immune system, depression, anxiety, hair loss, dizziness, allergies, insomnia, moodiness, deregulated blood pressure and cholesterol, headaches, migraines, shortness of breath, and muscle and joint pain.

Internal stressors, such as inflammation, also contribute to thyroid disorders. If the adrenal glands are imbalanced, there may be an imbalance in Cortisol levels. T3 only gets into the cells if there's enough Cortisol. Hyperthyroidism, or an overactive thyroid, can cause symptoms such as nervousness, anxiety, rapid heart rate, sweating, fatigue, heat intolerance, hyperactivity, increased appetite, eye disorders, tremors, and weight loss. For this reason, the high quality lab Diagnos-Techs includes Gliadin testing (a derivative of gluten), in the saliva/adrenal test. Most natural practitioners carry these take-home tests in their offices.

SOME COMMON CAUSES OF THYROID IMBALANCE

Low levels of iodine, and other nutritional deficiencies, as well as certain drugs can cause the conversion of T4 (thyroxin), the lesser active thyroid hormone, into T3 (triiodothyronine), the necessary active form, to become blocked. T3 is about three times more potent than T4. Clinical symptoms, the entire endocrine system, and nutrition all need to be evaluated. It is possible to have a subclinical condition, which is difficult to detect.

Nutrient deficiencies, medications, including birth control pills, and diet all play a role in an inability for thyroid hormones to convert to their active states. Pesticides, fluoride, mercury, and lead are among the strong factors. Certain foods can be contributing factors to the alteration of T4 to T3 conversion. Soy is a food that is associated with blocking this conversion and reduces the ability of the thyroid to function. The artificial sweeteners sucralose (Splenda) and aspartame also create weaknesses in organs such as the liver that diminish nutrients needed by the thyroid.

Thyroid disorders are commonly found in those with autoimmune diseases. In one study 14% of those with celiac disease (severe gluten allergies), were also found to have autoimmune thyroid disease, 10.3% with hypothyroid, and 3.7 with hyperthyroid (C.E. Counsell, et al, Celiac Disease and Autoimmune Thyroid Disease, Gut 35:844-846, 2005).

Inflammation lowers the body's ability to convert T4 to T3. The solution is to be sure the patient is getting T3 along with T4 (see below under "balancing the thyroid").

We discuss the genetic mutation of the MTHFr gene in the chapter four. This can cause the thyroid to become hypothyroid. Testing for this may be helpful.

Environmental toxins affect the thyroid. The thyroid is the gland that filters radiation. We must protect its health in the coming years due to worldwide exposure and the fallout from the earthquake in Fukoshima, Japan, in 2012. We must also be aware of fluoride accumulation in the thyroid. It can alter the ability of the thyroid to function. Do not drink fluoridated water, or ingest fluoride in anyway.

A weak or congested liver will cause hormone imbalances that affect the glands, including the thyroid and the parathyroid. Additionally, if the adrenals are weak then the thyroid will begin to suffer.

BALANCING THE THYROID

The three needed elements to convert T4 to the active form T3 are selenium, iodine, and L-tyrosine. There must be a sufficient amount of each in the body to enable the conversion process to take place properly. Iodine is one of the most needed nutrients for the thyroid, (see Hashimoto's below for iodine levels that may be too high). Zinc, vitamins A, C, D, E, B12, B5, B6, and alpha lipoic acid are all crucial components as well. Omega-3 fatty acids increase thyroid hormone transfer to the brain. If you remember we talked about the liver and the gallbladder needing to work properly to convert the needed essential fatty acids and alpha lipoic acid as a key component in detoxification. When these are effected the body cannot utilize these nutrients and it trickles down to the thyroid. There are also many things that prevent the necessary hormone conversions to take place.

To help the body with the conversion of T4, buy one of the most helpful prescriptions called natural, desiccated thyroid hormone. This is a swine thyroid glandular derivative. It is the closest known human glandular form. It naturally contains both T4 and T3. One of the most common synthetic prescription medications is Synthroid, which is only T4. Be sure not to get generic forms of this medication because the results are not consistent.

Dosages in any form must be correct. If symptoms continue after taking medication change brands, dosage levels, or, if on a synthetic, add an additional prescription of the active form T3 to assist with balancing the entire process. No two people are the same. Dosages and prescriptions are on an individualized basis.

Natural thyroid hormone can work more effectively because it contains both T4 and T3. I personally had much better success with the natural form Nature-Throid I received from my naturopath. It is free of fillers. Other natural forms, such as Armour Thyroid, contain fillers such as cornstarch and talc, which are both common allergens. Never take calcium with thyroid medication because calcium will inhibit its absorption.

Do not take calcium within an hour of taking any thyroid medication as it will inhibit the absorption of the thyroid medication.

HASHIMOTOS DISEASE

Hashimoto's Disease is the term used when there is an autoimmune reaction causing the immune system to attack the thyroid. It causes hypothyroid or low thyroid function but it has the addition of the autoimmune reaction.

Every autoimmune illness has three necessary triggers:

1. Genes
2. An environmental gene trigger, including stress. When the adrenal glands sense stress they weaken the thyroid. They

cause the thyroid to slow down by reversing T3. Gluten can be a trigger too.

3. Intestinal permeability-leaky gut (gluten causes intestinal permeability).

In the case of Hashimoto's adding iodine can make the problem worse, not better. It is important to do an iodine test to know that you are low before supplementing with it. (See iodine testing below.)

Hashimoto's is known to have a connection with celiac and gluten sensitivities. Going gluten free can actually reverse thyroid problems. People with Hashimotos also have low stomach acid. GERD or acid reflux is a common symptom as is loss of hair and fatigue. Contrary to common belief those with acid reflux are actually in need of more hydrochloric acid (HCL). Too little HCL can inhibit the absorption of vital nutrients such as B vitamins and iron causing additional fatigue. The toxic alcohol, acetaldehyde, released from candida prevents T4 from becoming T3.

Cleaning up the gut (this book will show you how) and being gluten free are great ways to assist balancing the thyroid. The supplement Metagest from Metagenics or any quality product containing betaine and pepsin will assist in building HCL. This will also help reduce fatigue and dizziness after meals. Betaine with pepsin can be found at most health food stores and on at many online sites such as www.pureformulas.com. Digestive enzymes are always a good idea too. They are discussed in detail in chapter eleven.

DETECTING THYROID IMBALANCE

Doctors are taught in medical school that a blood test is the best way to detect a thyroid problem. Unfortunately, this is often inaccurate and the common reason why so many thyroid disorders go undetected. Blood tests detect less than 5% of hypothyroid conditions. When these tests come back normal, a thyroid condition is ruled out and the patient does not get the help they need. The reason blood tests are usually inaccurate is because thyroid hormone is utilized inside the cells of the body. Blood tests measure just the thyroid hormone levels outside of the cells.

Basal Body Temperature

The self-test for detecting underactive thyroid is taking your basal temperature (underarm) first thing in the morning. Keep a thermometer next to your bed and before rising, first thing in the morning, place the thermometer under your arm for 15 minutes. Do not move while you are doing this, as movement can alter the reading. Do this for at least 5 days and keep a record of your readings. A temperature of 97.6 F or lower may indicate an underactive thyroid, or subclinical or borderline condition, especially if the readings are consistent.

Test Thyroid Stimulating Hormones (TSH)

Testing for levels of thyroid stimulating hormone (TSH) will help indicate thyroid health. If the thyroid is healthy the level should read *below* 2.5. you can get a copy of your own test to read for yourself. Note: TSH does not always show Hashimoto's.

Thyroid Peroxidies Antibodies and Thyroid Globulin Antibodies

Thyroid Peroxidies Antibodies (TBA) and Thyroid Globulin Antibodies (TGA) show if your thyroid is under attack from your immune system.

Iodine Tests

One way to test for iodine deficiency is to place a two inch by two inch square of nascent iodine on your body and see how long it takes to fade. If the iodine fades in less than two hours it means you are iodine deficient. The faster it fades, the more deficient you are. There is also a urine test from ZRT Labs that you can order and do in your home to determine iodine levels. Sometimes the problem is that iodine is too high. High iodine levels can trigger hypothyroidism too. You can find these tests at www.zrtlabs.com.

Regardless of test results, the numbers may or may not indicate thyroid imbalance, but symptoms do indicate it. Natural thyroid medication can be safely regulated by your doctor. Re-test thyroid hormones about every three months to detect patterns in your body and adjust dosages, if necessary. For more information, there is a helpful website called, www.stopthethyroidmadness.com.

TONSILS

Tonsils are part of the lymphatic system. They are also interconnected with the teeth and dental pathology. Energetically, they are part of the liver meridian. Weak tonsils breed bacteria and viruses. They also create neurotoxins for the brain. They should not be overlooked. Homeopathy and neural therapy do not seem to effectively treat them. Pathological issues with the tonsils may require a tonsillectomy. For more information on tonsils please visit, www.klinghardtacademy.com.

SKIN AND DETOXIFICATION TECHNIQUES

The skin is the largest organ of the body and an excellent source for detoxification. There are several ways to assist the body with detoxification via the pores in the skin.

- Magnetic clay baths can be purchased online at stores such as www.magneticclay.com, and www.amazon.com.
- Hot baths will cause the body to sweat and they also open the pores and allow for absorption. By putting about eight cups of baking soda into bath water, it will also become an alkalizing agent for the body as it is absorbed. Remember that the skin will absorb anything put on it, so be careful about the health and beauty products you use. Soaps, lotions, shampoos, and sunscreens are many of the chemical filled toxic substances people use daily on their skin. Hot showers and baths also open pours to water containing chemicals such as chlorine and heavy metals. See the chapter on environmental toxins for more information.
- Infrared saunas are extremely beneficial for detoxification and overall health. They can be rented, usually in thirty-minute increments, at local spas, or purchased and put into your own home. One website that has a quality product is www.infraredsauna.com.

- Dry brushing the body will also stimulate and free toxins. Use a large soft bristled brush that is made for this purpose. They are sold in healthfood stores everywhere.
- Sweating releases toxins through pores and exercise stimulates sweat, as do saunas.

MORE ABOUT DETOXIFICATION

When detoxifying, it is important to know that toxins are either natural or synthetic. Natural toxins, such as mold, are negatively charged. Synthetic toxins are positively charged. In order to disable toxins, the detoxifying agent must be the opposite charge.

For example, to detoxify mold, a natural toxin from the body, an agent such as cholestyramine, which is synthetic and negatively charged, can be used. To remove synthetic toxins, such as daily chemical exposure or pesticides, the natural agent's chlorella or magnetic clay can be used.

ADDITIONAL DETOXIFYING TECHNIQUES ARE:

- Enemas and colonic irrigation help to remove additional toxic waste in the large intestine and stimulate the liver.
- Liver flushing.
- Drinking enough pure water daily helps the body flush out toxins. We need six to eight glasses per day. Dehydration causes thickening of the blood and causes the cells to lose their water. Without proper fluids the cells lose their energy and cannot function.

Heavy metal detoxification is discussed in its own chapter.

ANTIOXIDANTS AND OTHER HELPFUL SUPPLEMENTS

Antioxidants are an important part of detoxification. They are discussed in detail in the chapter "Nutritional Supplementation." Helpful detoxification supplements include:

- chlorella
- vitamins C, D, and E
- beta-carotenes
- lipoceutical glutathione
- glycine
- cysteine
- taurine
- sulfate
- alpha lipoic acid
- Beta sitosterol by the company Pharmax (binds neurotoxins).
- Garlic and cruciferous vegetables such as broccoli are helpful detoxifying foods.

SUMMARY

The liver is the main organ of detoxification. Most children on the autism spectrum have a weak, congested liver, and therefore, poor detoxification. There are many good choices to assist the health of the liver such as Liver Life by Bioray which contains milk thistle and other natural ingredients to boost the immune system.

Along with the liver there are additional organs to help keep our bodies in balance, and that must be cleansed and healed in order for balance to be restored to the body, and brain. These additional organs include such as the kidneys, colon, lymphatic system, thyroid, and adrenal glands. Resources are given to help with these, as well.

The products found in this chapter can be found at http://naturallyhealingautism.com/a-healthy-home/

CHAPTER 6

DIFFERENT TYPES OF PATHOGENIC MICROBES

I had no idea how many different things could be going on in my son's gut that could affect, not only his health, but his behavior too.

There are several possibilities for children to have an imbalanced gut, weak immune system, or chronic inflammation. The first place to begin is the gut. For whatever reason, past antibiotic use, a diet containing alcohol, sugars, and processed foods, or extremely stressed mom who already had Candida overgrowth (too many bad bacteria) in her system prior to and during pregnancy. Pathogenic microbes such as Candida and its toxic by-products will cross the placenta and affect the development of the child. Fathers of children with autism often have abnormal gut flora or chronic inflammation, as well.

A mother's acidity and Candida overgrowth will affect her baby. Studies show that obesity in women is lessened later in life if a woman takes probiotics during pregnancy. This is likely due to the assistance that probiotics give in maintaining proper microbial balance.

Candida likes the hormone progesterone. Progesterone levels rise during pregnancy, so it causes an increase in the growth of Candida. The fetus is given Candida in utero and born with it.

When the baby is born, he already has a compromised immune system. He continues to receive Candida and other microbes from the mother's breast milk. When weaning begins, we commonly offer grains such as rice, starchy vegetables, and fruit. These tend to feed pathogenic bacteria, as they turn to sugars in the body, and he gets worse. The main food sources for pathogenic microbes are sugars and carbohydrates. This is often when we begin seeing more physical and emotional symptoms in our child.

A newer study released by decode Genetics found that children born to fathers age 40 or older were at higher risk of developing autism and schizophrenia. Although the finding showed the range of only 2% this is due to the genetic mutations that happen with age. The father's exposure to toxins during his lifetime would have increased also. This study said that the age of the mother had no consequence on the risk to the child, and that developmental and psychiatric problems genetically originate in the sperm and not the egg. Men need to remove mercury amalgam fillings and detoxify just as women do.

At about the age of one year most children are weaned from breast milk altogether. Western societies commonly do not support women breastfeeding their babies much after their first year. The still developing immune system and neurological system are still benefitting from the incomparable nutrients that only come from mother's milk (still the best choice over any formula). Two years of age is a better timeline for weaning due to its benefits.

When we add viruses and heavy metals from vaccinations into the mix we overload the undeveloped immune system. This, in turn, overloads the delicate and still developing neurological system.

The hepatitis B vaccination often contains yeast. Mercury, contained in many vaccines, is not only neurotoxic, but yeast and mercury are friends. This makes Candida overgrowth even harder to balance because mercury prevents the body's natural ability to remove Candida or yeast from the system, and helps it grow.

BIOFILM

One of the first pieces of this puzzle that must be addressed is biofilm. Biofilm is a strong protective matrix or shield developed by a microbe to protect it from harm. Biofilm protects bacteria, viruses, mold and other toxins, including heavy metals. When a microbe senses danger, such as an antibiotic or antifungal agent, it will pull from the body anything it needs to build this protective matrix. Commonly blood cells, heavy metals, starches, and proteins are used. Biofilm also contains calcium, magnesium and iron which it takes from its host. This is one reason why waiting to use vitamin and mineral supplements until after the pathogenic bacteria are eradicated is important. Biofilm also has a strong fat component so it is best to avoid fats and fatty foods during the initial stage of pathogenic eradication.

Microorganisms can mutate within their biofilm and become vaccine and antibiotic resistant. Microorganisms that live in biofilm are 100 to 1,000 times more resistant to treatment from antibiotics and other bacterial and antifungal fighting agents. These colonies can then continue to reproduce.

The most dangerous factor to the host is not from the bugs themselves, but from the response of the immune system. All of this pathogenic activity begins creating an inflammatory response which then turns on the immune system. The inflammation continues and so the immune system stays on. This creates an overactive immune system which causes autoimmune diseases, neurological damage, and more. Immune modulation must be addressed to restore balance.

Commonly known bacteria that are capable of building their own biofilm are K. pneumoniae, E. coli, H. pylori, Candida albicans, and the Lyme bacteria Borrelia burgdorferi.

If the pathogenic bacterium called Strep Mutans dominates oral biofilm it becomes the cause of dental cavities. It is common to see children on the autism spectrum or those with intestinal issues to have multiple cavities.

DESTROYING BIOFILM

Biofilm must be destroyed to minimize the risk of pathogenic organisms hiding or rebuilding. There are few products capable of doing this, but they do exist.

Products that destroy biofilm are: (Note: I used the top two listed below with great success.)

- Dr. Ohhira's probiotic strain TH10 that is in both his original and professional formula probiotics. It is found in healthfood stores and at www.crohns.net.
- The enzyme product Interphase by Klaire Labs is effective against biofilm. It is sold at www.pureformulas.com. I personally had great success with this product.

- Biofibrin is a blend of five ingredients essential in the destruction of biofilm. The first four are enzymes. They are 1. Serrapeptase which reduces inflammation and mucus, 2. nattokinase which dissolves the biofilm and the coating on cysts, 3. papain which helps eliminate toxins, and 4. bromelain for the prevention of clotting and the conversion of fibrinogen to fibrin which builds biofilm and cysts. It signals the body to build its own fibrous enzymes which dissolve fibrin tissue and scar tissue. Lastly, this product contains grapeseed extract which dissolves cysts and biofilm, is anti-bacterial and anti-viral. NOTE: If your child has an allergy to pineapple have him muscle tested to be sure the bromelain does not cause him a reaction as it is a derivative of pineapple. He can also be desensitized to the allergen; see the chapter on Alternative Therapies.) Biofibrin can be found at www.inspirednutrition.com.
- Cistus tea is helpful to destroy the biofilm, fight Candida, and H. pylori. Cistus tea also helps to fight the oral bacteria Strep. Mutans responsible for biofilm and plaque in the mouth. Cistus will assist in whitening the teeth. It is rich in polyphenols which are antibacterial. Cistus tea is also antiviral and repels ticks. Yes, you can even put a tablespoon of it into your dog's food for tick repellent. Cistus tea is a bit hard to find. Two online sites that carry it are www.fransussman.com, and www.retailbiopure.com. Steep for ten minutes and re-use the same tea three times to pull all of the necessary properties out of it.
- Grapefruit seed extract: 10 drops, two times per day in a beverage, varies with size and weight.

MOLD BIOTOXINS

Although there are many peer reviewed references published in PubMed, **www.pubmed.com,** one of the least known, and extremely common, health issues today is chronic illness due to exposure to mold. There is an actual genetic disorder contained by almost 25%

of the population that renders them helpless to dispel these biotoxins from their body. You can have these genetics but not be ill if they have not been triggered by stress, or an illness, etc. If this gene has been triggered then when exposed to mold a cascade of inflammation is set off in the system, but the body is not able to get rid of the toxins created within them.

This results in chronic inflammation which over activates the immune system. This often leads to many health problems. The most common health related problems are pulmonary and neurological.

Molds are one of the most commonly found allergens. It comes into many of our lives on a daily basis. Water damaged buildings such as homes, schools, and office buildings are common places to find mold. Their spores, dead or alive, can be contaminating the air we breathe. Small amounts of mold around the average person can be detoxified by the body within a couple of days. This genetic susceptibility renders some individuals more prone to the dangers of it.

WHAT'S GOING ON?

There is a gene, or protein, called transforming growth factor beta-1, or TGF beta-1, that is found throughout the body. It is one in a family of cytokines whose job it is to affect the growth and activity of cells. TGF beta-1 is important in fetal growth and development, the formation of blood vessels, muscle tissue and body fat development, the healing of wounds, the regulation of bone growth, and the functioning of the immune system.

When TGF beta-1 is inside of cells it remains inactive. It must be triggered via chemical signals to shift into its active form. One cytokine can trigger multiple cytokines. This can produce a cascade of inflammation. These levels are often extremely high when the body is undergoing high levels of inflammation. If the inflammatory response becomes unregulated it may result in chronic inflammation. The potential health problems associated with a defect in this genotype are due to this chronic inflammation. The immune system is constantly fighting issues triggered by ongoing inflammation in multiple systems of the body. This is why symptoms may be so varied.

MELANOCYTE STIMULATING HORMONE (MSH)

Chronic inflammation can suppress melanocyte stimulating hormone (MSH), and its pathways. MSH regulates the pituitary, and therefore, your hormones. It also has anti-inflammatory functions. Lowered MSH reduces the production of melatonin which affects sleep. The production of endorphins is suppressed which can lead to chronic pain. Further, lowered MSH can cause leaky gut which inhibits the absorption of nutrients from food, weakens and deregulates the immune system. The regulation of cytokine response by white blood cells which lowers the body's ability to fight infections. Your level of MSH usually correlates with your level of energy. Usually, the lower your levels of MSH are, the lower your energy is. Low MSH can also result in lowered resistance to Staphylococcus bacteria colonizing in the nasal pathways (see Staphylococcus below).

The symptoms of the mold biotoxin illness, or chronic inflammation, mimic many other autoimmune diseases. Individuals are often misdiagnosed with chronic fatigue syndrome, Epstein Barr virus, Fibromyalgia, Parkinson's, Muscular Sclerosis, rheumatoid arthritis, or some other autoimmune disease.

TYPICAL SYMPTOMS (due to chronic inflammatory response):

The most common symptoms are neurological, pulmonary, visual, dizziness, and stiffness and or pain in the back of the head and neck although they can vary greatly. This chronic inflammatory response can contribute to leaky gut, hormonal imbalances, intolerance to carbohydrates, gluten, dairy, and sugar.

Chronic inflammation in the brain can cause behavioral problems, learning difficulties, lack of focus, and hormonal problems. Other symptoms may include:

- Wake exhausted, never really getting a good night's sleep
- Chronic fatigue
- Flu-like symptoms
- Cough
- Respiratory issues, hard to take a deep breath

- Chronic pain in various parts of the body
- Stomach aches or pain
- Pituitary dysfunction/hormonal problems
- Trouble focusing or concentrating
- Language difficulty
- Learning disabilities
- Poor memory
- Anxiety
- Anger
- Depression
- ADD/ADHD
- Cold hands and feet
- Hormone imbalance
- Weight gain
- Frequent urination (more than 3-4 times per day).
- Irregular menses with heavy flow and severe cramping
- Poor blood clotting such as nosebleeds and more
- Chronic headaches, including migraines
- Abdominal pain/GI problems
- Chronic Candida albicans
- Diarrhea
- Bed wetting
- High immunoglobulin E (IgE) triggering asthma
- Nasal Polyps
- Nasal infections, commonly Staphylococcus
- Redness on hands and feet
- Redness from one cheek over the nose to the other cheek
- Blurred vision
- Tearing

- Light sensitivity
- Sound sensitivity
- Red eyes
- Poor vision
- Sinus problems
- Dizziness when standing quickly
- Resting tremors (found in 45% of biotoxin patients)
- Extremely long limbs as compared to the torso
- Hyper flexibility
- Muscle cramps
- Bell's Palsy

Adults commonly have multiple symptoms, but children may only have one symptom present. **The most common symptoms in children with the triggered mold genotype are:**

- Chronic headaches that last more than one to two months
- Fatigue for more than two weeks
- Chronic abdominal pain
- Bed wetting in children older than six years of age
- Inattention and ADHD (once treated for the mold biotoxin illness children often no longer need Ritalin).

When treated correctly younger children get better faster. Testing for mononucleosis and H. pylori bacterium are important to rule out with symptoms of chronic fatigue and abdominal cramps, but it is important to remember that the mold genotype illness mimics these symptoms. Note if either of the child's parents had bed wetting issues as a child, or even as an adult as this is hereditary.

MOLD BIOTOXIN ILLNESS AND THE BRAIN

It is important to note that some of your child's behavioral and physiological issues may be caused by extreme inflammation possibly due to the mold biotoxin illness. The mold genotype illness inhibits the body from dispelling the toxins derived from exposure to mold such as in water damaged buildings. This creates chronic inflammation in the brain, as well as the body. Inflammation on the brain can cause pituitary dysfunction which we already noted lowers MSH, therefore causing a myriad of hormonal issues. Increased TGF beta-1 often causes deregulation of the blood-brain barrier. This allows toxins and other chemicals, good or bad, to enter or exit the brain without regulation. There may also be unwanted pruning of dendrites which assist messages to get transferred in the brain.

Chronic inflammation is neurotoxic and create multiple cognitive disabilities. Depression is quite common in people with the mold biotoxin illness. The inflammation depletes dopamine creating problems with fine motor control and mood disorders such as depression. The common prescription for depression is serotonin reuptake inhibitor medication (SSRI's). Typically, SSRI's do not work on mold patients and often make them worse. The part of the brain called the prefrontal cortex is commonly damaged by chronic inflammation. This causes a loss of executive control leading to irritability and anger issues.

Possible neurological symptoms to look for:

- Absence of executive inhibition or impulsivity
- Issues with learning and memory
- Trouble with fine motor coordination
- Reclusive behavior
- Lack of enjoyment in things that should be enjoyable
- Language trouble such as comprehending and articulating words
- Tics
- Obsessive compulsive disorder
- Depression type symptoms
- Anxiety and panic issues
- Atypical seizures

A new MRI type of software called Neuroquant precisely measures brain volume. It is capable of detecting shrinkage in specific areas of the brain. Neuroquant is most helpful in gauging changes over time. The good news is that the brain can and does heal once toxic exposure is eliminated and proper treatment is given. For more information on Neuroquant go to www.radnet.com, or call 800-975-4674.

HOW TO DETECT YOUR CAUSE

First you must remove the cause. Environmental Protection Agency studies show that indoor levels of air quality are ten times more contaminated than outside air. Thirty million homes are known to have significant problems in the U.S. Homes with crawl spaces underneath them, improper duct ventilation and leakage for heating and air conditioning, fiberglass infiltration from the attic, leaky windows or ones that show water condensation, walls and baseboards are all sources of problems. Mold illness is caused by water damage to a building that affects the area indoors.

Often a child has abdominal pain during the week at school but not on the weekend when at home. Most people assume this is due to nervousness regarding stress that school may bring to the child. Typical "nervous" symptoms of abdominal cramping, headaches, and anxiety are also typical of mold contamination. Ask the school maintenance people to inspect for water damage. They may already be aware of it. If any building has a flat roof you can be sure there is past water leakage and mold contamination. Sometimes it is as simple as noticing that when you go away from your home (or school or business), for a few days you feel better only to find that you begin to feel tired and ill upon returning. Many homes do not show signs of contamination to the naked eye but may be a big source of the problem.

To detect hidden mold in your home you can purchase a test called the Environmental Relative Moldiness Index or ERMI test. The samples test thirty six species of molds. The ERMI can distinguish away from other fungi to detect the DNA of those that describe "the relative mold burden" from water damaged buildings. The ERMI runs on a scale range from negative ten to positive twenty. Homes scoring in the negative range (below 0), are less threatening than those with higher numbers, especially those above five. The absolute worst number would be twenty. The variables of the ERMI test are often measured against where the levels of your blood markers are. Some people are so high in TGF beta-1 that only a small amount of mold will give them symptoms.

Standards for this test come from the sleeping areas and the living areas even if the water damage is in a distal part of the home such as the basement. These spores, dead or alive, are capable of causing extreme illness to those with the mold genotype. They circulate in the air and settle everywhere in the home.

The ERMI test can be purchased at www.mycometrics.com. It comes with specific instructions which require attachment to a vacuum, or a different type that tests hardwood floors. Commonly a three foot by six foot sampling area on the floor is marked off and vacuumed for five minutes. This is done in the bedroom of the person being tested and the most used living area.

The ERMI test is necessary. If you or your children are suffering from a mold illness the home is the first place to check. The ERMI test is about $300.00. If finances are an issue there is another test called the HERTSMI-2 test. It is a shorter variation of the ERMI, and is half the price. To order these tests you will need to call Mycometrics at (732)355-9018. If your home or other places of possible exposure are not properly checked your child's asthma, autism and more may never recover. Many more dollars will be spent in the long run trying to figure out what is wrong and what can be done to help him without possibly ever finding the right treatment.

There are certified contractors who know exactly what to look for and will find mold and water damage where others will miss it. They have the proper diagnostic equipment. When found, mold must be taken out properly by specialists so that no remaining spores are left to continue breeding.

The company Wondermakers, www.wondermakers.com, trains and certifies contractors in all hazardous chemicals such as asbestos, lead, and mold. Any willing contractor can be trained and certified through them. Wondermakers trained individuals or those trained by Dr. Shoemaker's people are the only ones you would want to have help you fix the damage. Spraying bleach or cutting out the area in the wall will not stop the contamination. It is common to have to move out of a contaminated home, school, or workplace until the damage is properly taken care of. To find one of these certified contractors call Wondermakers at (888) 382-4154, or contact Dr. Shoemaker's staff at www.survivingmold.com.

When one of these certified contractors are used to repair the home properly it often improves energy usage as well. In this case, grants may be available through your local gas and electric company toward fixing the damage. I live in California and Pacific Gas and Electric may pay up to $4500.00 for repairs in their Energy Upgrade California Rebate Program.

TESTING AND TREATMENT FOR THE MOLD GENOTYPE

To either detect this or rule it out it would be wise for all children on the autism spectrum and those with asthma, ADD, learning disabilities or any other behavioral or physiological health issues to be tested for this genotype. Because this is genetic, parents should also be tested. It is a way to rule out one great potential antagonist. I myself tested positive. After blaming extreme fatigue on the thyroid gland for so long I was shocked to discover I carried this gene that had become defective. I also had extreme muscle pain in my right shoulder. I always attributed it to years of volleyball and baseball. Once treated for mold the pain diminished substantially.

There is a benign cholesterol binding agent called cholestyramine (CSM) that is capable of binding to the mold biotoxins to remove them from the body. You need a prescription for CSM, so contact one of the doctors on the surviving mold website for testing and treatment (see below). I have also found the homeopathic remedy called Enviroprotect from Apexenergetics to be helpful in alleviating my symptoms. Most natural healthcare practitioners carry Apex products in their offices. It can also be found at www.pureformulas.com.

Homeopathic treatments are also being used for those who cannot well tolerate the cholestyramine. The lab Real Life Labs has a test that is mold type-specific to determine which mold spores an individual is reacting to so it can be treated accordingly.

Detection of this genotype and whether or not it has been triggered to cause multiple susceptibilities such as health issues caused by its chronic inflammation is most accurate using specific blood tests using particular laboratories. There are only a small handful of trained doctors who are properly educated to treat this illness with its very specific protocol. They can be contacted for initial phone consults if you live at distance, but travel if necessary. They can order the blood tests for you with proper test codes. Then, if positive, you would work with one of the certified doctors. This is a very specific protocol. Do not let your regular doctor tell you that he can take care of this for you. Many important health issues can be missed and there is likely to be inaccurate treatment. Contact information for the certified doctors can be found at www.survivingmold.com.

VISUAL CONTRAST SENSITIVITY TEST (VCS)

The first test to do is the visual contrast sensitivity test (VCS). This is not a regular eye exam. It is used as an initial screening method to show possible levels of sensitivity in your neurological system. Failing the VCS test and having multiple symptoms is a good indication that lab testing should be done. With that said, adults who fail the test are usually positive, but teens and children who pass the test may still be positive for the mold biotoxin illness. Younger people may still pass the VCS test even when they are positive for mold biotoxins. The VCS test is an inexpensive way to check, but ultimately, you may need to get the blood work done. A VCS test is available at www.survivingmold.com, for $15.00.

Dietary changes will not fix TGF beta-1, and antibiotics do not help inflammation. This is a multisystem, multi-symptom illness that the body has acquired due to exposure from water damaged buildings. People may look fine, but feel awful.

NOTE: The protocol will not correct the antigliadin,(gluten allergy), but once the system is balanced and free of biotoxins and chronic inflammation your child can be treated by a natural allergy desensitization practitioner to see about clearing it (see the chapter on Alternative Therapies for allergy desensitization).

AT-HOME MUSCLE RESPONSE TEST FOR MOLD BIOTOXIN ILLNESS

While you should still do the blood work necessary and the visual contrast sensitivity test, this at-home muscle response test can be a helpful addition of information.

Muscle response screening:

1. Arms are extended straight out in front of each shoulder. Simultaneously press downward on each wrist to test for individual arm strength.
2. Again with arms extended straight out turn hands so palms face each other. Have the person being tested squeeze your hands, and note their strength of right verses left.
3. Relax arms at sides and lift shoulders upward while the person testing presses downward on them.
4. Same as step 1; arms extended out separately, test for strength in each arm by simultaneously pressing downward on each wrist.
5. If their dominant arm comes up weak in step 4 it is most likely that they have chronic inflammatory response.

BIOPURE PROPOLIS VAPORIZER

Biopure propolis vaporizers help eliminate mold spores and other air pollutants from your home office, school, car or other indoor area. Propolis is a resin-like substance derived from bees. It contains several strong bioflavonoids. Propolis vaporizers heat a small capsule of propolis and diffuse microscopic particles of bioflavonoids into the air. When inhaled, these flavonoids quickly enter the cells via the bloodstream. Propolis is known to be anti-inflammatory, anti-bacterial, anti-viral, anti-fungal, and anti-tumor. These flavonoids are known to reduce type one allergy. By killing microbes in the air it helps make homes safe for children.

Propolis has immune-regulating properties. It is great for those with a weakened immune system. These vaporizers are known to be great for people with mold allergies, asthma and any other respiratory issues. They are all-natural and free of chemicals.

The active flavonoids in propolis vary due to the regions in which the bees travel. The propolis sold by the company Bee Healthy Farms, www.beehealthyfarms.com, is certified to contain the necessary active flavonoids. They also carry a variety of vaporizers. The Biopure propolis vaporizer is small and can travel with you. They even make a car model that plugs into the cigarette lighter or power source in your car. They are very reasonably priced.

MOLD CLEANING AGENTS

The product concrobium prevents the regrowth of mold without any bleach, ammonia, or volatile organic compounds (VOC). As it dries it leaves an invisible anti-microbial barrier that prevents further mold growth.

Concrobium works on just about every surface. It is sold in home improvement and hardware stores everywhere, www.concrobium.com.

An additional alternative solution to killing mold without bleach and other toxic cleaning agents is a solution of ten to twenty drops grapefruit seed extract mixed with water. I have great success with this and use it to clean my home.

MOLD TREATMENT PROGRESS

1. Educate yourself about the chronic inflammatory response mold genotype.
2. Get tested by a certified doctor
3. Comply with all treatment, including having your home inspected for any mold by a certified mold clearing contractor and following exact protocol given to you by the doctor.
4. Track your symptoms with the doctor.
5. Do only one new thing at a time. Don't be eager to jump ahead before it's too soon.
6. Get support.

Not following any of the above steps will result in treatment failure!

PARASITES

It is crazy how many different parasites and pathogens can be in the gut. It is estimated that eighty percent of the American population have parasites, and most do not know it. Many children on the autism spectrum have parasitic problems. Most parasites live with us harmoniously, until the gut flora weakens to the point that they become a problem. Common ways we get them are from inhaling them from the air we breathe, in the food we eat, drinking water, swimming in contaminated water, and through our skin. Lesions in the skin, especially on the feet, allow for easy entrance into the body. Animals carry different parasites that they may pass onto humans. Poor hygiene plays a big role too.

The problems caused by parasites do not come from the bugs themselves but from the existing co-infections in the body. Parasites bring with them bacteria, viruses and fungi. Viruses in the nervous system often come from Staphylococcus and lungworm (see below). When parasites are present the immune system is even weaker and the child more susceptible to bacterial and viral infections. Leaky gut allows the parasites to enter the bloodstream and make their way to organs including the brain. Parasites often live inside the mucosa of the intestinal lining, but are capable of living outside of the intestines. See more on clearing viruses in the chapter on vaccinations.

People may go decades without symptoms while parasites feed on them. Common symptoms are intestinal discomfort, bloating, gas, diarrhea, nausea, dark circles under the eyes, skin rashes, and sinus congestion. They are many of the same symptoms of those with food allergies or leaky gut. It is also commonly seen in malnourished children as a failure to thrive. Two other lesser known symptoms of parasites are nail biting and bruxism, otherwise known as teeth grinding. Emotionally, parasites can cause impulsivity and even suicidal behavior.

Conventional methods of eradicating parasites are short term, at best. This is due to traditionally used antibiotics, such as flagyl, only killing some of the adult parasites. The eggs that have been laid will eventually hatch and the infestation returns. When you initially feel better and the tests all come up negative it misleads you to believe you are clear. Treating the parasites alone will not treat the cause of the whole problem.

We are all exposed to parasites on a regular basis. The question arises as to why some contract parasitic infections where others do not? The main reason why parasites are not eradicated is due to a weakened intestinal tract, an overly acidic diet, and a congested liver. If the liver is congested with gallstones (see detoxification and the liver), then the digestive tract is already weak. Toxins in the blood and lymphatic system become absorbed by the body. This allows for parasites which are passing through to harbor and create infection.

In order for parasitic infections to be cleared the liver must be cleansed and the intestinal tract must be healthy. A continued diet follows that is rich in alkaline foods to help prevent lingering infections. Please read the information on cleansing the liver and liver support in the chapter on detoxification. See testing and treatment for parasites below.

STAPHYLOCOCCUS

The most common bacteria living outside of the intestinal tract is Staphylococcus, commonly referred to as "Staph. infection". Staph. commonly lives in the nasal passages. It is estimated that 25% to 30% of the general population is infected, along with those recovering from Lyme disease. The percentage rises to 85% of those with the mold biotoxin illness due to chronic inflammation and the lowered MSH hormone. A nasal swab test will indicate if this is positive or negative.

Referred to as MARCoNS, Multiple Antibiotic Resistant Staph epidermis, staphylococcus in the nasal passages often travels to the hypothalamus and suppresses melanocyte stimulating hormone (see MSH). Common symptoms are extreme fatigue, ringing in the ears, sinus issues, headaches, visual problems, migraines, and dental issues.

My son and I tested positive for the mold biotoxin illness or gene, so we both needed to test for the nasal staph. My test came up negative, but my son tested positive. An effective and easy-to-use product used to eradicate staph in the nasal passages is known as BEG nasal spray. BEG stands for Bactroban, Edetate disodium, and Gentamicin. It is an antibiotic-resistant coagulase that is effective against antibiotic-resistant bacteria as an antibiotic and calcium chelator. The calcium chelator is used to help break down the protective biofilm. (See www.survivingmold.com, for more information). One bottle of the spray took care of this for my son. We retested afterward and he was free of the MARCoNS.

Jacob had been getting cavities even though he had been taking good care of his teeth. After the staph had cleared, his first dental checkup was good. His fatigue had improved also, but we still had mold in the home that needed to be removed to stop his exposure.

If staphylococcus bacterium is systemic, the product Monolauren has been shown to kill 100% of bacteria, including MRSA staph. (See "Lyme disease" for details on Monolauren.) It must be used in conjunction with biofilm agents (see biofilm above). I suggest getting the help of a qualified professional to assist you.

STREPTOCOCCUS

Additional bacteria found in many with parasites or mold issues are streptococcus, otherwise known as strep. Many people are familiar with the term "strep throat," and up to 95% of children have chronic strep. It can also be related to compulsive behavior.

It is common for strep to live in the tonsils. I was plagued with strep throat on a regular basis during high school. It got so bad that I was finally taken to a specialist. Eventually, at age 21, I had my tonsils removed, and I never had strep throat again.

Treatments for strep throat include Monolauren, Bio-fibrin, Dr. Ohhirra's probiotics, and cistus tea. Dr. Klinghardt has a much more detailed protocol on his website for treating streptococcus at www.klinghardtacademy.com.

I have personally found that the natural supplement Congaplex from Standard Process is very effective at fighting Streptococcus in the body and bronchial infections such as bronchitis. Their product, Spanish Black Radish, is also very effective for most common bacterial infections. They can both be purchased through many natural practitioners and at www.amazon.com. Muscle test for dosages (see Chapter Two) or ask your healthcare practitioner for guidance.

WORMS

The most common parasite living inside and outside of the intestinal tract is the lungworm. As its name would imply, they live in the lungs and can cause asthma. They also live in the mucosa of the small intestine. They are able to penetrate the upper and lower intestinal walls and travel back and forth from the lungs. We all get worms throughout our lives.

Lungworms mate and lay eggs that hatch and attach themselves in the bowel. They then absorb and enter the circulatory system. They are able to quickly multiply. Once you have them, they are there for life unless properly eradicated. Lungworms can be extremely dangerous for those with lowered immunity.

Symptoms range from skin rash, itching, wheezing, and coughing, to leaky gut and other intestinal problems, including ulcers.

Diagnosis can be difficult. The amount excreted by the body varies greatly, so it is relative to the amount excreted during a test. All children on the autism spectrum should be dewormed. As you are deworming your child, go through the process yourself at the same time. It is more than likely that we all have these microbes within us.

Deworming is simple. There is an Ayurvedic herb called mimosa pudica that is 30 times stronger than any medication. I purchased mine from www.biopure.me, 800-801-6187. We started with one-half teaspoon, twice per day, two days per week and worked up to one teaspoon per day for three months. Children may start at half that depending on age and weight.

An additional and necessary product is Intestinal Complex from Pharmax Nutriceuticals. Intestinal Complex contains slippery elm which will prevent the eggs of the worms from attaching to the bowel wall. This can be purchased at health food stores and at www.pureformulas.com. Treatment should continue for at least three months, preferably longer.

Mimosa pudica has a very bitter taste, so I encapsulate it for my kids. If your child will not take pills, you can add it to a smoothie for them.

WORMS AND CEREBRO-SPINAL VENOUS INSUFFICIENCY (CCSVI)

Lungworm may create an additional problem known as chronic cerebro-spinal venous insufficiency (CCSVI). This is a narrowing of the veins that return blood from the head back to the body. This is often found in people on the autism spectrum. There can be constant buzzing in the head, ringing in the ears, eye floaters, and other problems with vision, migraines, headaches, sinuses, and dental issues. It is possibly related to seizures and can cause lesions in the brain.

As is the case with most cranial problems, it can take time for the inflammation to affect the tissue enough to create symptoms, usually creating scar tissue. In craniosacral work, we often see the effects of whiplash about three years after the accident.

With CCSVI each therapy is individualized for the patient. Dr. Klinghardt recommends their Cranial Stimulation unit (see below) to help the children with this issue as well as the Bemer Mat for microcirculation for children with autism and adults with detox issues including lyme disease, blood and lymph, parasite therapy, and to increase effectiveness of protocols. These mats are used at home daily. Call the Academy for details, features and differences of recommended models. You can also ask for information here: http://www.bemer-partner.com/bemerGroup/DHS/your-partner/contact-form.

Cranial Stimulation System is a good option for resetting the brain when used 20 min. mid-AM & PM. Clipped on the ear. It helps to undo what EMFs are doing to the brain for neuro issues, sleep help, mental fog, depression, brain connectivity and enhanced feeling of wellbeing throughout the day. It is recommended for Autism support and Insomnia. Call the Klinghardt Academy at 908-899-1650 for resource.

TESTING AND TREATMENT FOR PARASITES

An increase in healthy "good" bacteria in the GI tract will naturally eradicate many parasites. The gut cleansing program in this book along with the right probiotic supplement will build the numbers of good bacteria which will chase most parasites out naturally. Use probiotics and the diet for at least one month before testing to see what pathogens, if any, remain to be treated with additional supplementation.

As I mentioned earlier, parasites do not show up in many tests because they are able to make themselves invisible. This may be misleading because your test results may read negative, even if you do have them. Some laboratories are more accurate than others. These laboratories are Genova, Diagnos-Techs, and Doctors Data. They all carry a Comprehensive Stool Analysis with Parasitology Test. They are superior to many others that often do not detect all of the pathogens, and they can be purchased online without any doctor's appointment needed.

Genova Labs grows out the strains of bacteria to find what the strength of it is and what can be done about it. The result sheet comes to you with a number scale. This scale tells you the strength of each strain. The greatest benefit I found was being given a scale of several natural products that were tested against the strains of bacteria that came up for me. The sheet told me what particular natural product would work best to eradicate my problem. The best option is given per individual.

The product that came up for me to use is commonly known in the holistic health field. It is called Tanalbit. Tanalbit is made from plant tannins. It is antifungal, helps restore normal GI function and is very helpful in naturally eradicating parasites. It is able to reach and eliminate yeast in their deepest hiding areas. It is highly effective because it survives stomach acid and gets into both the small and large intestine. An added benefit is that yeast and bacteria do not build up a resistance to this as they do with many other products.

Tanalbit is safe and effective and has been used for over 20 years. It reduces fatigue, allergic food reactions, and helps remove toxins. It will not contribute to die-off. One important note is that Tanalbit contains casein. If there is casein sensitivity in your child, you need to avoid this. It is best taken away from food. It can be purchased at www.crohns.net and www.pureformulas.com.

I purchased a comprehensive stool analysis panel from Genova Labs through www.crohns.net. If you purchase your test kit through them, you will also have the advantage of their licensed acupuncturist, Pamela, who is available to go over the results and offer assistance if needed. Pamela is a specialist in working with the issues of the GI tract with over 30 years experience.

The test kits for Diagnos-Techs can be found in most holistic health practitioner's offices, www.diagnostechs.com (425) 251-0596. Mainstream doctors, if willing, can order these tests for you also. The Doctors Data tests are sold online at many sites such as, www.labtestingdirect.com.

I personally have had exceptionally positive results when including the bacterial strain Saccharomyces boulardii to my protocol. It is very helpful in eradicating both yeast and parasites. The company Klaire Laboratories has a high quality product, www.klairelabs.com (888)488-2488.

While continuing on the Candida diet (see the chapter on "the diet"), and taking the accompanying supplements Tanalbit, and S. boulardii, I also added the product Interphase by Klaire Labs. Interphase and the TH10 strain in Dr. Ohhira's probiotics both help with destroying biofilm.

One of the parasites I had was H. pylori which is known to have strong biofilm. Interphase is commonly used to help eradicate this organism. Lastly, I took Candiclear5. It is also helpful in removing parasites. See the chapter on Candida for more information on this product.

I know this all seems like a lot but it is a protocol to destroy all aspects of the pathogens. Remember that by doing the gut healing diet in this book you will have naturally eradicated many invaders.

THE FULL MOON ERADICATION PERIOD

Interestingly, the moon, specifically a full moon, "awakens" parasites. They can become more active during this time; therefore, they are the most vulnerable to eradication. It is wise to span two full moon cycles during a parasite protocol.

HELIBACTOR PYLORI (H. PYLORI)

H. pylori are bacteria that are found in the stomach and duodenum (upper GI). We all carry these microbes in our GI tract. These otherwise harmless microbes become problematic when our gut flora becomes imbalanced and the cells of the stomach are damaged. Candida overgrowth is a direct cause of H. pylori problems.

Liver congestion is another culprit. When bile and toxins are frequently pushed back into the stomach, the cells become injured and weak and are then more susceptible to damage from pathogenic microbes such as H. pylori, which in this case can even cause ulcers.

H. pylori is also spread through saliva. Remember this when sharing food or kissing your child on the lips, especially if his gut is weak and he has Candida. By the age of six months, many babies already carry H. pylori.

H. pylori are strong, acid-resistant bacteria. Its resistance is so strong that it can survive stomach acid. This makes the stomach produce more acid, which damages the stomach lining. Their corkscrew shape also bores holes in the stomach lining. These factors cause non-stress induced ulcers.

Symptoms are often the same as those who experience stomach ulcers. The most common symptom is stomach pain, but other symptoms may include chronic migraine headaches, fatigue, lack of nutritional absorption, nausea, vomiting, weight gain due to the rise in cortisol, depression, anxiety, bad breath, sinus problems, joint pain, headaches, and lack of mental clarity. As you can see, these symptoms are many of the same that come from Candida albicans.

Tests for H. pylori are available through your practitioners, but I would urge you to use either Genova Labs or Diagnos-Techs lab for this. These give the exact level of detection of the organism, and they are very thorough laboratories. You may request that your practitioner use these companies. These labs will send test kits to your doctor.

Genova Labs microbial tests can be purchased at www.crohns.net (877) 240-7528. There is an additional fee, but if you call and ask for the add-on code, H. pylori can be added to any other test kit to be done at the same time. See the chapter on "Laboratories" for more information.

There are natural products to eradicate H. pylori. To assist the gut flora and relieve stomach pain, either break open into a beverage or chew on one to three of Dr. Ohhira's probiotic capsules. How many you use will depend on the weight of the individual. By opening up the capsule before swallowing, the probiotics are released directly into the stomach. For other purposes, such as getting the probiotics fed directly to the lower GI or colon, it is best to swallow them, but either way still works.

The solution is to balance gut flora and build the good bacteria, decongest the liver, and eat a healthy diet. These are in the healing stages of this book. However, if additional help is needed to eradicate H. pylori, the following supplements are extremely helpful.

One enzyme product made to eradicate H. pylori is Interphase from Klaire Labs, which gets beneath the mucosa where H. pylori lives. Be sure to take this product on an empty stomach. Interphase used with probiotics and the yeast strain Saccharomyces boulardii have been known to be very helpful in fighting H. pylori.

Saccharomyces boulardii also acts against Candida albicans. The same products used in the Candida cleanse, also help to eradicate H. pylori. They can be purchased at www.pureformulas.com. S. boulardii needs to be refrigerated, so shipping can be more costly. Check with your practitioner to see if they can get a better price for the entire purchase with shipping than you can.

Saccharomyces boulardii can also be helpful in cases of diarrhea. I used this myself as an addition to assist removal of parasites. I used the product made by Klaire Labs that has 3 billion CFU's (colony forming units). Muscle test to see how many pills your child will need per day and look at the dosage per capsule. They are best taken away from food. Usually one is taken in the morning and one at night. He may need a lot more or a lot less than originally assumed to help eradicate the pathogens. Always start slowly and work your way up to avoid die-off reactions.

Muscle testing is a good way to also check for the dosages needed. (See the chapter on alternative therapies to learn how to muscle test.) What is recommended for most is usually too much for our sensitive kids and those with an inflamed GI tract. To the contrary, sometimes we need a bit more good bacteria when treating an imbalanced gut.

When muscle testing, ask if a full packet per day is right, or a half of a packet per day, and go down to one eighth of a packet per day or every other day to begin. Individual needs vary greatly and will change over time as they heal.

MY STORY

My mother told me that when I was 15 months old I had caught a cold. The doctor told her that there was this wonderful new antibiotic called penicillin that could help me. At that time, it was combined with sulfa drugs. I was given a dosage and sent on my way.

The next morning, my mother she said there were bruises all over my body, and I looked as though I had been beaten. I was rushed to the doctor and found that I had had a severe allergic reaction to the antibiotics. I was never to be given penicillin or sulfa drugs again.

Once we have taken antibiotics, our immune system is weakened. Unless we are fully educated on probiotics and a proper diet to heal the gut, we fall into the category of those who fight Candida ongoing.

I've craved sugar my whole life. As a consequence of a weakened immune system, I would get sick frequently. In high school, I had Strep. throat on a regular basis. Each time I was given a new course of antibiotics. This, of course, weakened my system further. Years later I would find out what all of this weakening of my gut would create and allow to enter into my own body.

I love to travel. I have a history of traveling in foreign countries, although anything can be picked up in one's own country, and somewhere I had gotten parasites. I had suffered from digestive issues for years and could not figure out what was wrong. I took a test through Diagnos-Techs laboratories and discovered I did have parasites. I thought I could easily eradicate them with some antibiotics. Although I have a strong resistance to taking antibiotics, it seemed apparent that I should take them. Diagnos-Techs actually contacted the practitioner I got the test through and told them to be sure I took care of it immediately as the particular host I carried could bore holes in my liver. This scared me into taking all measures. I also realized that I may have been more susceptible to getting parasites due to a past with Candida and leaky gut. When our immune system, specifically our gut, is weak we are far more susceptible to many pathogens.

The first two-week round of horrid antibiotics did not work. They asked me to take them again. I had felt so awful the first time that it was like asking me to take poison again, but I relented. I wanted the parasites gone. A second round was taken and once retested I found that they were still with me. I spent some time rebuilding my gut and immune system. Through much research, I found a person who was said to be a specialist in parasites. His herbs were from South America, and he *almost* guaranteed this to work.

Three months of taking countless pills throughout different times of day and $700 later, I re-tested again. Much to my amazement the parasites were still there. Once again, I spent months rebuilding my system.

Almost a year later, I decided to see what my naturopath had to offer. I was given a homeopathic remedy called Unda 39 by Seroyal, specifically for parasites. My system purged. I thought this was working and so did she. Along with the Unda I was given a specific antibiotic for the particular parasite I carried. This was likely the best idea I had been given yet—something specific. It took me multiple pharmacists to find the one who could order it for me online because it was so rarely used in the United States. Apparently, this antibiotic was commonly used in Asia where this parasite is often found. I had been to Asia almost 20 years previously. Had it been from all the way back then that I had these parasites living in me?

Multiple questions ran through my mind. Could it have been then that I picked up this host on that trip to Asia? Was it the trip I took to Mexico in 1983 when I came home so sick? Had I carried this around for all of these years and not known it? Did I have these parasites when I was pregnant with my children? Could this have been the cause of trouble initially for my kids too?

I took this antibiotic for an entire month as recommended by my naturopath. Once finished, I strengthened the system before re-testing. I waited two months so there would be no false markers that are sometimes caused by inflammation or parasites still dying off.

At the end of this time, I re-tested again. Much to my amazement everything was still there! It was as though they were never going to leave me. I wondered if I had strengthened their ability to live in me from so much attention. My gut was probably so out of balance at this point that the strength of my system wasn't enough.

The naturopath was equally amazed. She said she had one last thing she could try. I was to take three doses per day of colloidal silver, Argentyn 23, the type without heavy metal possibilities. This is like a natural version of an antibiotic. It too will destroy the bad, but it does not discriminate either. The good bacteria would be destroyed also. I ordered about $300 worth of silver hydrosol and took it for the month.

When I finished this dosage, my belly was bloated twenty four hours a day. I began having almost constant diarrhea, and I was often fatigued. Even my good health habits weren't working.

I am a person who exercises every day. I also know how to eat. I stay away from processed food, eat low glycemic index foods, and try to eat as healthy as I can with plenty of protein. Yet my belly was big no matter what I did. I began gaining weight regardless of what I did. My thyroid showed low, likely due to fatigued adrenal glands. The internal stress had been hard on my body.

I had all of the symptoms of Candida. My hands and feet were dry to the point of cracking, my belly was bloated, I had extreme fatigue, lack of mental clarity, and I would wake in the middle of the night with anxiety. I returned to the diet but needed something for the Candida.

I put myself on a very strict diet of broth and protein without any sugar or starches. I also took the products listed in the gut cleansing and gut healing chapters. The diarrhea and bloating were better, but not gone. I tried to eat vegetables, but the fiber was too much for my GI tract to handle. The diarrhea returned and my intestines ached.

Due to my past history with Candida, I had tried many of the available resources, even those that claim to be the best. My problem was that the Candida never seemed to go away completely, and it would come back all too quickly.

Luckily, due to my extensive research for this book, I had looked deeply into many companies and their Candida products. One company stood out because it contained information on its products that had been researched, but also had frequencies infused to help with eradication at a far deeper level. The company is called Get Healthy Again, www.gethealthyagain.com. Candida is so important, especially for people on the autism spectrum that I have gone into much greater detail for you in the next chapter.

SUMMARY

We all carry microbes within us. They are tiny organisms that are too small to see without a microscope. Some of these microbes are good and some of them are bad. When they cause the body harm, they are known as pathogenic. These include, but are not limited to, Staphylococcus, Streptococcus, tuberculosis, and Escherichia coli.

Some microbes are always harmful, while others become harmful only to those with a weakened immune system. Air, water, soil, and physical contact with an infected person or a contaminated object are all common ways in which to become infected.

It is essential first to remove pathogenic bacteria and microbes from the body. If the bacteria in the gut is restored to balance, many of the pathogenic bacteria will diminish and not be problematic. A healthy GI tract will not allow for pathogenic overgrowth.

All children on the autism spectrum must be tested, and if needed, treated for parasites of other pathogenic bacteria first. The pathogenic bacteria will disrupt the immune system and allow for secondary infections such as bacterial, viral, and fungal infections. There are different types of parasites and bacteria and related disorders associated with them

Often parents will notice a change in their child as soon as weaning begins. Some common solid foods first introduced to a child are rice and starchy vegetables. They can even be organic, but if the child was born with pathogenic bacteria in his gut, then the starches feed them.

Pathogenic bacteria feed on starchy foods, even starchy vegetables. These starches turn into sugars in the gut. Pathogenic bacteria bore holes in the lining of the intestinal tract. The gut ends up with holes in it that leak undigested foods into the bloodstream where they find their way to the brain.

Cereals made from processed oats ground down to a fine powder and formed into a circle are an extremely poor choice. These starches help feed the pathogenic bacteria.

As breastfeeding decreases, the suppressed immune system weakens further. The pathogenic bacteria are fed the foods that help them grow. Eventually the child begins having physical and emotional problems due to the toxins invading his blood and neurological system.

If the child is vaccinated, their immune system cannot handle the invasion of viruses and toxins which also pass along to the still-developing brain.

The products found in this chapter can be found at http://naturallyhealingautism.com/a-healthy-home/

CHAPTER 7

IDENTIFYING THE UNDERLYING ISSUES

Of all the chapters in this book, this one took the most concentration, research, and personal trial and error. Candida is a very important factor and a tricky one. Statistics say that 90% of autistic children have gastrointestinal disorders. I think that number is incorrect. I would easily say there is sufficient gut dysbiosis in 100% of these children. Scientists estimate that 70% of all people have an overgrowth of Candida.

WHAT IS CANDIDA?

In our intestinal system, we have what are known as "good" bacteria. They work hard to keep our gut lining and our immune system in good health to fight off infection and disease.

Candida, also known as yeast or fungi, is some of the normal bacteria we all carry in our gut. The problem arises when Candida's numbers grow too high and get out of control. When the bad bacteria grow to a higher count than the good bacteria, we have what is known as an overgrowth. This is often referred to as a yeast infection or Candida albicans.

These bacteria have a delicate balancing system. This balance can easily be thrown off by such things as physical injury, poor diet, toxins, emotional stress, and the use of antibiotics. Fungus, such as Candida albicans in the gut, can easily be inhaled through oral secretions and affect our respiratory pathways and lungs. Fungus in the body is unknowingly tied to many allergies and can also mimic symptoms of a heart attack.

CANDIDA/YEAST IS SYSTEMIC

When most people hear the word "yeast," they think only of vaginal yeast. It is much, much more than that. In fact, if a practitioner thinks to test for yeast, they may only swab the vaginal area. If it is not found, they may tell you that you do not have it. This is not often the case.

Yeast is systemic. This means that it is present throughout the body and wreaking havoc in the organs, tissue, joints, and central nervous system, *including the brain.* Meninges are layers of tissue that cover the brain and spinal cord. Yeast/fungus is known to cause inflammation of the meninges, therefore, causing inflammation in the brain and the rest of the central nervous system. This is what is referred to as meningitis.

Candida is present in both males and females. For many, it is that large "Buddha belly" we see in so many people. This is a strong indication of Candida. For others, they may simply have behavioral problems, fatigue, or headaches that no one seems to be able to account for. This may be in a child that does not have the typical big belly associated with Candida. Other important factors to look at are gluten intolerance or other food sensitivities or allergies.

The GI tract is often damaged so severely by Candida that holes have been created in the lining of the intestines. The spores or babies of the yeast have legs on them that bore holes through the intestinal lining. This causes leaky gut.

This "leaky gut" allows undigested food and toxins to reach the bloodstream. These toxins flow to any organ or tissue they can. Leaky gut also causes food allergies. The undigested food is seen by the body as a foreign agent and antibodies are created against them. Foods once tolerated suddenly create allergic reactions. You may have already become aware of foods that seem to create symptoms in your child.

COMMON EMOTIONAL SYMPTOMS

- Hyperactivity or other behavioral problems.
- Excessive irritability
- Decreased cognitive function (brain fog)

- Depression
- Anxiety

Many people on antidepressant or anti-anxiety medication can have their symptoms disappear after a proper GI program that rebuilds, strengthens, and balances the good bacteria in their gut.

COMMON PHYSICAL SYMPTOMS

- Headaches
- Joint pain
- Ear aches and infections
- Tonsillitis
- Skin rashes (can be anywhere, but are commonly on the backs of the hands)
- Itchy skin
- Large protruded belly (indicative of allergy-inflammation due to yeast overgrowth)
- Cravings for sweets and carbohydrate foods
- Dark circles under the eyes (can also be due to food allergies which coincide with leaky gut)
- Chronic diarrhea
- Constipation
- Gas, bloating
- Low energy
- Chronis sinus congestion
- Itching in the vagina or anus
- Stuffy nose (fungi live in the nasal passages)
- Trouble breathing and/or wheezing

ADDITIONAL TESTING FOR CANDIDA/YEAST

How To Tell If You Have Candida - The Free and Accurate Candida Spit Test.

THE TEST: In the evening, put a clear glass of water by your bed. The first thing in the morning, briefly rinse your mouth, swallow, and then gather some saliva in your mouth and spit into the glass of water. (Be sure to spit out saliva, not mucus.) Keep an eye on the water for half an hour, especially the first few minutes. If you have Candida overgrowth, you will see one or more of the following:

1. **Strings (legs) hanging down from the saliva.**
2. **Heavy-looking saliva at the bottom of the glass.**
3. **Cloudy specks suspended in the water.**

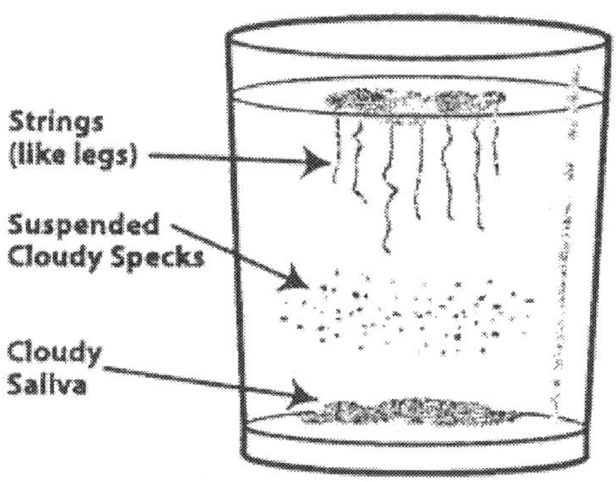

If you see "strings" hanging down within three minutes after spitting into the water, cloudy specks showing up in the water, or "debris" sinking to the bottom, you most likely have extensive overgrowth, which will require more Candida-fighting action on your part.

If it takes longer than a few minutes for anything to show up, the Candida is not as serious.

If the saliva just floats on top and the water stays perfectly clear, you most likely ***don't*** have Candida overgrowth.

The logic behind the test is simple.

If you have Candida overgrowth, it will show up in the saliva, a friendly environment for yeast. When you spit into the glass, the aerated saliva is lighter than water. However, Candida is heavier than either. Whether it sinks as "legs," falls to the bottom, or floats around in the water, these are all indications of Candida. The more you see and the faster you see it, the more systemic the infection.

MUSCLE TESTING FOR CANDIDA

Muscle testing is helpful in testing for Candida (see chapter on alternative therapies). Place the back of your hand directly over your child's belly button and muscle test him. If the muscle is weak, then their Candida is "up".

In my personal experience, it is easiest to look for some of the basic symptoms listed, do the saliva test, and use muscle testing. If you are still unsure and you want more thorough results, get a Genova Labs test from www.crohns.net. Children on the autism spectrum, with ADHD, ADD, asthma, food allergies, and beyond, all have imbalanced gut flora that must be treated. Treating for yeast is not harmful but helpful when done naturally without the use of drugs and their side effects.

An additional option that is helpful in giving you information is testing the first morning urine with litmus paper. This tells you how much acidity is in the urine and gives you a guideline to assist in giving you information from the beginning to the end of the Candida protocol. Higher acidity usually means higher microform growth. It is also a good indication of the amount of stress on the liver. Upon waking, prior to eating or drinking anything place the litmus paper under a stream of urine. The litmus paper will turn a color that you will match to the product's guideline. Be sure your litmus paper is one that moves by 0.2 such as 6.2, 6.4, 6.6, and not one that jumps by 0.5, such as 6.0, 6.5, etc. Look for the paper to go from yellow to green. Yellow is more acidic. There is not a perfect number, but essentially you are looking for something in the 6.4 range. This is simply a way to help track your progress. Litmus paper can be purchased at www.crohns.net.

A meridian stress (MSA) practitioner (discussed in the chapter on alternative therapies), can also test your child for his levels of

Candida, and more. They can also test the products you choose to use and give exact dosage levels.

CANDIDA INDUCED ALCOHOL POISONING

Candida requires sugar as food. This can come in the source of any chemical that ends in "ose" such as glucose, fructose, or sucrose. Carbohydrates such as bread and pasta are also converted by the body into sugars that act as another food source for the yeast. When glucose (from sugars and carbohydrates) is digested by Candida, it creates the alcoholic chemical ethanol and its extremely toxic byproduct, acetaldehyde.

Candida and this alcohol, acetaldehyde, are transferred via the placenta to the developing fetus and are capable of doing harm during development. After birth, the baby continues to receive alcohol through the mother's breast milk.

Alcohol can cause malnutrition by preventing the body from digesting proteins. Many liquid herbal tinctures contain alcohol. Be sure supplements are alcohol free.

Associated problems from alcohol:

- Aggressive and violent behavior. Alcohol causes damage to areas of the brain that can increase aggressive behavior to violent behavior.
- Anxiety
- Lethargy
- Impaired co-ordination, speech, and memory loss.
- Liver damage causing a lowered ability of the body's detoxification processes.
- Damage to the intestinal lining reducing the ability for proper digestion and absorption of nutrients.
- Inability of the hormones released by the thyroid to become activated. NOTE: The thyroid may produce an acceptable lab test because it is releasing the proper hormones. The problem is that, once released, the hormones cannot do their jobs due to acetaldehyde inhibiting the working sites needed by those hormones.

- Malabsorption and malnutrition due to inhibition of pancreatic enzymes and reduced ability for the stomach to produce hydrochloric acid.
- Altering the bodies' ability to utilize vitamin B6 which assists in the production of neurotransmitters for the brain.

WHY IS YEAST SO HARD TO GET RID OF?

We take antifungal agents to fight Candida, but the lesser-known truth is that they just build up resistance to these products and the yeast becomes stronger over time. This makes it harder to get rid of. When the yeast feels threatened by one of our yeast programs, it has the ability to hibernate in tissues where it is kept safe and sheltered from our anti-Candida program. Some is killed off, and we feel the effects of the die-off, so we believe it is working.

Candida also releases spores which are its "babies." These spores are also able to hibernate when they sense danger such as a yeast cleansing program or a strengthened immune system. When we feel better and stop our yeast cleanse, the spores come out of hibernation and recolonize in our gut, laying their own new babies, except now they are even stronger. In this case, the Candida problem returns usually worse than it was before.

SPORES

Yeast also releases spores which are like their babies. These spores can actually bore themselves into the tissues of our bodies and go into a sort of hibernation when they sense they are in danger. This keeps them safe from most yeast cleansing products.

During a Candida cleanse, these yeast and their spores do their best to stay safe. Since this is the case, it makes sense to find a product that can kill both the motherlode and their hiding babies. Otherwise, we begin feeling better, think we are yeast-free, end our eradication program, and soon find ourselves back where we started. The spores will come out of hiding, and begin breeding a whole new colony of yeast. It is frustrating to spend the money, and take the time, to go through the process and not make the progress hoped for.

Obviously, their behavior is a huge indicator of what is happening. Remember that things may get worse for a few days before they get better. Eventually, their appetite will likely increase for the right foods, their skin may clear up, asthma clears, and their stool will give you indications that the yeast is leaving their body.

When checking the stool, look for orange-colored mucus, and sometimes hair-like consistency. I know it sounds a bit gross but it can be a good physical indication that the body is excreting the Candida. There will usually be a strong odor that accompanies it.

THE YEAST/MERCURY CONNECTION

Mercury will slow down the removal of yeast. It is wise to continue the use of probiotics after Candida has been eradicated, during heavy metal detoxification, and after its removal. This ensures any remaining Candida has been removed and that mercury is not holding any of the yeast in the body and resisting its removal. Afterwards, continue on a maintenance dose. Probiotics will be continued daily for the rest of your child's life. Think of them as insurance against gut imbalance and immune deficiency. We all need them daily.

Yeast and mercury are friends. One reason why Candida can be so challenging to get rid of is because there is still mercury in the system. I have found that if we get rid of the mercury, Candida seems to go away more easily, but first we must heal and strengthen the gut. The toxins released from heavy metals and fungus lower the body's ability to turn the food we eat into energy. See the chapter on heavy metals for excreting mercury and other metals from your child's body.

With conventional sulfur-containing, heavy metal chelating methods, such as DMSA, one must exercise caution to be sure the liver is supported first, and that the gut has more balance prior. Sulfur may likely disturb the already weak GI tract. These drugs also deplete the body further of important minerals.

Mercury is known to inhibit the human body's ability to kill Candida. It does this by preventing a type of white blood cells called neutrophils from killing the Candida fungus. These cells normally destroy microorganisms and foreign matter in the blood. Two common sources of mercury are from vaccinations and mercury amalgam dental fillings.

When mercury is being excreted from the body, yeast will act up. By acting up, I mean that it will move around the body, get into the blood stream and organs, and create chaos. Hopefully, the yeast is dying off. Look for hyperactivity and behavioral issues to spring up for a few days while heavy metals are excreting. It makes sense that heavy metals may move around while yeast is being killed off.

A NOTE ABOUT HEAVY METAL DETOXIFICATION AND CANDIDA CLEANSING

I advocate healing the gut and getting the intestinal bacteria in balance *before* beginning a heavy metal detoxification. Even a few weeks into the Candida program will be helpful for the strength of your child's body prior to the natural product I suggest.

This Candida program also has a product called Candiclear5 that assists in the gentle removal of mercury along with the Candida cleanse. The recommended program for candida cleansing is in Chapter 26.

ANTIFUNGALS: WHY NOT?

Antifungal products have been used for years to help eradicate Candida albicans. I have found that they have been helpful in conjunction with other products but do not take care of the imbalance completely when used alone. Some of the products I mention below are helpful for the immune system or for short-term relief. However, Candida learns how to hide away from these types of products and lay their spores, only to come out of hiding once we stop the cleansing program.

The worst part is that Candida builds up a resistance to antifungal agents which make the yeast stronger.

COMMONLY USED ANTIFUNGALS:

- Oregano oil
- Caprylic acid: a fatty acid found in coconut oil
- Black walnut
- Garlic

- Olive leaf extract
- Pau d'arco
- Malic acid, found in apple cider vinegar
- Grapefruit seed extract (GSE): GSE inactivates pathogens and is effective against such bacteria as E. coli, salmonella, and staphylococcus. It is extremely antibacterial and more effective than chlorine bleach, colloidal silver, tea tree oil, or iodine at killing yeast (*The GSE Report,* Volume 1, Issue 1, pg. 6). If making your own product, use caution to follow directions on the bottle and guidelines from a practitioner. You can purchase a bottle of Citricidal grapefruit seed extract from www.crohns.net, or www.pureformulas.com to make your own tinctures or natural household cleaning agents. (Yes, that's right; it makes a great cleaning agent.) The company Citricidal also sells already prepared ear drops and nasal spray made with GSE available at www.pureformulas.com (800)383-6008.

I have to share my personal story of using grapefruit seed extract with you because it was an amazing experience. I had been treating myself for Candida (luckily for you I keep manifesting everything I write about, so you get more research and trials done), and one day my left sinus completely stopped up, and my throat felt thick and scratchy. When most of us would think it was only allergies, I knew otherwise. I could have muscle tested to be sure, but my gut told me that it was a Candida flare-up, and I felt all right otherwise. (Note: the sinuses are connected to gut issues.)

I drank 5–15 drops of grapefruit seed extract in 5 ounces of water, 1 to 3 times per day. I also purchased a small, 3-ounce bottle with a nasal spray top. I placed a drop or two of the extract into the bottle with pure water and sprayed it into my nose 1–3 times per day to kill off the fungi and bacteria in the nasal passageways.

Garlic and coconut oil are important foods to add to your regular diet. Both are naturally antibacterial and antiviral, and garlic is well-known as an aid to the immune system. Coconut oil is also one of the good fats that help our brain to function, and it contains caprylic acid which breaks down the cell walls of Candida.

If you choose to look into them further, antifungal tinctures, either individually or in combinations, can be found in healthfood stores and at many online websites such as www.pureformulas.com. A product by Pharmax called garlic freeze dried is one example. The company Brainchild Nutritionals has many of these products and they specialize in products for autism spectrum disorders. Their products can be found at http://naturallyhealingautism.com/a-healthy-home/. Please be sure to use the code "naturallyhealingautism" to receive 15% off all of their products.

SULFATE-REDUCING BACTERIA

Sulfate is a natural form of sulfur, and 95% of children with autism show a deficiency in sulfates. Sulfates are an important part of the body's detoxification process. Sulfate helps give glutathione antioxidant strength and assists in detoxification by attaching to toxins and helping to eliminate them from the body. It can be very helpful for children on the autism spectrum, and it is beneficial for those with repetitive behavior. Sulfates also assist in the metabolism of neurotransmitters for the brain.

Pathogenic, sulfate-reducing bacteria in the gut, are responsible for turning the sulfate from foods we eat into their toxic form called sulfites, therefore depleting the body of the much-needed sulfates. The lack of sulfates also causes food to putrefy in the gut. This is the cause of that rotten egg odor that accompanies the stool and flatulence. When the pathogenic bacteria are eradicated from the GI tract, healthy food can be absorbed, and this should provide the needed sulfates.

A note about sulfur: Sulfur may help kids with the removal of heavy metals and other chemicals. It is contained in DMSA, the medical form of heavy metal removal, but it may disturb the gastrointestinal tract by increasing yeast growth. For this reason, use caution if Candida/yeast is a problem. Talk to your healthcare practitioner. Foods that help increase sulfur content are asparagus and garlic. Epsom salts supply the body with sulfate. Epsom salts baths calm the system via skin absorption.

LEAKY GUT

Yeast can attach itself to the wall of the intestines, creating holes that allow undigested foods and other toxins to enter the bloodstream. This is known as "leaky gut."

It is essential to protect the gut and keep it healthy since it is the main source of our immune system, and it filters out toxins from the environment, including foods. Antibody producing cells line the intestines and secrete a substance called immunoglobulin A or IgA. IgA protects the lining of the intestines by preventing bacteria from binding to it. This prevents the bacteria from passing through the intestinal wall and entering the bloodstream. Candida weakens IgA production.

Beware of using any non-steroidal, non-inflammatory medications (NSAIDS), like aspirin or amphetamines. They are known to weaken the gut lining. Cow's milk should also be avoided or minimized since it is known to promote leaky gut.

If any food gets into the bloodstream intact, it can be very toxic to the entire system, especially the brain. This lowers resistance to infections and leaves us vulnerable to greater susceptibility of food intolerance and allergies. This is something we see commonly in children with autism.

Immune reactions of this sort cause the body to be in a continual fight for health. When the immune system is constantly in the "on" position, it can become depleted, leaving us even more vulnerable to infection disease and autoimmune illnesses. It also depletes the body's serotonin levels, which contribute to anxiety, depression, and sleep disorders. (More on this in the chapter "Supporting the Brain")

Some examples of illnesses caused by Candida and larger molecules passing through the gut lining are rheumatoid arthritis, asthma, food allergies, celiac disease, cystic fibrosis, skin disorders such as eczema, and pancreatic dysfunction, which reduces the body's ability to produce enough enzymes needed for digestion of food and for many necessary cellular reactions.

Stress, too many sugars (including bad carbohydrates), fruit, processed food, and alcohol can all repopulate the "bad" bacteria. Just when you think everything is under control, it comes back. Yeast is ongoing if you let it be.

Once the holes in the gut heal, the parasites are eradicated, and the good bacteria are restored to balance, the persons' susceptibility to these issues diminishes. However, if parasites are detected, the Candida diet will help to eradicate many of the pathogenic bacteria, but the parasite issue must still be addressed.

LYME DISEASE

In this segment, I have listed multiple remedies for eradicating Lyme. This bug does not leave easily and multiple systems are affected. Antibiotics alone have been disappointing in the treatment of Lyme disease. A broad-based treatment that affects all co-infections and assists the body on multiple levels is necessary. Energetic frequencies, nutritional therapies, and the occasional need for anti-parasitic medicine and antibiotics all need to be reviewed so that you can make educated decisions for your child.

You will need help. Not all doctors are fully informed on the proper treatment of this disease. To find an educated Lyme doctor in your area, visit the International Lyme and Associated Diseases Society website at www.ilads.org.

WHY ARE WE TALKING ABOUT LYME DISEASE?

The prevalence of Lyme disease is on the rise. This is likely to continue due to increasing global temperatures. Microbial-carrying insects flourish in a warm environment. One in every four children on the autism spectrum tests positive for Lyme infection. It is the fastest growing vector-born infection with 300,000 new cases per year, and this number is said to likely be an underestimate. It continues to be under-diagnosed due to the Center for Disease Control's inadequate established bands or markers used for detection in blood tests. Those who have had the Lyme vaccination will often come up with a false positive. Blood must be tested several times due to dormancy of the bacterium and cysts. Additionally, blood tests can still be unreliable because the bacteria can divide into undetectable strains.

Lyme infection is usually caused by a tick bite which releases the bacteria from its saliva. We now know that other insects may carry the disease such as some spiders, biting flies, and mosquitoes. Lyme disease can also be transmitted during sexual contact, through breast milk, and in utero via the placenta. Maternal blood often has no evidence of spirochetes, but the baby may have them, often in the liver. In babies, it is common to have brain, nerve, spinal cord, and heart problems.

COMMON SYMPTOMS OF LYME DISEASE:

- Lyme disease can mimic other disorders such as:
- Attention deficit disorder (ADD)
- Learning difficulties
- Obsessive compulsive disorder (OCD)
- Depression
- Alzheimer's
- Schizophrenia
- Multiple sclerosis
- Chronic fatigue
- Fibromyalgia
- Heart conditions
- Bell's Palsy

LYME'S AFFECT ON THE BRAIN

Lyme's affect on the brain tends to:

- Shrink the putamen, involved in learning, and the release of GABA and acetylcholine, which affect the nervous and muscular systems.
- Enlarge the thalamus, which is responsible for the comprehension of language, sending and receiving all sensory signals, regulating the sleep-wake cycle and conscious awareness.
- Weaken the cerebellum, which is involved in motor coordination, attention/focus, and language.

There is a software imaging program called Neuroquant that takes images of the brain and shows the volume measurements of its different structures. This is a tool that can be used to measure the health of various parts of the brain. For some, it has been useful before and during Lyme treatment for assessment and to note changes. It is very inexpensive (about $96) compared to other imaging. This can be a useful tool. For more information visit www.radnet.com/neuroquant.html or call (800) 975-4674.

The four bacteria that cause Lyme infection are borrelia, ehrlichia/anaplasma, babesia, and bartonella. Common symptoms for each are:

- Borrelia: mixed symptoms starting with flu-like symptoms, arthritis, fatigue, occipital headaches (back of the head) with neck stiffness, emotional, bull's eye (circular) rash. Usually there are four-week cycle symptom flare-ups.
- Babesia: a common co-infection includes fever, headaches, sweats, trouble breathing, and severe fatigue. Symptoms cycle every four to seven days.
- Bartonella: most symptoms are from the neck up with anxiety, sleep disturbance, and enlarged lymph nodes in under arm area. Bartonella live on cats and can inflict humans in contact.
- Ehrlichia/Anaplasma: muscle pain, headaches with sharp pain behind eyes, elevated liver enzymes, high white blood cell count, trouble remembering names or words mid-sentence.

TYPES OF BACTERIAL FORMS IN LYME'S DISEASE

Borrelia is responsible for the initial spread of the infection. These bacteria have the ability to transform itself into three different bacterial forms: spirochete, cell wall deficient, and cyst. Spirochetes are mobile and can penetrate any area of the body including bone. When it senses danger, it can transform into cyst form.

1. Cell wall deficient (CWD) is more dangerous than the spirochete form and harder to treat. Its name is what it implies; that it has no cell wall. This can make it very difficult to eradicate, as it can transform with the use of antibiotics.

Those suffering are often deficient in vitamin D as CWD converts it into an immunosuppressive hormone known as 1, 25-D. CWD also causes autoimmunity. Common symptoms from CWD include paralysis, multiple sclerosis, mental disorders, and chronic fatigue.

2. Cysts lie dormant, unaffected by antibiotics, pH changes, hydrogen peroxide, or temperature changes. It will convert back to spirochete form when safe to do so. this form can remain asymptomatic for years.

TREATING LYME

The bacteria that cause Lyme disease can keep changing form and re-infect. Each must be treated specifically. Multiple infections suppress the immune system, so multiple systems must be treated. Lyme decreases immunity so secondary fungal, bacterial, and viral infections appear. This happens even easier if heavy metals and toxins are in the system.

Do not use traditional methods of heavy metal detoxification such as DMSA or EDTA when Lyme is present. Mercury can inhibit Lyme. If a heavy metal detoxification process allows reabsorption of toxins back into the body during the excretion process like these chelators do, then the mercury released into the system may activate the Lyme disease.

Lyme has multiple co-infections. It is systemic, gets into the intestines, and makes you intolerant of carbohydrates and sensitive to gluten, casein, and sugar. These compounds are not able to digest and drop into the lower intestine. Instead, they remain in the upper GI to feed pathogenic bacteria. For this reason, IVs are best for treatment with magnesium and other supplements as spirochetes use it in the gut to flourish.

The areas most infected are the brain and face, including the teeth, ears, and sinuses. Next, due to lowered immunity and fungi, the parasites invade the other systems of the body, including the immune system.

ASYRA TESTING

Effective testing with blood is minimal. The standard "blot" blood test often shows a false negative, especially when the immune system is weak. Asyra is an effective test for Lyme. It is a non-invasive bio-energetic screening and is known as the world's number one, bio-energetic screening test. One appointment gives you the answer. You can learn more at, www.asyra.co.uk.

One resource for ASYRA in the U.S. is in California at, http://www.immunematrix.com/joomla-dist/index.php?option=com_contact&view=contact&id=1&Itemid=71

EFFECTIVE HERBAL TREATMENT

A known effective treatment protocol for Lyme is The Lee Cowden Lyme Protocol with Nutramedix. It is an herbal Lyme protocol. You can learn more at, www.nutramedix.ec/nc/cowden-support-program.

TRADITIONAL ANTIBIOTIC TREATMENTS FOR LYME

When antibiotics are used, it is critical that very specific and different types of them are used in rotations or the bacteria will hide and transform themselves, becoming resistant. Lyme bacteria builds biofilm, therefore the biofilm must be destroyed to minimize the risk of bacteria receding and returning. Biofilm has already been talked about in detail earlier in this book. There are many different treatment protocols.

I have spoken with people whom antibiotics have helped and those who did not respond to them. Different treatment options are available for those who wish to do alternative treatments first or for those who have not had success with antibiotics. Chronic illness may remain even after antibiotic treatment. This may be due to the body's inability to remove biotoxins.

Without a doubt, the most critical part of Lyme treatment would be to find a specialist in this disease. Your regular doctor cannot help you eradicate this illness the same as someone who specializes in it.

Consult a "Lyme Literate Medical Doctor" ("LLMD"), typically a clinician who is a member of the leading organization for Lyme called ILADS (International Lyme and Associated Diseases Society), www.ilads.org.

One lab that solely focuses on Lyme and its co-infections is www.igenex.com. They are better than other labs at positively detecting, although not always 100% accurate.

THE MARSHALL PROTOCOL

The Marshall Protocol is commonly used for chronic inflammatory diseases often known to be bacterially caused. It is a way to activate the immune response. Pulsed low-dose bacteriostatic antibiotics are used on a specific schedule along with olmesartan (brand name Benicar). Olmesartan is a general hypertensive agent that stimulates the innate immune response. Olmesartan is increased over time, while antibiotics may be reduced or even eliminated. When the Marshall Protocol first began, antibiotics were routinely used. Today, more is known about the recovery process and less or none may be needed.

This process minimizes immunosuppression. The premise of the Marshall Protocol is that by activating the immune system and increasing inflammation, it actually assists in killing the bacteria and bringing recovery. The protocol enhances the effectiveness of the antibacterial properties but is not immunosuppressive. It is able to destroy cell wall-deficient bacteria, therefore having the ability to cure Lyme disease. The pulsing of dosages also reduces biofilm and reaches the dormant bacteria.

For further information and to find a physician skilled in the Marshall Protocol, go to www.mpkb.org. Bryan Rosner has also written several books on Lyme that include information on the Marshall Protocol. Bryan's information can be found at www.lymebook.com.

ENERGETIC FREQUENCIES

RIFE

One treatment that uses energetic frequencies instead of antibiotics is known as Rife. An American inventor by the name of Royal Raymond Rife created an energetic resonance frequency machine. Rife passed away in 1971, after many years of successfully working with cancer patients. His device was criticized by conventional medical doctors, so it was not until the 1980s that the Rife machine began getting due notice. Books were written about it that educated the layperson and began further interest and use. It became known as an affective alternative therapy.

The energetic resonance frequencies in the Rife machine are programmable by computer. These frequencies disrupt, weaken, and destroy microbial pathogens. This does not induce conversion of spirochetes into other forms. It also treats cysts.

Bryan Rosner has several books and has CDs available written from his own experience with Lyme. He has researched both conventional and alternative therapies and has a ton of information to offer. Bryan has an entire book on the Rife machine and another titled, *The Top Ten Lyme Disease Treatments*. This book offers everything from rotational antibiotic treatments, homeopathies, Rife, and more. For more information please visit www.lymebook.com.

INDIGO BIOFEEDBACK

An additional energetic treatment for Lyme and its co-infections is the Indigo Biofeedback machine. It is discussed in more detail in "Chapter 8: Alternative Therapies."

NUTRITIONAL ASSISTANCE

There is a product called Monolaurin made from lauric acid which is derived from coconut oil. It prevents the reproduction of bacterial cells, including Borrelia. Monolauren is found in breastmilk in the highest concentration. It is capable of killing fourteen viruses, including MRSA Stapholococcus. It contains the same size lipid fat molecules as the pathogens, which makes it inevitable for penetration of their walls. The Lyme bacteria Borrelia have soft outer membranes allowing Monolaurin to penetrate them. Once inside the cell Monolauren will disrupt its reproductive cycle, and eventually rupture the cell wall killing it. It also kills spirochetes and the common co-infections of Borrelia.

Monolauren is commonly used to fight flu viruses and bacterial infections. Lauric acid is commonly used to treat Candida. It fights only the bad bacteria, but not the good. It has also been used against shingles, hepatitis C, herpes, and measles. It is available at www.inspirednutrition.com. They have descriptive usage information on their website. Muscle test for dosage.

Additional help:

- PEKANA Homeopathic-Spagyric Medications, www.bioresourceinc.com.
- Iodine disrupts cell walls
- Niacin for mental/emotional support
- Enzyme combinations
- Freeze dried garlic
- **Lyme builds biofilm. See the chapter on Different Types of Pathogenic Microbes. The biofilm** must be dissolved in order to kill the spirochetes.

A COMPLETE PROGRAM

One protocol that mixes East and West is from Dr. Deitrich Klinghardt. Dr. Klinghardt is one of the foremost authorities on autism. He is a medical doctor who practices both traditionally and alternatively. He combines Eastern and Western philosophy and specializes in many fields including pediatrics, chronic illness, and chronic pain. Dr. Klinghardt has a very specific protocol for Lyme disease. The entire protocol plus more is available on his website and on DVD at www.klinghardtacademy.com.

LYME AND MOLD BIOTOXINS

When chronic illness remains even after full treatment where spirochetes and other protozoa have been eradicated, it is likely due to the body's inability to remove biotoxins. Lyme symptoms and the mold genotype overlap, including Staphylococcus in the nasal passages. Are they Lyme positive and live in a tick area? If they are positive for the mold genotype Lyme treatment will not work, especially if you are living or working in a water damaged building.

EXERCISE

Exercise is important to increase blood flow, increase oxygenation throughout the body and to assist with lymphatic drainage.

REMEMBERING TO ASSIST DIE-OFF

Die-off reactions, known as Herxheimer's, are caused by the toxins from the bad bacteria that are released as they die. When this happens faster than the liver can keep up, there may be reactions such as fatigue, headaches, and flu-like symptoms. To assist with die-off be sure to take some liver support. Liver Life by Bioray, or Liver Support and Detoxification from Pharmax can be very helpful. Both are available at healthfood stores and online at sites such as www.pureformulas.com.

Additional support for decreasing the toxic load on the body is:

- Lymphatic drainage via homeopathic remedies, Craniosacral therapy or other specified bodywork.
- Dry brushing the body.
- Far infrared saunas are very helpful and can be found locally at spa centers for rent. They can also be purchased and put into your own home. One quality source is www.infraredsauna.com.
- Alkalizing baths of baking soda, Epsom salts, or alkalizing bath salts are available at www.biopure.edu.

When die-off has balanced (via reduced symptoms), slowly begin your needed protocol or protocols. This may include protocols for parasites, mold, Lyme, Candida, or a combination of these. Lyme and mold protocols are often begun immediately and with the assistance of a qualified healthcare practitioner.

Last, beta-sitosterol by Pharmax may be helpful to bind and excrete neurotoxins. It also helps to stop re-absorption of these toxins. Antioxidants and other necessary supplements may be helpful now. Remember to muscle test first. *Only add one new product at a time.* Let the body adjust and be sure you know what causes any behavioral or physiological changes for the better or worse.

LYME PREVENTION

The nymph tick is as small as a poppy seed. We often do not realize when we have been bit. Ticks tend to live in grass, leaves, and shrubs closer to the ground. They do not jump, but if brushed against, they will cling to you.

Wear light-colored clothing so you can see them. Do not do yard work without wearing gloves, tuck your pants into your socks, and avoid tall wet grasses and piles of leaves. Remove them using tweezers. Do not touch ticks with your bare hands or use alcohol, bleach, or a burning cigarette as a means of removal as these decrease your chances of becoming infected.

(See Appendix A for Lyme resources.)

PROTOCOL NECESSITIES FOR ALL PATHOGENIC ERADICATION

Gut restoration, including liver, bowel support, and immune support should all take place in a specific order. Multi-vitamin supplements and antioxidants need to wait until parasitic eradication has taken place as they will feed the parasites if given too soon. The gut is often not able to absorb them yet either.

Gut restoration comes first. Follow the guidelines for pre-Candida diet supplements (noted in Candida's diet chapter: probiotics, gut healers and inflammation fighters, and liver support). Slowly introduce the cleaner Candida diet and watch for symptoms of die-off. (Note: There should be three weeks of gut restoration and bowel support with probiotics before starting any multi-vitamin, multi-mineral, or antioxidant supplements as they will feed the parasites.

SUMMARY

The most common problematic microbe for children with autism is candida albicans. This bacteria is commonly referred to as yeast or fungi. Candida can grow to detrimentally high numbers through such avenues as poor diet, and the use of antibiotics.

If a pregnant woman has an overgrowth of candida she will pass this on in utero to her unborn child. The gut makes up as much as eighty percent of the immune system, therefore the child is born with compromised immunity. Yeast or candida creates extreme toxicity. It gets into the blood stream and effects many systems of the body including the central nervous system and the brain. More detailed information on treating candida is given in chapter 25.

An additional pathogenic microbe that can be passed from mother to child in utero is Lyme. Lyme causes multiple co-infections and inflammation in the body. It is tricky to detect and to treat, as many people are antibiotic resistant. Several options to eradicate Lyme are given in this chapter.

The products found in this chapter can be found at http://naturallyhealingautism.com/a-healthy-home/

CHAPTER 8

BASIC NUTRITION AND SUPPLEMENTATION

As parents, there are many basic facts to know about nutrition. Most people are confused about what to eat and when to eat it. There actually is a lot to know. It is simple once you have learned the concepts, but they will be ultimately helpful for your child's digestion, absorption of nutrients, and his overall immune system. I am developing an app for your phone that will help simplify this information.

Take from the following information the general facts and then decide what your child needs. There are many great companies who make nutritional supplements with those on the autism spectrum or poor digestion in mind. They have been given to you in the following chapters.

Do not begin multiple vitamin and mineral supplements before his gut is healed. If there are parasites, they will use them as their food and make things worse. It is likely that his gut has very poor absorption at this time anyway. We will go into this in greater detail.

Research over the past two decades has shown that proper nutrition may have the greatest effect on protection from disease. By strengthening the body's defenses nutrition can override many of genetic triggers, whether they are chemical or environmental. The reverse effect of this can come from negative signals such as the genetic susceptibility to juvenile diabetes (Type 1), often occurs after exposure to a virus, cow's milk, or the excitotoxins monosodium glutamate (MSG). These can turn on the signal for the diabetes gene. Without a trigger, the disease may never arise.

One study showing that genes can be changed by diet comes from Waterland et al. Agouti mice, often fat and yellow in color, were fed folic acid, vitamin B12, choline and betaine. This affected their genes and they gave birth to skinny, brown offspring.

PROPER NUTRITION

Proper nutrition can create defenses against toxic impact, including those from heavy metals such as mercury, and assisting in its excretion. Nutrition also protects the nervous system in many ways by keeping cell membranes strong or strengthening weak ones, protecting DNA, improving the production of energy within the cells, and reducing inflammation. Proper nutrition also protects the enzyme systems that detoxify the cells and the liver.

What the average person, and the average professional, thinks good nutrition is are often vastly incorrect. Many Americans still think the french fry is a valid, nutritious vegetable and we eat from boxes and cans. A compromised digestive tract does not allow the nutrients from fresh foods to absorb into our cells and fulfill our body's needs.

Read your labels. Know what to look for. Our foods today are poisoned routinely by large manufacturing companies that choose to add ingredients that are chemical in nature. Many of these foods actually make us crave more food. They also contain sugars and toxins that will invade the central nervous system—this means your child's brain!

How we grow, feed, and prepare our food is another issue altogether. Conventional food is grown in soil that is so depleted of nutrients to feed the growing crops that when the crop is mature enough to eat, it lacks sufficient quantities of nutrients. We eat food thinking it is giving us the nutrition we need. Most grains, fruits, and vegetables are genetically modified and are grown in toxic pesticides. Our livestock is fed grains grown in these same pesticides, and they are fed antibiotics and hormones that remain in the meat we eat. This means more toxic overload.

Time magazine's August 31, 2009, issue entitled "The Real Cost of Cheap Food" explains some of the issues that endanger our health due to inhumane and unsafe feeding practices of our livestock resources. The book (and movie), *Food, Inc.*, also explains these practices.

Another good eye-opener is the documentary titled, *Supersize Me.* This story takes a perfectly healthy individual who decides to eat only fast food to show to others through his film what could happen to the body if we eat a poor diet, especially fast foods, on a daily basis. In less than a month, his liver begins to shut down. He cannot make it up the stairs to his home any longer, and he experiences extreme fatigue. He is told by doctors to stop his experiment for the movie and begin eating properly or he could die.

Children with autism, ADD, food intolerances, or an improperly working digestive system are already deficient in vital nutrients that their growing brains need. It is never a deficiency of just one nutrient—when one vitamin or mineral is lacking, additional deficiencies develop. These children are usually not absorbing the nutrients from the good foods they eat, and they have a breakdown in the metabolism of nutrients as well. We all need supplementation along with good nutrition, but these children especially do.

Another very important aspect is that our food sources are severely depleted of nutrition due to over-use of soils, therefore limiting them of vital nutrients. Seeds for grain are mutated, often to the point that our bodies do not even know how to digest them. These same grains, also laden with chemicals, are given to the animals that we eat, along with hormones that have been ingested and injected.

When we put this into our bodies, we not only lack what we need for good nutrition, but we ingest so many chemicals ourselves that we need supplementation to combat the toxicity. Growing evidence shows that there are exceptional long-term gains to adding nutritional supplementation to your diet.

We need seven to ten servings of fresh, quality fruits and vegetable every day. Not many people actually get that. Supplements should not take the place of fresh foods in our diet, but because our diets do not include all that is necessary we must be sure we are getting what we need daily.

FREE RADICALS AND ANTIOXIDANTS

Good nutrition also supplies the body's defenses by feeding it antioxidants. Antioxidants do just what they say—they prevent oxidation. Oxidation is a common daily process we are all familiar with. A banana, once peeled, is exposed to air and starts to break down. This brown coloring we see on the fruit is oxidation.

We need oxygen to live, but if our cells start to oxidize, it is incredibly destructive. Due to a daily and ongoing attack on the body's cells from free radicals (destructive particles that eat away at our cells), we need antioxidants.

Free radicals can easily damage any part of the cell they come in contact with. Once the cell is attacked, not only is the entire cell in danger, but so are all of the tissues in the body. This is likely the basis for autoimmune diseases.

Free radicals can destroy DNA (the cell's director), the cell membranes, and the proteins within the cells. Many cellular proteins are enzymes that enable thousands of necessary chemical reactions to happen. Damaged enzymes cannot do their job properly, and the cell becomes weak.

Cell membranes protect everything inside of the cell. They also contain the mitochondria, which is the cell's vital energy source. The membrane passes along messages of instruction to the cell. If the message center does not function properly, vital connections are not made. Many of these can be neurological connections. Cell membranes are made up of fatty molecules that, if damaged, lead to something called lipid peroxidation. Lipid peroxidation happens in almost every disease known.

Lipid peroxidation largely affects organs that are made of fat. The brain contains 60% fats, therefore it is highly susceptible to the damage that can be done by lipid peroxidation and to toxins from lipid-soluble substances such as pesticides and mercury.

See the chapter on nutritional supplementation for specific antioxidants.

CAUSES OF FREE RADICAL DAMAGE:

- inflammation
- stress
- environmental toxins
- ultraviolet radiation
- x-ray radiation

- magnesium deficiency
- excitotoxins
- activation of the immune system
- metabolism (byproducts of)

Some examples of free radical toxins known to cause damage in brain tissue are from aluminum, iron, lead, mercury, and cadmium. Even fluoride, yes the same fluoride most people brush their teeth with daily, is extremely toxic and some cities have added it to your drinking water. My children do not use toothpaste that contains fluoride, and their teeth are very healthy.

These environmental toxins, natural or man-made, cause great free radical damage within tissues. This could be a major contributor of many neurological disorders.

One effective method of treating many infections and inflammations is through heavy use of antioxidants. Improvements have been seen in illnesses such as Lyme disease, viral hepatitis, rheumatoid arthritis, Alzheimer's disease, Lou Gehrig's disease (ALS), multiple sclerosis (MS), lupus, and encephalitis. The more I researched, the more I found that many of these types of illnesses have much in common with autism and ASD's.

The common link seems to be an increase in the metabolic rate due to ongoing inflammation in the body. This causes the immune system to attack its own host. The immune system releases a mass of free radicals to fight the infection. Our metabolism then leaves behind free radical by-products that can weaken and even destroy our cells. The many possible causes of this happening will be covered later in the chapters on heavy metals and prevention.

WHO IS AT RISK OF FREE RADICAL DAMAGE?

We are all at risk; however, our children, because they are young, along with those with compromised immune systems, are more vulnerable to environmental toxins. If you know that your child is already battling a neurological or physical disorder of some kind, then it is essential that the greatest care is given to the food he eats, the water he drinks, and any medications taken. His system will not be able to fend off more than it already has going on.

An overload will be seen as behavioral, whether in a tantrum or additional "stimming" (rocking back and forth), etc. Due to the overload on the immune system, sometimes a cold or virus will appear, or a skin rash will appear. There are many possibilities. More than anything, you do not want *additional* damage done to the immune or neurological system.

FOODS KNOWN TO INCREASE FREE RADICALS

- monosodium glutamate (MSG)
- aspartame (found in NutraSweet, Equal, and others)
- carrageenan

These are known to damage the brain, especially the area that controls memory and fine motor coordination. There will be more information on this later; an entire chapter has been dedicated to excitotoxins, artificial flavorings, and colorings.

GENETICALLY MODIFIED FOODS

A genetically modified food is one that has had its DNA changed within a laboratory. This is often done to crops to make them grow faster, resist pesticides, or alter their nature to create a different sort of plant altogether. This is common of wheat. In order to force the grain to contain a higher gluten content, due to the increase in its requirement by processed foods. Gluten is "glue" and it holds things together. This has made our wheat crops about 90 percent higher in gluten than it used to be. This bioengineering, or genetically modified product becomes one that the human body cannot process well. This unnatural alteration produces foods are linked to allergies, neurological disorders, depression, fatigue, loss of mental clarity, nausea, and even cancer. GMO's effect sulfur metabolism which also effects the body's ability to detoxify, and to make the important "feel good" neurotransmitter serotonin, and the natural sleep chemical melatonin.

Genetically modified foods are in everything including baby formula (especially soy-based), farm-raised fish, grains, and dairy. Soy products are incredibly high in GMO's. GMO soy has been linked in studies to anxiety and aggressive behavior. Many people who are vegetarian or have allergies to dairy use soy as a substitute. This is a poor alternative, unfortunately dairy is not good either.

Beware of dairy that is *not* labeled with the words "from cows not injected with rBGH/rBST". These are genetically engineered hormones that are commonly injected into cows. GMO grains including corn are often fed to beef cattle as well as dairy cows. When we eat this meat we are eating these hormones, genetically modified meat, and often the added antibiotics too.

In research done with rats it was found that those that were fed with GMO foods were antisocial, irritable and aggressive. Those who were fed with non-GMO foods were calm, and did not express these behaviors. Similar results were observed with livestock including pigs. When their food was switched back to non-GMO feed the behaviors reduced significantly.

The Lancet is the world's leading general medical journal. In 1999 it published a study on rats that were fed potatoes loaded with GMO. In as little as ten days the lining of their stomach and entire digestive tract was much thinner and weakened. Similar evidence has been seen in livestock fed with GMO feed. These are comparable to the symptoms of children on the autism spectrum. Since the lining of the digestive tract is so weak it may be easily permeated, and be connected to one reason why leaky gut is so common among them.

Lack of knowledge relating to GMO foods was partly due to some governments trying to hide the information from the public. Large food manufacturing companies, many subsidized by the American government, did not want the public offered the knowledge regarding which foods were genetically modified and which ones were not. The reason for this was simply financial. The less people know, the more money the companies and the governments often stand to make.

HOW TO DETECT GENETICALLY MODIFIED PRODUCE

While over 40 other countries, including all of Europe and China, label their genetically modified foods for consumers the United States does not. More than 80% of the US food supply contains genetically modified organisms (GMO).

Mandatory labeling of genetically modified foods was put on the November 2012 California ballot. Lack of awareness along with advertising from wealthy companies who sell GMO foods helped to prevent this measure passage. Most people do not know what the numbers on the label on a piece of fruit mean.

What do the numbers on your produce mean?

- If this number has four digits, it means it is conventionally produced.
- If it is a five-digit number starting with "8," it means that the food is genetically modified (GMO).
- If the number on the fruit has five digits, but starts with "9," it means that the food is organically grown.

If the consumer is unaware of the information within these numbers, they mean nothing to them. People are purchasing and consuming foods they do not know could potentially harm their bodies and their children.

PESTICIDES, ANTIBIOTICS AND HORMONES IN FOODS

Pesticides and herbicides are used to kill unwanted insects and plants by causing their tissues to create highly concentrated levels of free radicals. The Environmental Protection Agency (EPA) reports that the average American consumes four pounds of pesticides each year, and over 3,000 chemical additives can be found in our foods. Many of these chemicals are known toxins and are harmful to the neurological system. (This means your brain.) They can also cause cancer and many other diseases.

Pesticides are cumulative from the time we are in utero. A study in California revealed that the children of women exposed to a type of pesticide known as organophosphates were sixty percent more likely to be diagnosed with an autism spectrum disorder than those who were not. This likelihood increased the closer the mother lived in proximity to pesticide sprayed fields during pregnancy. Various neurological disorders and ADHD are also among diagnoses after pesticide exposure. Biology capabilities and detoxification differs per individual. Exposure continues to cumulate from exposure in schools near farming locations, the workplace, and pesticide residue on foods. To learn more about how you can determine the pesticides on different foods that you eat check out, www.whatsonmyfood.org.

Dozens of pesticides can still be found on foods even after washing. The percentage of Americans who were tested by the CDC for metabolites of neurotoxic insecticides (organophosphates) in their urine was over 93 percent. If you are going to have to eat foods that are nor organic there are fruit and vegetable washes sold in health food stores that can help the end result far better than using water alone. The best choice is to eat organic.

WHAT TO EAT; ORGANICALLY GROWN

Conventionally grown foods including animals carry antibiotics, hormones, viruses, and a lot of other toxins that our children's delicate system cannot handle. Children on the autism spectrum often have a congested liver. If we choose foods covered with pesticides and filled with hormones and antibiotics, it is likely to overwhelm their system as their liver will need to filter out the added toxic load.

The price you pay for foods sprayed with pesticides is much higher than you think. Children with autism are more sensitive than the rest of us, but toxins are harmful to everyone. The one thing you have the most control over are the foods you eat. A child with autism may be a very picky eater, so begin with one baby step at a time.

It is best to buy food from organic or local farmers whom you trust not to use harmful toxins. More and more foods are available that are pesticide and hormone-free, but they must say so on the packaging. Be careful of packaging that says "natural". Natural does not mean anything when it comes to food labels. Try to get 100% organic and grass fed if at all possible. You don't want the contaminants of conventional meat or farmed fish.

Farmer's markets are a great choice. They are also quickly increasing in numbers due to the growing knowledge and concern over our food's safety and freshness. Ask if they use pesticides or herbicides, and decide if you believe them if they say that they do not. Unfortunately, some of them will flat-out lie to you. After time you will become familiar with the local growers and know whom to trust. If their sign says "organic," then by law it has to be organic. These people are regulated by the government. Many are not *certified* organic but do not use pesticides and will be honest with you about their practices.

It is almost impossible to find healthy wheat products in the United States. I try to stay away from them completely. Alternatives are nut flours such as almond and coconut flour. Instead of soy as a dairy substitute try coconut milk. Natural and unsweetened it has less sugar than milk anyway, and it tastes good. Many people like almond milk too. Try different brands until you find the ones you like.

PROTECTION FROM FREE RADICALS

In the case of ASD's, the body is already busy defending itself on a fairly constant basis. When this happens, the body becomes deficient in antioxidants and cannot defend itself, which causes greater damage to the immune system.

Good old vitamin C, vitamin E, and omega-3 fatty acids are always helpful and important when fighting free radical damage; however, there are a few antioxidants that are far and above any others: chlorella, lipoceutical glutathione, and alpha lipoic acid. Antioxidants work best if given in combinations. (See the chapter on nutritional supplementation for more information on antioxidants.)

SUMMARY

Every individual is unique and has different needs throughout life. In order to heal and maintain proper health and functioning of all organs and systems the body needs a balance of good, essential nutrients such as healthy fats and alkaline foods, with minimal bad fats and acidic foods. Combining the right foods together in a meal allows for better absorption of nutrients and less possibility of ill effects such as ill regulated hormone levels, and imbalanced blood sugar which can lead to diabetes. Attention must be paid to eating for your own personal metabolic type, and varying health needs.

The products found in this chapter can be found at http://naturallyhealingautism.com/a-healthy-home/

CHAPTER 9

BALANCING THE BODY'S CHEMISTRY

GOOD FATS VS. BAD FATS:

Cells are made of fat, and the brain is 60% fats so make sure you are eating enough of the right kinds of fat. The key is to eat the good fats and avoid the bad ones.

GOOD FATS

Many people have come to fear anything with fat in it. The diet industry says to avoid all fats. This is false information. We need fats in our diet, but we need the right kind of fats. There are good fats that are vital to feeding organs that need them, such as the brain. Without the right kind of fats in our diet, our brains will not be able to function properly and can even be harmed.

Between 1910 and 1970, Americans went from eating 83% animal fats down to 62%. During this same time period, the consumption of sugars and processed foods increased 60%. The consumption of butter went from 18 pounds per person per year down to 4 pounds. We have been falsely taught that all fats are bad for us. Unfortunately, this caused vegetable oils and refined oils to increase by 400%. Margarine, not butter, is linked to building bad cholesterol and heart disease. Butyric acid from butter is very beneficial fueling the integrity of the GI tract. Only eat organic butter.

There *is* such a thing as good fats. In fact, good fats are essential to our health in many ways. We will talk further in much detail about omega-3 fatty acids, but in general, good fats like saturated animal fat and polyunsaturated fat from fish oil are best. They assist the brain, strengthen the immune system, and reduce inflammation.

One essential or omega-3 fatty acid is DHA (docosahexaenoic acid). It is particularly important in brain health, synapse health, assisting the brains circuitry, and in its ability to function properly. Several studies have shown that low levels of DHA fats increase depression and that increasing its intake relieves it. (Weidner, Conner, Conner and Hollis, "Improvements in hostility and depression in relation to dietary change and cholesterol lowering." *Annuals Internal Medicine* 117(1992):820-823.)

Mother's milk contains 50% fat, mostly saturated. Brain development relies on saturated fat and cholesterol. Why would the American Heart Association begin recommending low fat and low cholesterol diets for children? It's just plain wrong. Many baby formulas are also low in saturated fat. Avoid these products. One study has shown failure to thrive in children with low fat diets. Just be sure to give your children the right fats, not the wrong ones.

Animal and vegetable sources of saturated fat provide sustained energy, building blocks for cell membranes, hormones, and other chemical processes in the body. They also assist in the absorption of the necessary fat soluble vitamins A, D, E, and K.

Animal fats (organically grown) are essential to health. Vegetarians do not like to hear this, but it is difficult to supply the brain with enough essential, non-synthetic B vitamins and healthy fats on a strict, animal-free diet. Saturated fats are not the cause of heart disease or cancer. Eating good fat does not affect your cholesterol or contribute to excessive weight gain. You actually need cholesterol to maintain liver health.

Short chain, saturated fatty acids such as butter and coconut oil are easily absorbed for quick energy, do not need bile salts to break down, and contribute the least toward weight gain. They also have antibacterial and antifungal properties.

Monounsaturated and saturated fats are best. Too much polyunsaturated fats are bad. Some good fats are found in butter, fish, avocados, coconut oil, macadamia nut oil, and olive oil.

ANIMAL FATS

Broth from homemade meat or fish stock is exceptionally healing for the gut. Animal fat contains the nutrients that nourish the cells of the gut lining which helps to heal it and keep it healthy. It also helps to reduce inflammation in the gut. With that said, a diet that is excessively high in saturated fat is not healthy either. Processed meats such as bacon will kill off bifidus, the good bacteria in the gut.

Eggs are a fabulous food source of nutrients. The entire egg, white and yolk, are both healthy sources of protein, vitamins such as B, D and E, minerals such as zinc, and the amino acid tryptophan. Tryptophan helps to build the neurotransmitter serotonin which assists in a calming mood.

MORE GOOD FATS

- Olive oil: cold pressed and organic
- Coconut oil: natural, non-hydrogenated
- Avocados
- Flaxseed oil
- Walnuts and walnut oil

When the liver and gallbladder are congested, so is the pancreas. (See the chapter on organ weakness for liver/gallbladder cleansing.) These organs help digest fats. This, of course, means the good fats and the fat-soluble vitamins all necessary for proper health.

There are a couple of great choices to assist with the digestion of fats. Pharmax makes a product called Pure Pancreatin which assists with the absorption of oils into the blood. It is found in most healthfood stores and at www.pureformulas.com. Remember that our omega-3 fatty acids are oils and they need to be properly absorbed to get to the brain. Take Pure Pancreatin with your omega-3 fatty acids or krill oil for best results. Houston Enzymes also makes a product called Lypazyme that can be helpful in the digestion of fats. Houston makes additional blended enzymes that help with the digestion of fats, carbohydrates, and proteins all in one product. They are of the highest quality and are sold in most healthfood stores and many online stores such as www.houston-enzymes.com, and www.pureformulas.com.

BAD FATS: Trans fats, hydrogenated or partially hydrogenated fats

Trans fats are hydrogenated or partially hydrogenated fats, also known as plastic fats. These chemicals were created in the 1920s to help prevent food from spoilage. Spoilage lowers profits. Unfortunately, these chemicals also preserve the cells in your body. They create a plastic film around the cells making them ineffective. When the body signals that it is hungry, glucose and insulin are released. When they reach the cell membrane, it has become impermeable to the glucose and insulin due to its plasticity. The cell continues to send messages of hunger but receives nothing. This is why people who eat trans fats continue to gain weight. This causes insulin resistance which leads to Type 2 diabetes.

Trans fats also cause the liver to become like plastic; it cannot properly remove toxins coming through it. This causes immune system failure and chronic diseases such as fibromyalgia. The liver also makes bile which is responsible for the digestion of fats. Bile is stored in the gallbladder. Without enough bile, you get nauseous. In order to repair the liver, you must eat good fats, about 75% saturated animal fats and 25% polyunsaturated fats such as fish oil. The liver must be able to handle these fats coming in to heal.

If nausea occurs with fats, you will need to repair the gallbladder and the liver. The gallbladder is backing up due to a weak liver. To do this, we must take bile supplements with every meal until health is restored. One of the best products on the market to assist with bile and the gallbladder is AF Betafood by Standard Process. They are small pills that can easily be crushed down with a pill crusher. Muscle test for correct dosages. Standard Process also makes a product in liquid form called Phosfood Liquid that will assist the gallbladder. They are both sold by most natural healthcare practitioners and at www.amazon.com. Liver Life by Bioray is also a great product to assist the health and repair of the liver and can be found at www.pureformulas.com or www.amazon.com.

Remember that all the cell membranes are becoming plastic, including brain cells. New cells are built from surrounding materials. You can offer your body plastic or healthy fats to do so.

Trans fats can lead to depression, chronic fatigue, attention deficit, and foggy thinking. These bad fats can impair the body's ability to build and maintain adequate amounts of neurotransmitters which regulate such things as mood. According to Public Health Nutrition, those who ate more pastries and fast food were 41% more likely to develop depression than those who ate none.

Lower your intake of polyunsaturated omega-6 fats. We get more than we need in our daily diets, and they battle against omega-3 fatty acids, often winning. When too many omega-6 fats are in the system, they will deplete the good omega-3s from the body. We need omega-3s for brain health among many other necessary body functions.

The bad, omega-6 type fats include corn oil, safflower oil, sunflower oil, peanut oil, soybean oil, and canola oil. These oils promote inflammation and suppress the immune system. Most restaurants, especially fast food restaurants, use the bad fats for cooking and frying.

Cook only with animal fats, including butter, or non-hydrogenated coconut oil as they will not alter their chemical form under heat as other oils will. When the beneficial cold-pressed oils such as olive, flaxseed, or avocado are heated, they change from unsaturated fatty acids to trans fats.

CANOLA OIL/RAPESEED

We have been fooled in our society to believe that canola oil is safe and good for us. It is not. We know peanut oil comes from peanuts, olive oil comes from olives, but where does canola oil come from? The word canola is actually a made up word from "Canada" and "oil" or Canadian oil. The Canadian government paid the United States Food and Drug Administration (FDA) $50 million dollars to put canola oil on the GRAS list, Generally Recognized As Safe." (Source: Young Again and others.)

Canola is a genetically engineered plant developed in Canada from the rapeseed plant. It is part of the mustard family which is considered toxic and poisonous. Rapeseed oils have been used for many years to make industrial oils, lubricants, and synthetic rubber bases. It is toxic to humans and animals. Even insects won't eat it.

Rapeseed has a cumulative affect and may take up to ten years for symptoms to manifest. In studies on rats, they developed fatty degeneration of heart, kidney, adrenals, and the thyroid gland. When canola oil was removed from their diets, fatty deposits dissolved, but scar tissue on all vital organs remained.

Some common and possible side effects of canola oil are:

- negatively affects the respiratory system, and is shown to cause lung cancer
- damage to heart muscles
- growth retardation
- anemia
- constipation
- irritability
- loss of vision
- reproduction issues
- adrenal problems
- inhibits proper metabolism of food
- inhibits normal enzyme function
- causes cancer
- destroys the myelin (protective sheath) of the nerves.

Here is a good review article on the toxic affects of canola (rapeseed oil) and its toxic affects from a Swedish Medical journal: Physiopathological effects of rapeseed oil: a review; Borg K; Acta Med Scand Suppl (1975)585:5-13 ISSN: 0365-463X.

Read your labels. Canola oil is found in many commercial items, especially salad dressings.

For more information go to www.askjeeves.com and type, "Where does canola oil come from?"

ACID VS. ALKALINE

DIET: THE FIRST PIECE OF THE PUZZLE

The most important piece of the puzzle again is getting the GI tract into balance with proper diet. The gut flora or friendly bacteria must increase, and the bad bacteria must decrease. The lining of their GI tract must heal. A diet high in organic meats, eggs, poultry, chicken, beef or fish broth, non-farmed, non-contaminated fresh fish, and good fats will heal the body the quickest. Adding quality probiotics into this mix is essential. See "Candida: Diet and Supplements" for more on this.

ACID REFLUX OR GERD

It is interesting that when people have acid backup (GERD) or digestive issues, they tend to take antacids. This actually exacerbates the problem because it further alkalizes the gut. What these people need is more stomach acid or hydrochloric acid (HCL). Supplements of hydrochloric acid can be somewhat helpful short-term but the real problem exists in the liver and gallbladder. Too little hydrochloric acid production does not allow for the food in the stomach to digest properly and move downward. Instead, it remains there too long and begins to ferment. The remaining product begins to back up into the esophagus. Another common symptom of low HCL is the feeling of extreme fullness and bloating after eating any size meal, even a small one.

Additional causes of heartburn may be overindulgence of food or alcohol, eating excessive amounts of animal fats, eating spicy foods, smoking cigarettes, drinking coffee, drinking cold beverages, dehydration, stress, taking anti-inflammatory drugs such as aspirin, X-rays, and Candida albicans. This backup is caused by a build up of gallstones in the liver and gallbladder that create congestion there and prevent bile from doing its job.

The best thing to do is a liver and gallbladder cleanse like the one described in the chapter about supporting the organs of detoxification. If this is not fully possible, then assisting digestion with enzymes listed under "liver," and supplementing with hydrochloric acid may be helpful. Take them just prior to eating as you would digestive enzymes. Some good products are Metagest by Metagenics, Zypan by Standard Process (both of these are in pill form but can be crushed) or Betaine

HCl with added pepsin. All are sold at most healthfood stores or for a good price at www.pureformulas.com and www.amazon.com.

Another common instigator of acid reflux is Candida albicans. The overgrowth of Candida or yeast in the gut will release toxins. This toxic waste effects digestion and the ability of the gut to produce hydrochloric acid.

There is a product that can help with the removal of the toxic waste from Candida, and therefore, the acid reflux that comes along with it. It is called CandiClear5 by Get Healthy Again. The product is found online at www.gethealthyagainstore.com or 800-832-9755. It is even more helpful to take with their product Candelim. Wait to take Candida cleansing products until after gut restoration has taken place with the diet and support supplements for three weeks or more. See the chapter on Candida for further information.

Disease, Candida, and tumors all thrive in an acidic environment. Candida is covered in greater detail in its own chapter in this book.

The only time we are vulnerable to germs is when our body is acidic. An acidic body also overloads the immune system and can cause problems ranging from headaches and allergies to adrenal and liver trouble.

An easy way to check acidity is through first morning urine. Upon waking, prior to eating anything, use litmus paper for a clear reading. You can purchase litmus paper from your local healthfood store, pharmacy, or online from www.crohns.net. Use the paper to check first morning urine. This is also a good indicator for stress on the liver which is very common with children having ASD or ADHD. If your child turns up to be acidic, it is likely that they also have microform overgrowth. See the chapter on Candida for what to do to combat microform overgrowth.

Weakened cells finally break down and become bacteria, yeast, and fungus. Excreted waste from the organisms lead to further toxicity and breakdown in the body. Remember that the tainted blood gets into your child's organs and brain where it really causes havoc.

Those common behavioral outbursts are often due to the effect of these toxins on the brain and the central nervous system. Have some sympathy next time your child or you are having a tantrum. Just think of what it feels like to have all of those organisms invading your body and brain. Haven't you ever felt like you wanted to jump out of your skin? That's what they feel like. No one enjoys a tantrum.

WHAT CAUSES ACIDITY

The most common cause of an acidic body is poor diet. Poor diet leads to poor digestion, which only makes the system even more acidic. Emotional stress also plays a role.

Once you have brought balance back into your child's system, it will not be necessary to have tests done. The extreme change in behavior is usually enough of an indication, but keep watching over time. As stress invades and diet falters, do all the things you know how to do to get them back on track.

CREATING AN ALKALINE ENVIRONMENT

Most harmful organisms cannot live in a healthy alkaline environment. One way to create an alkaline body is by eating the right foods.

Some good alkalizing foods are asparagus, broccoli, almonds, lettuce, squash, most fruit, spinach, cucumber, carrots, garlic, onions and brown rice. Almond butter is very tasty. Beets and all kinds of greens, eggplant, and seeds are also good.

Some acidic foods are red meat, sugar, corn, cow's milk, and cow's milk cheese. Yogurt is neutral. Fish, beans, poultry, and tofu are still somewhat acidic, but are far better choices than beef or pork, which are highly acidic. Limiting tofu is a good idea due to it being a high allergy food and its effects on hormone levels.

The concentrated liquid product Cell Power helps balance acid levels, boost immune system response, oxygenates cells, and feeds enzymes, amino acids, and trace minerals through nanotechnology. This reaches the cellular level. It also assists in the removal of toxins, and kills bacteria, fungi, and viruses. It can be found at most healthfood stores and at www.brainchildnutritionals.com.

FOOD COMBINING

One way to maximize the absorption of the foods you eat is by knowing how to properly combine, and not combine, certain foods. As you read the following guidelines, it is easy to see why so many people have digestive problems, especially in the United States. The typical Standard American Diet or SAD defies all of the rules of proper digestion and absorption.

Food combining is both helpful and healthful. When we eat meat together with vegetables, the alkalinity of the vegetables help to balance out the acidity of the meat. An added benefit of eating meats with vegetables is that meat helps our bodies absorb iron from green leafy vegetables. If you pour some healthy, cold-pressed organic olive oil on your salad, the oil will provide your gut and your immune system the fat they need for their health.

Note: It is important to be sure that your child's GI tract is ready to digest vegetables. Vegetables contain a lot of fiber, and it may be a few days or weeks before vegetables can be added to an initial gut-healing diet. The same is true of fruit.

Once diarrhea, constipation, or abdominal discomfort are gone, try to add a tablespoon or two of cooked vegetables and see how they do. If all goes well, try adding a little bit more each day. Although raw vegetables contain more enzymes, they are harder to digest. You be the judge when it's time to offer them and when it is time to temporarily remove them. Generally, raw vegetables should be added last.

Note that eating fruit with meat can interfere with digestion as meat digests slowly and fruit digests quickly. The meat will cause the fruit to stay in the stomach longer than its normal transit time and it can ferment and become rancid. It is best to eat fruit at least 30 minutes before or an hour after eating high protein foods. I tend to like fruit with my yogurt. Most of the time my stomach is all right with this, but there are times when I notice my digestion is disturbed by it. I usually will notice acid reflux. During these times, I will take a day or two to strengthen my digestion with more broth and enzymes before trying it again. The enzymes usually help a lot, and I am able to eat the combination again with no problem.

HYPOGLYCEMIA OR LOW BLOOD SUGAR

Hypoglycemia is a condition that comes from low blood sugar or glucose. Behavioral outbursts, anxiety, and lack of ability to think clearly come from the brain being starved of its energy supply. When it has been too long since our last meal or snack, blood sugar drops and our brain cannot function properly. If we eat too many sugars and refined carbohydrates, our body responds by releasing large amounts of insulin to counteract the effects of all of the sugar. This is especially hard on the liver and can cause it to become congested creating further physical and behavioral problems.

Hypoglycemia or low blood sugar can trigger many unhealthy reactions in our bodies. Excess insulin secretion can contribute to many severe disorders including allergies, asthma, alcoholism, cancer, heart disease, chronic fatigue, depression, diabetes, and more.

Parasites and leaky gut can contribute to hypoglycemia or low blood sugar. This is just one more reason to eradicate any parasites and heal the gut. Hypoglycemia causes stress on the body, which reacts by triggering the adrenal gland to release the stress hormone cortisol. The stress hormone rises and registers stress to the brain. Insomnia can be associated with this at night as your body begins to have more trouble going longer periods of time without food to keep the blood sugar balanced. We already talked about this in Chapter 7. One supplement that helps balance cortisol regulation is Seriphos by Interplexus available at www.pureformulas.com.

The remedy to restoring blood sugar back to balance is to eat. The best choice would be a healthy snack or meal including protein and plant-based carbohydrates. Complex, or plant-based carbohydrates such as whole grains, vegetables, and fruit do not affect your body in the same way as refined carbohydrates such as sugar, pasta, cookies, and crackers. With this said, remember that all grains are carbohydrates. This means they break down in your body to become sugars. Wheat breaks down into sugar faster than other grains. The wrong fruit or too much fruit can give the same response as sugar. Eating before you get really hungry is the key to keeping blood sugar in balance. I carry almonds with me to have a healthy protein source available. See the glycemic index for more information on this.

SUPPLEMENTS THAT HELP TO BALANCE BLOOD SUGAR:

- omega-3 fatty acids, especially DHA
- COQ10 or ubiquinol
- alpha lipoic acid
- chromium picolinate
- gamma linolenic acid (GLA)
- berberine
- cinnamon
- vitamin D
- peppermint

Always eliminate soda and limit juices, refined sugars, and carbohydrates. Reduce fructose in your diet, even from fruits. Completely avoid high fructose corn syrup. Increase your amounts of good oils such as coconut, olive, and avocado. Get enough protein from whole food sources such as nuts, seeds, eggs, grass-fed meat, organic poultry, and raw vegetables (if tolerated by digestion).

LEPTIN RESISTANCE

A diet of sugary foods and refined carbohydrates can cause health risks for both you and your baby. Metabolic problems and insulin sensitivity begin in the womb. This can even create insulin sensitivity in the baby's eggs, therefore, affecting not only the fetus but its children as well.

Leptin is a hormone produced by fat cells. It regulates both appetite and weight loss. Leptin signals your brain regarding hunger and controls your food intake. It is crucial in weight loss because it tells your body when to burn fat. Leptin congests the liver and prevents it from receiving the necessary hormonal signals such as insulin.

It also helps regulate body temperature, regulate blood circulation, produce bone, and is important in reproduction. Women having trouble conceiving should have their leptin levels tested. Overall health and aging can be measured through leptin levels.

Leptin levels must remain stable and low. If they become too high, our cells become resistant to their messages. High leptin levels trigger stress hormones in your body and can create anxiety. Balancing leptin levels helps to control your hunger, cravings, and body weight.

Testing for leptin is done through blood work, but lowering leptin levels can be done through diet. The book, *The Rosedale Diet*, by Ron Rosedale, M.D. gives detailed information regarding leptin, leptin resistance, and contains the complete list of proper foods with a specific diet that teaches your metabolism how to burn fat. It is all of the same principles of the diet in this book.

The diet promotes the intake of good fats—yes, good fats actually help you burn fat. You eat a balanced amount of protein but not too much. High amounts of protein will not balance leptin resistance and can actually become toxic and unhealthy. Generally, protein allotments are between 50 and 75 grams per day with 15 to 20 grams per meal for the average female adult. Children would eat less, but it depends on their age, height, and activity level. About 10 grams of protein per day can be added for those with a high activity level. You may eat all the high fiber vegetables you want. It takes about 21 days to switch your metabolism and shift leptin resistance. During this time, no starchy or sugary carbohydrates are allowed at all. If you are insulin resistant, then you are usually leptin resistant. This means your body burns sugar instead of fat.

DIABETES

There are two types of diabetes: Type I and Type II. Type II diabetes is acquired insulin and leptin resistance due to poor diet such as one high in processed foods and refined sugars combined with a lack of exercise. If you are lucky you can balance Type II diabetes with the proper diet and exercise with no need for insulin injections.

Type I diabetes is more severe. It is an autoimmune disease caused by the immune system attacking the pancreatic cells that produce insulin. People with Type 1 diabetes need injections of insulin or they will die. Type I diabetes can be hereditary and triggered by many things.

COMMON GENE TRIGGERS OF DIABETES:

- Drinking cow's milk before the age of two is known to be one cause of juvenile diabetes (Vaarala O, Knip M, Paronen J, et al. Cow's milk formula feeding induces primary immunization to insulin in infants at genetic risk for type 1 diabetes. Diabetes 48(1999): 1389-1394). The milk proteins are quite similar to the proteins made by the pancreas which causes the body to attack its own insulin cells.
- Vaccinations: According to Dr. Donald Miller, Jr, M.D. there has been a 17-fold increase in Type I diabetes, from 1 in 71 hundred children in the 1950s to 1 in 400 today. This correlates with the increase in the number of vaccinations.
- Virus exposure
- Monosodium glutamate (MSG)
- Feeding grains to infants: Do not feed your infant grains. It is often the first food offered to babies in their first year. Grains are often processed, contain allergens, and feed pathogenic bacteria in their gut.
- Low levels of vitamin D: about 70% of children in the US have low vitamin D levels.
- Poor diet such as too many simple sugars causing the pancreas to become stressed to the point of exhaustion. When this happens, it stops producing insulin and there insulin injections are necessary.

DIABETES PREVENTION:

- Be sure vitamin D levels are adequate. One of the leading researchers in vitamin D, Dr. Michael Holick, has found that, "Children who receive vitamin D supplements from the age of one and on had an 80% decreased risk of developing Type I diabetes" (www.mercola.com).
- The omega 3 fatty acid, docosahexaenoic acid (DHA), reverses insulin resistance. It is also known to naturally activate cell receptors called peroxisome proliferator-activated receptors,

(PPAR's). PPAR's regulate gene activation that affect blood glucose levels. The medical industry uses drugs to activate these proteins for the prevention and treatment of diabetes. DHA is the effective, natural, and safe way to do this.

- Berberine balances blood sugar, increases good gut bacteria, gut function and metabolism.
- Low levels of magnesium can cause leptin and insulin resistance.
- Gamma linolenic acid (GLA) levels are often low in diabetics. It balances insulin and improves insulin functioning. Evening primrose oil and borage oil are good sources of GLA. Evening primrose oil is especially helpful with diabetic neuropathy.
- Test for gluten allergies as they are commonly related to Type 1diabetes.
- Use caution and be fully educated about vaccines.
- Breastfeeding is the best choice always!
- When weaning and beyond, a diet of healthy whole natural foods grown organically are best.
- Stay away from the standard American diet of sodas, chips, processed foods, and those sprayed with pesticides or grown with antibiotics and hormones.
- Fructose promotes insulin resistance and fat storage. This can be dangerous to your health. Be sure to avoid foods high in fructose, especially high fructose corn syrup.
- Chromium picolinate is mineral that is helpful in balancing blood glucose levels, reducing hunger cravings and improves the metabolism of carbohydrates. It can be extremely helpful with sugar cravings!
- COQ10 or ubiquinol decreases blood glucose levels by over thirty percent, increases metabolism, increases energy, is an antioxidant, and increases the level of glutathione inside of the cells.
- Zinc also helps to stabilize insulin.
- Research has found a possibility in assisting recovery from diabetes by using stem cells to replace pancreatic islet cells.

For more information visit: www.mercola.com/2010/5/13/5-reasons-why-diabetes-is-on-the-rise.aspx.

THE GLYCEMIC INDEX

The importance of knowing the glycemic index of your food choices is a preventative measure in your child's health and behavior. This will also help to prevent obesity and diabetes along with keeping his gut flora in better balance.

The glycemic index or GI is a way to measure the physiological effect that various foods have on blood glucose levels. Knowing this can help you control hunger and energy fluctuations during the day by eating better choices. This becomes very easy in a relatively short period of time. Once you begin to learn what foods are high and which are low, it starts to fall into common sense.

Based on scientific data, foods have been tested to show their effect on blood glucose levels. Foods with a low GI will have less of an effect on blood sugar than foods with a high GI. The foods we eat have a direct impact on how quickly our bodies are able to digest them. Slower digestion gives your body a chance to regulate the release of insulin better.

Many inexpensive, pocket-sized books are sold on the glycemic index. It is worthwhile to pick one up and learn how the different foods you are feeding your child will affect his blood sugar. If we look around at the childhood epidemic of obesity and diabetes, it is easy to see how it can be prevented by better choices of food. Some foods and their glycemic index are listed below. There are also many websites available.

- Foods with a high GI break down rapidly, releasing glucose into the bloodstream very quickly. This causes a rapid release of insulin, which starts to weaken the body's ability to balance blood sugar levels. This also weakens the adrenal glands (our stress handling organs), which then weakens the thyroid gland, which helps to regulate our hormone levels. All of this contributes to diabetes and obesity.

- Foods with a low GI will break down more slowly, releasing glucose into the bloodstream more gradually.
- Lower glycemic index foods will:
- Keep you feeling full longer
- Assist in weight loss (by reducing insulin levels it helps you burn fat)
- Assist in the prevention of diabetes, heart disease, and some types of cancer
- Help prevent hypoglycemia, which is associated with headache, fatigue, sleep problems, and lack of mental clarity
- Improve blood lipid profiles
- Assist in better cholesterol levels
- Help with metabolic syndrome (insulin resistance also known as Syndrome X)

Protein is a great choice because it is low on the glycemic index. When we eat protein, it takes a longer time for our body to break it down. The higher nutrient content combined with a low GI will also assist in satiation. Our body will be fed a source of food it can utilize and one that takes much longer to digest. This keeps us feeling full longer and does not have a negative impact on blood sugar.

It is vital to feed your children small amounts of protein throughout the day to minimize their body's cravings for carbohydrates, the very food that converts into sugar and feeds the Candida. Foods higher on the glycemic index also have a greater likelihood of creating hyperactivity and then a "sugar crash" with loss of all energy within an hour or two after consumption. We do not want to use protein in excess as too much can be hard on the liver. Small amounts that are spread out will suffice to keep blood sugar balanced.

Note: It has been found that if a recovering alcoholic eats foods lower on the glycemic index, and they keep their blood sugar level, their craving for alcohol is greatly diminished and they will have a greater chance at recovery.

Remember to eat protein first. When combining a high GI food and a low GI food, be sure to eat the lower GI food first. For example, if you were eating chocolate, it would be better to eat chocolate with almonds so that the protein in the almonds would help slow down the rapid digestion of the sugars in the chocolate. Apply this rule to anything such as fruit or high carbohydrate, high GI foods.

Eating some almonds or celery with almond butter on it at any time of day will help keep blood sugar more balanced. Eggs are a far better choice for breakfast than cereal or waffles, which are hard on blood-sugar because they are high GI foods. We want to curb those cravings for the wrong things before they get a chance to hit.

The glycemic index is based on 0 as the lowest and 100 as the high rating. Look for foods with the lowest numbers on the glycemic index rating. Many pocket size books are available at most stores such as drug stores, and grocery stores.

As an initial example of high glycemic foods, let's look at sweeteners.

- **Artificial sweeteners** should never be used. They are toxic to the brain and still affect the glycemic index.
- **Stevia=0**: An all natural sweetener from the stevia leaf. As a 0, it is your number one choice. There can be an aftertaste with most brands, but NuNaturals has one called NuStevia White Stevia Powder, with no bitter aftertaste. (Their NoCarb Blend does have a bitter aftertaste.)
- **Xylitol=7**: This one is my favorites because it tastes good, has no aftertaste, and this all natural product made from birch is actually beneficial in fighting cavities (see studies from Finland and www.xylitolstudies.com).
- **Agave=15-30**: Getting higher on the GI now.
- **Fructose=17**
- **Raw honey=30**
- **Organic sugar=47**
- **Corn syrup=75**
- **White refined table sugar=80**
- **High fructose corn syrup=87**
- **Glucose=100**

- Additional examples:
- White bread=100
- An average cola=70

LOWEST (BEST) GLYCEMIC SOURCES OF PROTEIN

- Meat (beef, lamb, buffalo)
- Poultry (chicken and turkey)
- Seafood
- Trout
- Eggs
- Nuts
- Seeds
- Dairy has a higher glycemic protein index due to its natural sugar content.

SAFER LOWER GLYCEMIC VEGETABLES

- Artichokes
- Asparagus
- Beans
- Broccoli
- Cauliflower
- Celery
- Cucumbers
- Green beans
- Lettuce
- Tomatoes
- Spinach
- Zucchini (although a starchy vegetable)

HIGHER GLYCEMIC VEGETABLES TO BE LIMITED

- Beets
- Potatoes (all kinds)
- Yams
- Carrots
- Corn
- Peas
- Winter squash

LOW-GLYCEMIC FRUITS

- Apples
- Apricots
- Blackberries
- Blueberries
- Cantaloupes
- Cherries
- Grapefruit
- Nectarines
- Peaches
- Plums
- Raspberries
- Strawberries

Berries are an especially good choice when it comes to lower glycemic fruits due to their high fiber content. They are also high in antioxidants. However, they can be high in phenol content due to their rich colors, which should be noted if your child is phenol sensitive. See chapter ten for more information on phenols.

HIGHER GLYCEMIC FRUITS

- Bananas
- Clementines

- Dates (any dried fruits)
- Grapes
- Honeydew melon
- Oranges
- Papayas
- Pineapples
- Raisins
- Tangerines
- Watermelon

A NOTE ABOUT JUICE

All juices are higher on the glycemic index because they are in liquid form. Your body does not have to break them down so they enter the bloodstream very quickly. Juices are also very bad for the teeth. Pure water is always the best choice.

TIPS TO HELP HIM DRINK MORE WATER

DRINK SIX TO EIGHT GLASSES OF WATER PER DAY!

Water is the healthiest choice of any beverage, but kids often want something sweet to drink. The number one food contributing to diabetes is soda. If your child wants juice, a good compromise is to pour a cup with a ratio of one quarter juice to three quarters water. This flavors the water enough that they enjoy it and are getting hydrated, and lowers the sugar content greatly. Remember to use 100% juice with no added sugar or high fructose corn syrup and stay away from juices that are canned due to the toxins in metals that are released quickly from the acid in the juice.

Sweet Leaf makes stevia liquid drops that are in an assortment of flavors. I like the root beer flavored one, my daughter likes grape the best. It only takes a drop or two in a glass of water to create good flavor with almost no effect on the glycemic index. These products are sold at most healthfood stores and at www.amazon.com.

LOW-GLYCEMIC STARCHES

- Ezekiel bread (any bread that is sprouted)
- Breads that are multigrain and/or high fiber
- Sourdough bread (yeast free)
- Bulgur
- Pumpernickel
- Wasa crackers
- Akmak crackers or bread
- Millet
- Low-carb bread
- Kavli bread
- Quinoa
- Amaranth

Regular breads will inhibit calcium absorption, whereas sprouted-grain breads will not. Sprouted breads also have the added benefits of vitamins B and C. Adding butter or olive oil is helpful when eating breads or starches because the fats assist in slowing down blood sugar fluctuations.

HIGHER GLYCEMIC STARCHES-TO BE LIMITED

- Plain oatmeal (not instant) steel cut or Irish are best
- Brown rice
- High-fiber cereals (no sugar added)
- Pita bread
- Spinach pasta
- Corn tortillas
- Peas
- Melba toast

HIGHEST GLYCEMIC STARCHES TO BE AVOIDED

- Bagels
- White bread
- Cakes
- Cookies
- Muffins
- Granola, granola bars
- Pretzels
- Rice
- Semolina pasta
- Cold cereals (except high fiber)
- Crackers
- Refined flours
- Rice cakes
- White sugar

BASIC RULES

1. Do not combine proteins and starches (e.g. meat and potatoes, eggs and toast, cheese and bread, fish and rice).

   WHY?

   Protein digestion requires acid and starch digestion requires alkaline. When eaten together, they neutralize each other. By the time the food is pushed out of the stomach and into the intestines, the protein has putrefied and the starch fermented.

2. Fruit should be eaten alone and on an empty stomach. After eating fruit, wait 20 to 30 minutes before eating a meal.

   WHY?

   Fruit digests quickly and rapidly moves into the intestines. If there is other food in the stomach, such as vegetables, proteins, and starches, this rapid movement is prevented causing the proteins to putrefy and the starches to ferment. This causes a toxic acid system.

NOTE: Melons, such as watermelon, cantaloupe honeydew, etc., should be eaten alone or before other fruit.

3. Vegetables can be eaten with anything *except* fruit.

   Note: It is acceptable to eat "vegetable fruits" with either fruits or vegetables. These foods are cucumbers, avocado, tomatoes, and peppers.

4. Do not eat sweets for at least hour after meals.
5. Drink 2 glasses of purified water 15 minutes to ½ hour before meals. Do not drink beverages with meals or at least 1 hour after meals.

Eating foods in this way will help to prevent purification or fermentation of your meal into your digestive track. This aids in optimal digestion and absorption of nutrients from the food and prevents additional toxins entering your system that you body will have to work hard to eliminate. These toxins can also get into the bloodstream where they cause further damage to organs and the central nervous system.

Do your best to follow the guidelines now that you know them. Any step in the right direction is a step well taken.

THIS MEANS YOU CAN:

1. Eat protein with vegetables
2. Eat starches with vegetables
3. Eat fruit alone
4. Eat melons alone
5. The four vegetable fruits can be eaten with vegetables or fruit; they are avocado, cucumber, tomatoes, and peppers.

HIMALAYAN SEA SALT

Contrary to popular belief, salt is very good for most of us (exceptions would be those with health issues such as kidney disease). It is most beneficial to eat a natural mineral salt that has some color to it, not the white, processed kind. The best is Himalayan salt, which is pink in color. This shows the rich mineral content, and it is naturally high in iodine.

Salt stops the bad microbes in the gut and assists the adrenals to function properly. Our sodium conversion can be so out of balance that although we are drinking enough water, our cells cannot absorb it, so we continue to be dehydrated. I add Himalayan sea salt to my food and drinking water daily, especially first thing in the morning and around 3:00 in the afternoon. It can help to give your body energy as it is also extremely helpful with adrenal fatigue.

FERMENTED FOODS

Fermented foods are foods that have been brined or soaked in salt, water, spices, and a probiotic starter. Many foods can be fermented such as fish, grains, vegetables, and dairy. The salt will stop the bad microbes that can spoil the food. This is why it was used for centuries as a way to preserve before canning existed.

Yogurt, sour cream, and kefir are the most commonly known fermented dairy sources. Homemade products are best because commercially made yogurt is often pasteurized after fermentation and many of its natural nutrients and enzymes are lost. Fermented vegetables and grains are much more tolerated by the digestive tract.

My personal favorite is a fermented coconut milk, kefir or yogurt made by New Earth Superfoods. Their products are organic, non-GMO, free of fillers and additives. It is also free of dairy, soy, and gluten. The company has a store near where I live and they make the kefir-like coconut probiotic product on their premises with a highly stabilized source of D-lactate free multi-probiotic formula, coconut powder, spring water and has a small amount of raw agave added. You could use stevia at home if you prefer it to agave.

The specific strains of probiotics they use can be found on their website. They are high quality probiotics that survive storage and stomach acid. These strains are important in healing your child's gut and balancing his biology. (We discuss the many necessities of probiotics in chapter eleven.) When coconut is added to specific probiotics they found that the greater beneficial properties of coconut are activated. Coconut oil is a protein fat and is one of the good oils for our body and brain. It is anti-viral, anti-bacterial, boosts immunity, has vitamins and minerals including calcium and potassium, and has a significant amount of electrolytes to help hydrate the system. It tastes really good too.

I was so happy to learn that New Earth Superfoods products are becoming available in stores nationwide. To find where their products may be available nearest you go to, www.newearthsuperfoods.com, or call (805)592-2450.

Fermentation foods are predigested and help make food easier to digest. They offer beneficial probiotic microbes, enzymes, vitamins, and minerals. The fermentation will help predigest some of the proteins and consume lactose in dairy products. Fermenting foods also creates lactic acid that kills pathogens. The bacteria from fermented vegetables help with detoxification and the removal of heavy metals.

Only small quantities are needed to assist digestion and gut healing. Sauerkraut is a common fermented food made from cabbage. As little as two tablespoons of the juice from sauerkraut is enough to be beneficial. Fermented foods made from adding salt, water, and probiotics are helpful at any time. Many recipes are available online on sites such as www.nourishedkitchen.com and www.gaps.me

If candida overgrowth is an issue it is best to either wait to add "wild" or naturally fermented foods to the diet, or only add a very small amount, such as about a teaspoon per day in the beginning of your cleanse. Too much naturally occurring fermented bacteria ingested too quickly may cause die-off reactions. As the bad bacteria die, they release toxins. When the toxins are released faster than the liver can remove them, fatigue, headaches, flu-like symptoms, and emotional outbursts may appear.

EATING FOR YOUR METABOLIC TYPE

The greatest importance of metabolic typing for you and your child is that it balances total body chemistry, and it has a tremendous impact on the nervous system. Metabolic typing addresses issues at the core, or the cause, and once in balance, it is used for prevention to keep you at optimum health.

The old premise that says in order to be healthy everyone should eat only a vegetarian diet or everyone should eat a protein diet is no more. There is a fabulous book called *The Metabolic Typing Diet* by William Wolcott and Trish Fahey that describes every aspect of this in length. There are 65 questions that take between 30 and 60 minutes to answer. For further discussion, go to www.metabolictypingonline.com or www.healthexcel.com. Detailed food plans are offered for each type.

Essentially there are three types of metabolism: carbo or carbohydrate types, protein types, and mixed types. Each of us falls into one of these categories, and we need to eat according to our type in order to stay healthy. It can be the reason why one person heals from an illness and another will not.

A protein type does best on a diet composed largely of proteins combined with good fats and very few carbohydrates. A carbo type does best if they eat mostly carbohydrates, and a mixed type can eat a balance of both. You can also determine if you are a fast or a slow oxidizer. This is the way your body metabolizes and utilizes fats and carbohydrates.

Note that children on the autism spectrum and those with seizures, ADHD, bipolar disorder, or other behavioral disorders most often do best on a diet high in the good fats with medium protein and very low carbohydrates. This is the diet in this book. The main reason is that this type of paleo diet is anti inflammatory for the brain. We will go into this further in the section on brain support.

Before we move on, I must emphasize that just because your child is craving carbohydrates does not mean he is a carbohydrate type. Often our children are craving these foods for all of the wrong reasons, such as a sugar source for the Candida in his system or gluten for the food sensitivity or allergy that has developed. The questionnaire in Wolcott's book will help you understand more.

WHY WEIGHT LOSS CAN BE SO DIFFICULT

Many mothers talk about their children, (or themselves), having trouble losing weight. Often it is due to combined factors beginning with a diet high in sugars and starchy carbohydrates, but other factors may be contributing as well. Sometimes they may be eating what they believe to be a healthy diet and exercising, but still remain overweight. When this happens I think of seven things; metabolic syndrome, liver congestion, thyroid imbalance, adrenal imbalance, candida, leptin resistance, and brain support.

Metabolic syndrome is an imbalance in your metabolism. Blood sugar levels cannot stabilize and it causes a myriad of other problems in the body. It can lead to type II diabetes. Metabolic syndrome is usually caused by a diet high in sugar and bad fats (corn, safflower, sunflower, peanut, canola, and soybean oils). This can also be inherited in utero from the mother's eating habits. It should be noted that monosodium glutamate or MSG, a flavor enhancer that is added to many foods, is toxic to the brain and contributes to obesity. Additionally, when the body has multiple toxins to remove the liver becomes congested.

The omega 3 fatty acid docosahexaenoic acid, (DHA), reduces the risk of metabolic syndrome. It reverses insulin resistance, is known to reduce stomach fat, decreases inflammation, and is a necessary component of brain health.

Most children on the autism spectrum are born with a congested liver. We have discussed this in detail in the chapter on detoxification and organ support. If the liver cannot detoxify quickly enough then it cannot do its job of helping to remove excess hormones and keep them in balance. After all, hormone levels are balanced by the liver. The amount of hormone issues a person has often correlates to the health of their liver.

Insulin is a hormone. It allows our body's cells to absorb glucose, or sugar, from our blood. Glucose stops the body from using fat as energy. A congested liver and fat deposits around this organ cause the liver to become insulin resistant, thus causing it to produce more glucose, raise blood sugar levels and further increase insulin resistance. To further aggravate the situation once all sugar stores are used up from the liver your cells will begin to break down protein from your muscles and bones to burn as sugar. You must reverse this process and re-train your body to burn fat.

This vicious cycle triggers the stress response on the adrenal glands. The adrenal glands release stress hormones adrenaline and cortisol. This triggers a spike in blood sugar and eventually trains your body to remain burning sugar instead of fat. This constant stress response over works the adrenal glands and causes us extreme fatigue. Eating sugar also triggers the stress response.

Today's modern diet and medically advised beliefs that eating less fat and eating more carbohydrate has caused an epidemic in obesity and diabetes. Remember that carbohydrates turn to sugar in your body. This is often seen as belly fat or fat around the waist or midline. The real health problem is that there is fat depositing itself around your internal organs and arteries that go to your heart.

Candida albicans or yeast can become overgrown in the gut. When this happens it not only effects the health of our gut, immune system, and brain but our blood sugar, as well. We will crave carbohydrates and sugar because candida uses it as its food supply. Candida also causes the gut to leak and allows for undigested food particles to enter the bloodstream causing food allergies. Enzyme production decreases and bloating increases. This all triggers an immune response that alerts the adrenals to have a stress response. Worse, because the lining of the gut is damaged it is not properly absorbing vital nutrients from the foods we eat. We then can become malnourished, even though we are eating a lot, and we remain hungry because our body and brain are starving for nutrition. For detailed information on candida see chapter 6.

Leptin is the main hormone that regulates both appetite and weight loss by telling your brain when to eat and how much to eat. Mainly it tells your body when to burn fat and when not to. When leptin sensitivity is balanced you will stop storing excess fat control hunger and food cravings and lose weight, normally. Cutting down on calories is an actual diet of long term self-defeat. This tells our body we are starving and further imbalances leptin keeping us fat.

We are not meant to use sugar as our primary fuel. This comes from a triggered stress response that causes our fat burning hormone, leptin, to become imbalanced. It is produced by your fat cells, and can become resistant over time. The body can be put into a stress response from factors such as improper diet, inflammation, food allergies, stressful environmental factors, toxins, or a brain imbalance that triggers ongoing anxiety. When this happens adrenaline is released. This contracts blood vessels which deplete the cells of water, sugar, and much needed nutrients. A lack of nutrients causes a feeling of excessive hunger. This signaling to the brain comes from the hormone leptin.

What you can do is eat plenty of food, just the right ones in the right combinations. The gut healing diet in this book will rebalance leptin levels and heal the gut from candida. Protein sources in moderation combined with lots of good fats, yes, that's right, and non-starchy vegetables. The good fats are avocado, olive oil, coconut oil, and nuts, (except peanuts).

It takes twenty one days to rebalance your leptin levels. After this time you may eat foods not on the diet, but within moderation. Once leptin is balanced you should continue to maintain your weight. Some meal examples are eggs with avocado, chicken with a green salad and olive oil, nuts such as almonds, cashews and macadamias. Maintain a reduction or elimination of bad starchy carbohydrates (cereal, cookies, crackers, etc), sugar, bad fats, monosodium glutamate, or sugar substitutes such as aspartame and sucralose. Also, see more on leptin in chapter 8, "balancing the body's chemistry".

For further information there is an excellent resource and diet book on leptin balancing offered by Ron Rosedale, titled, The Rosedale Diet.

HOW TO LOSE WEIGHT THE HEALTHY, NATURAL WAY

1. Have your thyroid levels tested by your health care practitioner.
2. Have a saliva adrenal test done through your natural health care practitioner. Be sure to get the test that measures saliva at four different times of day. Diagnos-Techs is an excellent lab for this. They also test your gliadin (gluten) sensitivities in the same test. Support the adrenal glands with Drenamin by Standard Process (for pill takers). For non-pill takers; Ribes Nigrum Gemmo homeopathic liquid by Seroyal is a good choice. Both products are available at www.pureformulas.com.
3. Balance the health of the liver with either liver flushes, (see chapter 4), or using Liver Life by Bioray, available at most health food stores and at www.pureformulas.com.

4. Follow the gut healing diet in this book, along with the gut healing supplements, especially the omega 3 fatty acid DHA, and probiotics. They will help to heal the gut lining and balance candida. Read more information on leptin from the book, The Rosedale Diet, by Ron Rosedale.
5. Helpful brain supplements: If anxiety is a problem then the supplement GABA can be very helpful. If satiety is an issue, especially around 4:00 P.M. when serotonin levels drop, get muscle tested for serotonin imbalance. (Serotonin can become low around 4:00 P.M. therefore, increasing hunger.) If needed, add 100 mgs of the supplement 5HTP to your regimen at this hour of the day. See chapter 21 for more information on 5HTP. Take magnesium daily as low levels of magnesium can cause leptin and insulin resistance.
6. Supplements that are helpful to balance blood sugar: Chromium picolinate is mineral that is helpful in balancing blood glucose levels, reducing hunger cravings and improves the metabolism of carbohydrates. It can be extremely helpful with sugar cravings! COQ10 decreases blood glucose levels by over thirty percent, increases metabolism, increases energy, is an antioxidant, and increases the level of glutathione inside of the cells. Zinc also helps to stabilize insulin.

SUMMARY

Many people have trouble losing weight, including those on the autism spectrum. Often blood sugar imbalance has been triggered by a diet high in sugars and starchy carbohydrates, but sometimes it is even more. Organ weakness in the liver and weak adrenal glands and candida contributes to the imbalance of fat burning hormones such as leptin. To balance leptin a diet of protein in moderation with plenty of good fats, and non-starchy vegetables must be included with the elimination of carbohydrates and sugars for twenty one days. Supplements to heal the gut are essential, especially the essential fatty acid DHA.

Every individual is unique and has different needs throughout life. In order to heal and maintain proper health and functioning of all organs and systems the body needs a balance of good, essential nutrients such as healthy fats and alkaline foods, with minimal bad fats and acidic foods. Combining the right foods together in a meal allows for better absorption of nutrients and less possibility of ill effects such as ill regulated hormone levels, and imbalanced blood sugar which can lead to diabetes. Attention must be paid to eating for your own personal metabolic type, and varying health needs.

The products found in this chapter can be found at http://naturallyhealingautism.com/a-healthy-home/

CHAPTER 10

COMMON NUTRITIONAL DEFICIENCIES

We often believe that because we are giving our children vitamins or feeding them healthy foods that they are getting the nutrition they need. Lack of absorption from an injured gut and poor quality supplements are just a couple of reasons why we need to learn more. This is commonly called "failure to thrive." The child may become hyperactive, or the opposite, lethargic. They may have difficulty with issues such as concentrating, learning, have extreme irritability, headaches, stomach aches, become sick easily, and more. They may seem like they are lazy and do not care but it is more of a neurological problem. Healing their gut is key.

When there are nutritional deficiencies and excesses, the greatest areas of dysfunction are the nervous system, the immune system, and the digestive system. When not in balance, there can be a downward spiral effect where one deficiency then creates another. Children with autism, intestinal issues, allergies, and asthma have greater needs than the general population, although the gap seems to be narrowing year by year. As more children have intestinal issues and toxic exposure, the needs increase.

As general nutrition and food productivity is altered, our bodies undergo many changes. Dr. Weston Price wrote and interesting book titled *Nutrition and Physical Degeneration*. Dr. Price's research indicates that as foods native to one's culture are changed, the body will often show signs of degeneration. Most commonly, the palate will narrow, often narrowing the face, and the teeth will crowd and decay. The book is an excellent testament of the negative effects that processed foods have on our health.

With any supplement, the proper dosage depends upon age, size, and protocols during treatments and any other indications present. As the gut heals, the need for supplementation will decrease. It is advisable to use the assistance of your trusted healthcare practitioner. Those supplements that specialize in helping specific symptoms have been listed in the chapters that pertain to them. These products can be purchased at www.naturallyhealingautism.com under "healthy home products."

It is recommended that three weeks of gut healing be done removing parasites and strengthening the gut lining with the recommended supplements in the chapter on healing the gut prior to starting other supplements such as multivitamins, minerals, and antioxidants. The intestinal lining is not ready to absorb properly, the liver is congested, and parasites will use them as food to strengthen themselves.

GENERAL SUPPLEMENTATION

There are many forms that supplements come in such as pills, capsules, sprays, etc. When the digestive system is compromised, as it is in children with autism, we want to use the most highly absorbable form possible.

Oral sprays are able to easily absorb into the bloodstream, losing little to nothing in the process since they completely avoid the digestive tract. Not all supplements are available in this form, so use them when possible. Be sure to get the correct type of vitamin you are looking for, such as Methyl B12, and be sure that you can get the dosage amounts that you need from that product. Sprays and liquids are also beneficial when your child will not take pills. They are very easy to use and offer better absorption.

For an overview program on how to improve the immune system please see the post, How To Keep The Immune System Strong, at www.naturallyhealingautism.com.

QUALITY FIRST

This is no time to cut corners trying to save money. The supplements you purchase should be produced by a highly reputable company. Quality control is the highest priority. Avoid anything with additives, dyes, and synthetic nutrients. Essential minerals are extremely important in addition to a multivitamin. You don't want to spend good money for something that has had so much processing that there are no nutrients left in it or one that has an inability to be absorbed by your child's delicate system.

Do not purchase any supplements that contain additives and fillers. One of the most commonly used additives is magnesium stearate. Magnesium stearate is used to prevent the ingredients from sticking to the equipment during production. It is dangerous for humans because it can prevent the absorption of nutrients, may be harmful to the intestines, and weaken the immune system. Read the entire label including the part at the bottom that says, "other ingredients."

First of all, I would not suggest purchasing your supplements from the average grocery store. The shelf life of the product is limited and the quality is often minimal at best. Cheaper

ingredients are substituted to keep the price down, but this also means that the quality is way down, and they often contain allergens and cheap fillers.

A quality local healthfood or nutrition store is a far safer bet, and some good online resources carry excellent choices. There are a few companies that are an even better way to go because they focus on the specific needs of children on the autism spectrum. This does not mean that they are not also a great choice for your other family members who may have their own specific needs.

One company that focuses on the specific needs of autism, ADD, and the very sensitive is Brainchild Nutritionals, www.brainchildnutritionals.com. Please be sure to use the code "naturallyhealingautism" to receive 15% off all of their products.

Another company I have found that carries only the highest quality supplements, and more, that is also a great online educational resource is www.crohns.net. Phone: (877)240-7528.

They specialize in everything from autism to celiac disease to inflammatory bowel disease, and more. They sell top quality products at great prices. I get all of my Dr. Ohhira's probiotics through them. They have the best prices I have found on them anywhere.

For a great multi-vitamin, antioxidant, flavonoid complex I also like Vita Power from www.herbprod.com. This is an excellent synergistic complex.

When looking for any specific individual complex or a combination complex of any kind there are two websites I like that offer quality products with good prices. These sites are www.swansonvitamins.com, and www.pureformulas.com. Pure formulas has the highest quality products and free shipping always.

The company Standard Process has excellent supplements. They produce products for just about every health need and are very high quality. They do, however, share equipment, so gluten contamination may exist. Standard Process supplements are sold through many healthcare practitioner's offices, so be sure and muscle test to know that the product is compatible with your child's body. Some Standard Process products are also now sold at www.amazon.com.

"STANDARDIZED" HERBAL FORMULAS

When purchasing herbal formulas it is wise to look for the word, "standardized." Authorities on herbal remedies have established a specific standard of excellence for herbal extracts. They must be of the highest quality with guaranteed consistent levels of each plant's medicinal elements to be labeled "standardized."

SPRAY VITAMINS

Why Spray Vitamins?

Because it's not how much you take, it's how much you absorb that matters.

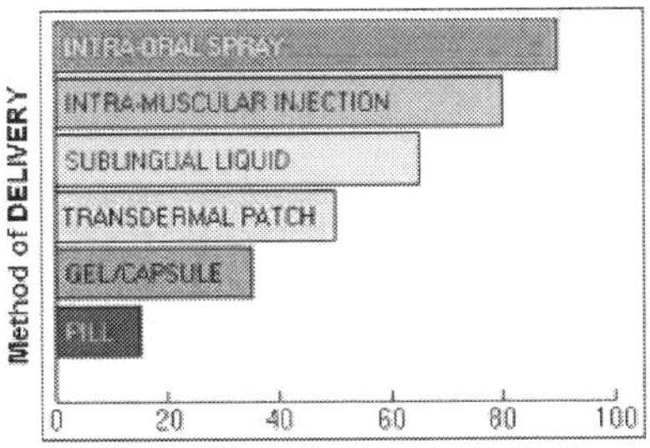

% ABSORBED into the bloodstream - As illustrated in the PDR (Physicians Desk Reference)

ORAL SPRAY CHART AND INFORMATION FROM WWW.CROHNS.NET

The greatest breakthrough in delivery of nutrients to the body since pills was invented over a thousand years ago. Oral spray is up to nine times more effective than pills or capsules, and is 1/5th the cost.

Oral absorption is the fastest, most efficient and convenient method (http://www.crohns.net/Miva/education/aboutsprays.shtml) to take a daily dose of vitamins, minerals, or other nutritional supplements. Spray vitamins should be held in the mouth for about 20 seconds, if possible, for best absorption.

Oral sprays deliver the purest form of vitamins, minerals, herbs and other nutritional supplements directly into the bloodstream. When sprayed into the mouth, micro-sized beads or droplets are instantly absorbed into the tissue through the capillaries, which lie close to the surface of the mouth lining. This allows the nutrients to be absorbed within seconds without causing any stress to the organs.

The sprays overcome the solubility and absorption problems accompanied by traditional nutritional supplements. They are ideal for people suffering with any digestive complaint such as Crohn's disease, colitis, gastritis, IBS, and more.

Spray vitamins can be found in healthfood stores and online at many sites, including those that specialize in digestive disorders and the autism spectrum such as www.nbnus.net, www.crohns.net, and www.brainchildnutritionals.com.

Many companies make liquid vitamins and mineral supplements. The company, Brainchild Nutritionals, www.brainchildnutritionals.

com, 877-253-5711, carries very high quality liquid (or capsule) forms and their products are made specifically with children on the autism spectrum in mind. Although their products are ingested rather than sprayed sublingually, they are high quality and well thought out. Their liquid formulas have been specially broken down for better absorption. Their staff is knowledgeable and helpful when needed. Their products are also sold at www.pureformulas.com, with free shipping.

EMPTY CAPSULES

Vegetable capsules contain no animal products and do not interfere with digestion or absorption of the ingredients they carry. Vegetable capsules do take 30 minutes to dissolve after ingestion; which means your supplement will not be released right away. If you need your product released quickly, as in the case of enzymes, you are better off to go with the gelatin capsule which dissolves immediately. Some people have allergic sensitivities to gelatin, so if you use it, be sure to have your child muscle tested ahead of time to be sure it is compatible with their system. If your child will take the supplement in straight powder form, it is better than encapsulating.

Any supplement can be sprinkled onto any food or beverage that you know your child will eat. If you have to do it, go ahead and mix it into pudding or a sweet food just for the sake of getting it down them. Otherwise, please minimize your amounts of sugary or processed foods.

FILLING YOUR OWN SUPPLEMENT CAPSULES

There are multiple options for giving your child the correct supplements in many forms. In fact, I hear from most moms that their child will not take a capsule so they need supplements in liquid or powder form and most do come this way.

My son will take any pill but will not drink anything I give him that has a less than good taste to it. Sometimes adding powders to juices will work but I want to tell you about encapsulating your own supplements. If you are in need of a way to encapsulate a supplement on your own, you can purchase"cap-m-quick" capsule filler for less than $20. They are sold at many healthfood and nutrition stores or a good online source is www.nowfoods.com. They also sell empty capsules in different sizes. Be sure to match your capsule size to the size your capsule filler is made for.

SUPERGREEN FOODS

Nutrients from plants are called phytonutrients. Supergreen foods are one of the richest and most concentrated forms of phytonutrients. They also provide the body with a concentrated form of detoxifying vegetables. It can be easier to get your child to drink a small amount of this powder in a beverage than to eat multiple plates of vegetables.

Supergreen foods are beneficial for increasing energy if you or your child has fatigue. They also help keep your body alkaline and are food based, so they have better absorption and quality. The grasses in these products are highly concentrated. Quality products with multiple grasses in them are much more alkalizing than what vegetables can do for you alone. They contain enzymes, coenzymes, phytochemicals, and are nutrient rich.

Supergreen food products contain chlorella which benefits the immune system, assists in removing toxins, and is helpful in excreting heavy metals during chelation. Spirulena is also usually a component in most supergreen foods and it is helpful to the nervous system.

There is one supergreen food sold in healthfood stores called Nanogreens with Nanosorb technology. This product boasts having a more highly efficient absorption rate than others. This can be good for an already compromised system that has limited absorption. It is always a good idea to muscle test your child for a particular product when you begin using it to be sure it is right for him. For many years I have personally used the product Supremely Green from www.herbprod.com (831)688-8706. Supremely Green is sold in bulk powder form. I add a hefty teaspoon to my morning protein drink. Children generally take about half that amount. Supplements in food form are more concentrated, so less needs to be taken. A quality supergreen food can fulfill most or all of the necessary daily vitamins, minerals, and antioxidants.

For your child, judge the dosage by their size and age. A small amount, such as an eighth if a teaspoon, can be good to start with. It's food, so it's safe, but always begin slowly. The company is very helpful if you have more questions regarding the product in any way.

Note: Gluten should be cleared (desensitized) as an allergen before using supergreenfoods as they may contain gluten "tags" and be seen by the body as an allergen. Gluten tags are particles in the product from barley or grasses that may trigger the immune system to gluten.

OMEGA-3 FATTY ACIDS

Omega-3 acids are essential fatty acids, which means they cannot be made in the body, so they must be ingested. The essential fatty acids derived from omega-3 oils are DHA (docosahexaenoic acid) and EPA (eicosapentaenoic acid). Where DHA helps to build and protect the brain, EPA helps with the functioning of the brain. We need both.

Omega-3 fish oils help reduce inflammation in the brain and the body which can be helpful in healing the gut, therefore improving the immune system. They help protect the mitochondrion which is like the insulation on a phone wire. This helps the transmission of vital information to get into the cell. They are necessary for neurotransmitters in the brain, and assist in cognitive ability and mood. Omega-3 fatty acids are commonly used for mood disorders such as depression, anxiety, and aggressive or violent behavior.

A study done by Dr. Gordon Bell at Stirling University in Scotland showed two thirds of children with autism showed a deficiency in omega-3 fatty acids. When the diet is supplemented with omega-3 fats, parents report less aggression, irritability, hyperactivity, and improved sleep.

The poor dietary habits including trans-fats and processed foods fill our bodies with omega-6 fatty acids to a point where they imbalance the trio of omega-3, 6, and 9. Omega-3 is a vital component to assist the brain and much more, but too much omega-6 in your diet will compete with omega-3 causing further deficiency. Omega-6 oils come from many of the bad fats such as corn oil, safflower oil, peanut oil, canola, and soybeans. They suppress the immune system and promote inflammation.

Most diets today are deficient in omega-3 fatty acids. Supplementation is necessary, especially for children on the autism spectrum or those with learning disabilities or behavioral issues. This is a vital and essential nutrient.

Three companies I trust to carry out the guarantee to be free of any fish oil contaminants, such as heavy metals and PCB toxins, are Nordic Naturals, Pharmax, and Carlson. They carry child's dosages of cod liver oil, but remember that children on the autism spectrum and with digestive disorders need more than the regular child's dosage. It may be best to purchase the adult formula. Nordic Naturals has their cod liver oil flavored in peach, strawberry, orange, lemon, or unflavored. Carlson has one in lemon, strawberry and unflavored. They come in liquid or softgel form. Liquids are easy to disguise in a cup of juice. They are all available at most local healthfood stores and for a good price at www.pureformulas.com with no shipping fee. Always keep oils in the refrigerator to avoid rancidity.

Vegetarians looking for a quality omega-3 essential fatty acid supplements can find one from Essential Formulas. Dr. Ohirra's vegetarian essential living oils come from NON-GMO seeds and plants. They are a balance of omega-3, 6, and 9. To learn more or to purchase, go to www.crohns.net.

Please see the chapter on "reducing inflammation; essential supplements," for more information on omega-3 fatty acids.

KRILL OIL

Most of you now have heard of the benefits of omega-3 fatty acids. The most commonly known source of these is fish oil, but there is an even better way to absorb them through krill oil.

As I began researching the benefits and the quality of krill oil, I saw a lot of inconsistencies. This is a common proponent to research, so I dove in deeper. What is important to those of us with children on the autism spectrum or anyone who cares about really getting the benefits of omega-3 is the quality content of DHA and EPA and its absorption ability.

In the chapter on "reducing inflammation; essential supplements," I explain in detail why krill is better than fish oil. Here is a snapshot: Krill has all the benefits of fish oil and a lot more. It contains all the benefits of DHA and EPA, but is more absorptive due to its phospholipid structure. The fats in our cells (including our brain) are phospholipid, which means that the fatty acids have the same chemical make-up as the cells in our body, This makes krill oil more bioavailable.

Captain's Krill oil is the freshest, the purest with no fillers or added ingredients, and it has the best price.The best places to purchase are either www.amazon.com or www.stillsmilin.com.

VITAMINS, MINERALS, AMINO ACIDS AND ANTIOXIDANTS

Adequate amounts of vitamins and minerals are necessary for many different functions in the body. Importantly, they build brain-cell energy and assist in brain-cell repair and brain protection. There are many vitamins and minerals necessary for proper health and absorption, and most will come in a multi-formula containing the essentials. Some, but not too many, will need to be purchased separately.

This is why I have mentioned the two companies above that specialize in autism spectrum disorders. Their products are for everyone but contain the essentials for the sensitive, the allergic, and those with greater needs. The company Brainchild Nutritionals is an excellent choice for highly bioavailable multiple vitamin/mineral products and more www.brainchildnutritionals.com (831)465-0104. Many of their supplements are available in liquid form. They are also great for your other growing children who may or may not have symptoms such as irritable bowel, low nutrient absorption, allergies, or hyperactivity. These products are comprise a well-thought-out, balanced program. Their website is extremely helpful in answering questions about their products, how to get started, and which one to start with. Their staff is also helpful by phone if you have more specific questions.

Always start out slowly. I did so with my son and found I still needed to back off from even a very low starting point. Just after starting the brainchild supplements, my husband and I noticed that my son had developed a slight tic or twitch. The supplement, at first, was too high of a dosage for his system. I researched and found that tics are also often related to low magnesium levels, among a few other things.

When we started the brainchild supplements, it overwhelmed his system. When I reduced the amount of multivitamin supplements and increased his normal magnesium dosage, the tics disappeared. Over the course of the next few months, I very slowly increased his dosage of the vitamin and mineral supplements while I watched for any symptoms. He adjusted well.

Watch your child for signs of tics, hyperactivity, or increased emotional behavior. Vitamin B supplements are absolutely necessary for many physiological needs, but remember that as the gut heals and absorption of nutrients from food increases, less supplementation may be needed.

MINERALS

Over 60% of children with autism are deficient in zinc, magnesium, B6, and omegas. Symptoms include fatigue, anxiety, sensitivity to loud noise and light, pale skin color, problems sleeping, not wanting breakfast, and prone to rages.

Those who already have neurological disorders usually have weaker neurons, lower antioxidants, and are deficient in selenium, zinc, calcium, and magnesium.

For children with ASD, minerals are as important, if not more important, than vitamins. Both are essential, however, the coenzymes in minerals are essential for a huge number of enzymatic reactions, neurological connections, and in neutralizing strong acids. They assist in alkalizing the blood and in keeping the cells properly hydrated. Most children on the autism spectrum are mineral deficient.

Minerals are best in ionic form. This charges them and makes them more absorbable. Individual and blended mineral supplements are found through many companies such as www.pureformulas.com. There are companies that make mineral supplements for children on the autism spectrum and those that are extra sensitive. A good company for this is www.brainchildnutritionals.com. A product my family uses daily is called Vital Minerals which consists of inland marine minerals from the Great Salt Lake. They are a blend of 84 ionic essential minerals, most as essential trace minerals that are found in blood plasma and are needed by the body. I purchase this through www.herbprod.com (831)688-8706.

HAIR ANALYSIS TESTING (FOR MINERALS IN THE BODY)

Tissue mineral analysis is done with hair analysis testing. Both minerals and many toxins can be evaluated with this test. Holistic doctors and nutritionists can do these tests for you, or you can save money and order the test yourself.

Test before supplementing and then test again about six months after they have been administered to see where the levels have moved to. This gives you a basis for adjustment of dosages. Remember, you are working to get your child's system working efficiently on its own, although there are supplements that all of us need on a regular basis.

Three companies that carry mineral hair analysis tests are:

1. www.labinterpretation.com, 775-851-3337
2. Dr. Ann Louise Gittleman's website: www.annloise.com or www.unikeyhealth.com, Phone 800-888-4353.
3. www.arltma.com/HairAnalysis.htm (screens for the level of 20 minerals and toxic metals in one sample of hair)

These companies have practitioners who will discuss the test results with you.

CALCIUM

Minerals such as sodium, potassium, calcium, and magnesium aid in eliminating acids from the body. If there is not an adequate supply absorbed from food or supplements, the body will recruit from its own resources, such as retrieving calcium from bones and magnesium from muscle. This leads to deficiencies in those areas and greater problems can result.

We know that calcium is crucial for strong healthy bones and teeth, but calcium has many other important functions in the body. Calcium is crucial to the healthy functioning of the brain. This is one of those chemical exchange situations in cells critical for cell signaling. It helps to activate cell functions and methylation. Calcium is also important for nerves, cells, and muscle contraction.

Additionally, heavy metal toxicity increases with deficiency of calcium. It allows aluminum and cadmium to become more toxic. Some sources of aluminum are vaccines, food, shampoos, lotions, and cooking in aluminum pans. Those with calcium deficiencies are also more susceptible to fluoride toxicity. It is best to avoid any form of fluoride, which is commonly found in toothpaste and drinking water. Proper amounts of calcium have been shown to reduce the effects of fluoride toxicity. The heavy metal cadmium is also known to alter calcium absorption. This is covered in greater detail in the chapter on heavy metals.

Most of us do not get adequate amounts of calcium in our diets, and poor liver function prevents proper absorption of calcium due to a lack of bile. For any person who is allergic to casein (the protein in milk) or who is lactose intolerant (does not make the lactase enzyme in their body), it is essential to take a calcium supplement. See the chapter on organ weaknesses for information on liver cleansing which will assist calcium absorption.

Calcium is best utilized in the body when it is combined with essential co-factors. Calcium needs magnesium, vitamin K2, vitamin D3, and the trace mineral boron present in the system. Magnesium is especially important for calcium absorption, but it is best if taken separately from calcium. The oils from omega-3 fatty acids help transport calcium to the blood. This creates a calming effect and is one of the reasons omega-3 is helpful with ADD.

No more than 500 mgs of calcium can be absorbed by the body at one time, some argue less, therefore it is best to divide dosages up during the day. Afternoon and evening can work well because calcium can have a calming effect. If your calcium supplement contains B vitamins, they should not be taken close to bedtime as they may stimulate the system. Note: Calcium supplements will inhibit thyroid supplementation, so avoid taking them within an hour of each other.

FOODS THAT CONTAIN CALCIUM

- Green leafy vegetables such as lettuce and broccoli
- Almonds
- Sardines
- Salmon
- Oranges
- Dairy products

Too much calcium can create trouble for the kidneys. The parathyroid gland regulates calcium absorption, so be aware of this if you have thyroid issues. The best sense is an absorbable form of calcium *for you.* Different forms resonate better for different people. Muscle test prior to usage and to determine dosage, unless otherwise guided by your physician. Remember, some of your daily needs are met by foods. The recommended dosages are 1,000 to 1,200 mgs for anyone over the age of eight.

There are several different kinds of calcium. Elemental calcium is the amount of calcium the product actually offers after absorption. Read labels to see how much is necessary to achieve your needed dosage.

Some good choices are:

- Calcium lactate is a good choice for kids, especially with the O blood type
- Calcium malate chelate is a combination of calcium and malic acid chelated. This process bonds the two for better absorption. There is a good one from Designs for Health, sold through www.pureformulas.com.
- Calcium citrate: This is a good choice.
- The product called Bone Strength Take Care from New Chapter makes a calcium supplement from a plant source. It is a whole food source, so it is dissolves easier, making it more absorbable. This is also in a capsule form that can be opened up and mixed with a food or beverage. It is gluten free, but does contain fermented soy. Usually fermented soy is all right

for those with allergies to soy because its chemical structure has been altered, however, it is best to check with your doctor or natural allergy desensitization practitioner.

- Calcium Absorption Formula from A. Vogel is a homeopathic sublingual product. This quickly dissolves under the tongue, so it may be easier to give to children.
- Calcium is also available in liquid form. Many different companies provide this at your local healthfood stores and online such as www.pureformulas.com.

It is best to avoid:

- Calcium carbonate: it is cheaper but harder to digest. This is not good for our kids with already low digestive absorption.
- Destructive amino acids such as glutamate and aspartate can create excitotoxicity. For this reason, I avoid calcium and magnesium from the same sources such as calcium aspartate or magnesium aspartate.

BORON

The mineral boron assists in calcium and magnesium absorption for bone health. It is also known to assist in the removal of toxic fluoride from the system. Purchase ionic boron such liquid ionic boron by Liquimins as it is the most absorbable form. This can be found at www.pureformulas.com.

MAGNESIUM

Magnesium is one of the most deficient and most needed minerals in the human body. It is crucial for protecting the brain and producing cellular energy. It is necessary for over 300 enzymatic reactions. Remember, our children on the spectrum usually have injured enzyme systems. Deficiency in this mineral is often the cause of tics (known to be part of Tourette's syndrome). Other common symptoms of magnesium deficiency are muscle cramps and weakness, blood clotting, heart weakness, bed wetting, hearing loss, imbalanced brain chemistry, lowered immunity, energy metabolism, insulin sensitivity, the body's use of glucose, issues with respiratory function, increases energy production, and the regulation of blood pressure.

Regulating magnesium levels can help with asthma or other respiratory issues such as chronic obstructed pulmonary disease (COPD). It also helps with ADD, strengthening the cardiovascular system, helping to regulate blood pressure, relieving blood clotting post-surgery, diabetes, fatigue, kidneys stones, migraine headaches, osteoporosis, PMS, and can even be helpful for toxemia in pregnancy and premature delivery. It also assists the methylation process.

Magnesium is also very calming to the system. Epsom salts contain magnesium. Bathing in a warm bath of Epsom salts will not only calm a child, but it has the additional advantages of being a detoxifier. Add one to two cups of Epsom salts to a hot bath.

Like calcium, a deficiency in magnesium allows heavy metals such as aluminum and fluoride to become more toxic. Magnesium deficiency is common in those with heavy metal toxicity. Magnesium supplementation helps due to its involvement in detoxification. Magnesium is also needed by the body in order to absorb vitamin D.

Some food sources of magnesium are green leafy vegetables, seafood, brown rice, tofu, and soybeans.

The best product for proper absorption comes from an ionic magnesium citrate by the name of Natural Vitality/Natural Calm. It comes in powder form. The powder is added to water that is warm enough to make it fizz. This fizzing action creates the ionization of the mineral which charges the magnesium to make it bio-absorbable. Natural Vitality/Natural Calm can be found in most healthfood stores and online sites such as www.swansonvitamins.com and www.vitacost.com.

You can also use an ascorbate form of magnesium. 500 mg per day is known to be helpful depending on age and weight. Start slow and work your way up to bowel tolerance. Magnesium is safe, but too much will cause loose bowels and digestive distress.

PHOSPHORUS

Phosphorus is well known for its role in strong bones and teeth, but it has other important functions too. It is important for children on the autism spectrum because it assists the kidneys in detoxification, and it is necessary in order for the body to make protein and process carbohydrates and fat. It helps with energy production and the storage of energy as well as nerve signaling and brain function.

ZINC

Zinc is commonly deficient in children with autism. When the body is deficient in all zinc, copper, and manganese, it cannot create the enzymes needed to neutralize many dangerous free radicals. Zinc is another metal that requires proper enzyme functioning to work properly. These enzymes are also destabilized by aluminum. Heavy metal toxicity, such as cadmium, increase with a deficiency in zinc. Zinc increases the ability of the liver to detoxify heavy metals through increased production of metallothioneins. These are a proteins and polypeptides that contain large amounts of metal and sulfur. They are found throughout the body. When mercury, lead or cadmium enters the liver, its cells begin producing large quantities of metallothioneins. Zinc should not be used in excess as it can increase the amount of toxicity from heavy metals. Usually 10 to 15 mg per day is plenty, depending on age and weight.

Zinc is crucial for the proper functioning of cognition and plays a vital role in many areas, including breaking down carnosine, a protein building block, strengthening the power of melatonin, and healing the gut. Zinc also enhances methylation. It builds metallothioneine in the body, which helps reduce damage from toxicity. Zinc is also needed by the brain, specifically the hypothalamus.

Zinc, like magnesium, is found mostly within cells. Inside the cell it can protect DNA and cellular proteins. Too much zinc in the body can displace copper, and too much copper in the body can displace zinc.

Zinc deficiency leads to weak adrenals. Weak adrenals lead to excessive copper, therefore throwing off the delicate copper/zinc balance. Stress can also create a zinc deficiency which leads to weak adrenals. Blood tests are your best bet for proper knowledge of these levels. There is also a test you can order from your home. No expensive doctor appointment is needed. For more information and to order tests, visit Dr. Shari Tenpenny's site; www.tenpennyimc.com.

COPPER

Autistic children tend to have too much copper in their systems. This can be neurotoxic. As mentioned above zinc and copper can displace each other in the body. Copper alone is a tricky one. Many kids have too much and some too little, so getting these levels checked is important. More often, copper is in excess and zinc is deficient. Weak adrenals allow copper to accumulate, and too much copper can cause the liver to be sluggish. If this happens, the liver's ability to remove toxins is impaired and so is its job in metabolizing hormones.

MANGANESE

Manganese is a trace element and an antioxidant. It increases energy production, helps with calcium absorption, and is necessary for many biochemical reactions in the body. It is essential for proper brain activity.

Supplementation is often needed. The enzymes needed by manganese are often unable to work due to aluminum in the system. When chelated (bonded) with amino acids, manganese has much better absorption.

MOLYBDENUM

Molybdenum is a trace element and an antioxidant assisting the liver. It is necessary in many biochemical reactions involving metabolism, such as those in the thyroid, kidneys, and adrenal glands. It is also helpful in building key enzymes that assist with the digestion of specific foods.

TAURINE

Taurine is often deficient in children on the autism spectrum. It is a necessary component in detoxification such as the methylation process. It is an antioxidant that stabilizes membranes, assists with structure and function of muscles including the heart, assists with calcium signaling, and is involved with the central nervous system and anti-anxiety, regulating the nerve sensory threshold. It also helps with fatty liver, regulation of high blood pressure, and protects against toxicity of lead and cadmium. Taurine assists with the bioavailability of many important nutrients such as magnesium, fatty acids, and vitamins A, D and E.

IRON

Beware of low iron in children. It is important in brain development. There may be many causes to their fatigue, lack of ability to focus, or ADHD, and low iron may be one of them. Our children often have heavy metals in their bodies and levels of lead may be also be elevated if there is a deficiency in iron. Proper enzymatic activity is critical and iron also helps assist the many functions associated with it. These enzymes are necessary for proper functioning of iron and are often not working properly due to the presence of aluminum in the body.

On the other hand, we do not want excess iron in the body because it can cause oxidation and inflammation. Yeast and intestinal bacteria can use excess iron to their advantage, and it can be overall immunosuppressive. Iron can help strengthen pathogenic (bad) bacteria in the gut. Studies have shown blood iron deficiency to contribute to restless leg syndrome. If iron levels are normal, then the supplement 5-HTP can improve, and even eliminate, restless legs.

Too much iron in the body can increase the damage from excitotoxicity due to glutamate. If your child has weak liver or kidneys, check with your healthcare practitioner regarding his iron levels as too much can be dangerous for him. Diabetics should also be very cautious with excessive iron.

ANEMIA

It is common for those with imbalanced gut flora to be anemic. Anemia is when there are a lowered number of red blood cells in the body. Our kids often look pasty white and can be lethargic and weak most of the time. One likely culprit is the lack of iron, but it takes much more than iron to balance anemia. Healthy blood needs almost all of the B vitamins, vitamin C, A and D, amino acids, along with multiple minerals, including magnesium, manganese, iodine, copper and zinc.

Getting meat into their diet is crucial. Red meat and liver carry the most iron. Get organic and grass fed meats. Remember, we do not want the contaminants of conventional meat.

Meat increases the absorption rate of iron from fruits and vegetables. Spinach and other leafy greens carry iron and vitamin C. The vitamin C in vegetables also increases the absorption of the iron from the meat. Remember that fruit is best eaten away from meat as their transit time is so different. Fruit digests quickly, but meat does not. The slow digestion of meat will cause the fruit to ferment in the stomach and become rancid.

SELENIUM

This is one mineral that is essential for children with autism and one I feel is critical in the turning point. Selenium is necessary for assisting in excretion of heavy metals in the body. It is a powerful antioxidant, aids the immune system, assists the thyroid gland, protects cell membranes, and is essential in metabolizing glutathione. Deficiency of this mineral can trigger autoimmune diseases such as with the thyroid.

Although this mineral is essential, as with most supplements, too much selenium can be dangerous. Generally, 200 mg per day is the maximum amount necessary for most adults. It is important to give supplementation depending on the size and weight of the child. Your child may need half this amount but rarely more. The brain also relies on selenium to build the enzyme glutathione peroxidase to protect it from free radical damage.

CHROMIUM PICOLINATE

Chromium picolinate is very helpful in balancing blood sugar levels and fighting off the cravings of sugar. Studies have found that 500 mg twice per day reduces blood sugar in adults, children may need half that. I personally take chromium after lunch, since the afternoon is when we usually have our greatest decline in blood glucose levels. Chromium deficiency is also related to Type II diabetes.

As beneficial as chromium picolinate is in keeping blood sugar in balance, it is wise to regulate the dosage as too much chromium picolinate can be hard on the liver.

IODINE

Iodine deficiency is common in today's society. Women are often deficient during pregnancy, so it is passed on to the fetus. This causes the baby to be born already needing this essential trace mineral. More and more research is linking children on the autism spectrum and those with learning disabilities to iodine deficiency. The thyroid gland requires the proper amount of iodine to function normally. Thyroid hormones affect the development and functioning of the kidneys and the liver in utero, two of our key detoxifying organs.

Iodine deficiency during pregnancy can cause the baby to have mental disabilities, mental retardation, deafness, and an inability to thrive. It is also linked to autoimmune diseases.

The body cannot make iodine on its own. Due to the increase in processed food, iodine deficiency has become commonplace. Healthy foods no longer contain enough, if any. Salt was once the best-known source but most today are not pure and do not contain the mineral. It is important to purchase salt that is iodized and has color to it. The best source is Himalayan sea salt. This has a slightly pink tint which notes its mineral content. Himalayan sea salt is sold in many stores today and for a good price at www.swansonvitamins.com.

THE IODINE TESTS

An easy and inexpensive test is the iodine patch test. You need to purchase nascent iodine. This is not the type you put on a wound but a liquid you could drink if you wanted to. I had to purchase it at the naturopath's office because no pharmacy or healthfood store carried it, but I did find it at www.amazon.com.

Paint a patch about 2 inches by 2 inches on any part of your body with the iodine. Watch the patch for disappearance over the course of 24 hours. If the iodine disappears within six to eight hours or less you are iodine deficient. For a final test, repeat this a day later using a different spot on the body and see if your results are the same.

If the test shows a deficiency in your body, add an iodine supplement and wait a few days before re-testing. If deficiency still shows up, slightly increase your dosage and re-test again in a few days. Continue until the patch does not disappear over the course of 24 hours.

There is also a urine test from ZRT Labs that you can order and do in your home to determine iodine levels. Sometimes the problem is that iodine is too high. High iodine levels can trigger hypothyroidism too. You can find these tests at www.zrtlabs.com.

I use a liquid iodine supplement because they are more absorbable than tablets. Many liquid products are available at healthfood stores and at www.pureformulas.com. Dosages will vary depending on age, weight, and personal needs.

VITAMINS

THE B VITAMINS

The B vitamins, which are water-soluble, are crucial for a variety of reasons. Nerves cannot function normally without them. B vitamin deficiency along with heavy metal toxicity is among the leading causes of irritability, anger, and violent episodes. It is also commonly a problem among those with anxiety and seizures. The B vitamins protect the brain from excitotoxicity, and a deficiency in B vitamins causes low taurine levels, reducing the body's ability to detoxify. B vitamins are essential or crucial to survival, but our bodies cannot make them, so they must be provided by dietary means. The B vitamins also increase cellular energy.

The B vitamins can be purchased in a form called pyridoxal-5-phosphate, or P5P. This is a more bioavailable (absorbable) form. Some people supplement with vitamin B6 and do not notice results. It is possible that this is because they are not using a quality bioavailable form such as P5P and it is not being utilized by the body. B vitamins also work synergistically, meaning they work better together because one often needs another in order to be able to do its job properly.

There is a multivitamin supplement with P5P available through Brainchild Nutritionals, www.brainchildnutritionals.com (831)465-

0104. Liquid forms are available. The company Pharmax also makes a high quality liquid vitamin B complex called CWS which contains vitamins B1, 2, 3, 6, 12, and folic acid. It is available in health food stores and many online sites such as www.pureformulas.com.

I had my N.A.E.T. practitioner (discussed in the chapter on alternative therapies) test my daughter for certain allergens. She is not on the spectrum, but was showing signs of hyperactivity and emotional instability that I was sure were food related. It turned out that she was having an over-sensitivity to B vitamins. The practitioner told me that it is likely many children today are having this same reaction because synthetic B vitamins are added to so many foods. Our practitioner desensitized her for this, and she calmed down almost immediately. See the chapter on N.A.E.T. practitioners and desensitizing for more information on this.

Natural sources of B vitamins, such as beta-carotene from vegetables, will not accumulate in the body the same way synthetic vitamins can. For this reason, I like to use supergreen food supplements. Some good choices are Nanosorb or Greens First, which can be found in healthfood stores. I use Supremely Green from www.herbprod.com. There are also practitioner grade supplements from a highly reputable company called Standard Process. They make natural "food based" supplements. Bee pollen is a great food with significant B vitamins, protein, vitamin C, DNA, RNA, amino acids and numerous flavonoids and carotenes. Generally, about a teaspoon a day is helpful, adults may take more.

VITAMIN B 1 (Thiamine)

Thiamine is another name for vitamin B1. Thiamine is involved in energy production, normal nerve functioning, and metabolism of carbohydrates and fats.

VITAMIN B 2 (Riboflavin)

Riboflavin is another name for vitamin B2. Riboflavin 5-phosphate is the active form of vitamin B2. Riboflavin is important in normal nerve functioning, building ATP, increases energy metabolism, carbohydrate metabolism, and assists in the production of glutathione. It is important for the health of the eyes, mucus membranes, skin, and fetal growth and development. Riboflavin is involved in converting vitamin B6 and folic acid into their active forms. It is naturally found in eggs, meat, and broccoli.

VITAMIN B3 (Niacinamide)

Vitamin B3 also comes in forms known as niacin and niacinamide. It assists the activity of GABA in the system creating a calming affect, metabolizes fat, and is commonly used in treating high cholesterol. Too much B3 may harm the liver, and cause skin sensitivities. Excess niacinamide also uses up methyl groups resulting in further deficiency in methylation. Keep dosages to 50 mg per day or less. It is naturally found in greens, meat, poultry, fish, and eggs.

VITAMIN B5 (Pantothenic acid)

Pantothenic acid is important in the production of energy and assists the adrenal glands. It is helpful for those with ADHD, autism, asthma, depression, diabetic nerve pain, and more. It is naturally found in meat, eggs, and grains. Generally, 25 mgs per day is helpful.

VITAMIN B6 (Pyridoxine)

Vitamin B6 is also known as pyridoxine and must be converted to pyridoxal-5 phosphate (P5P as noted above) to be properly used by the body. It is helpful for children with autism in doses up to 500 mgs per day. Vitamin B6 is important in nerve functioning and maintaining a healthy immune system, and also assists methylation. It is beneficial for the GI system, symptoms of nausea, and assisting with better sleep. Vitamin B6 also lowers blood and brain levels of glutamate. Higher dosages of vitamin B6 have been used in treatment with seizures. Generally, 25 mgs per day is helpful.

FOLIC ACID OR FOLATE

Since 2011, three studies have shown a correlation between using folic acid before conception lowers the risk of autism by about 40%. Folic acid is important in nerve functioning, DNA synthesis, and helps build vitamin B12. Methyl B12 builds methylation, so they are both essential components for proper immune function and antibody formation.

Generally, 400 to 800 mcg per day has been known to be helpful.

VITAMIN B12

Most children on the autism spectrum are deficient in vitamin B12. Mercury in the system is known to alter the body's ability to make its own B12, and when the gut is disrupted, it cannot absorb nutrients properly. Vitamin B12 blocks glutamate from the brain, preventing excitotoxic damage. It also revives methylation.

Vitamin B12 is necessary for digestion, food absorption, protein synthesis, DNA synthesis, protection of the myelin sheath (nerve tissue coverings), and metabolizing of fats and carbohydrates. It also assists the immune system by helping to build the master antioxidant, glutathione, and building red blood cells, which also helps to prevent anemia. Common symptoms of deficiency are depression, mania, and fatigue. It is also important in fetal growth and development.

Once your child's GI tract has healed, B12 will be more available to the body and more absorbable via the intestinal tract. The best food sources of vitamin B12 are beef, lamb, liver, fish (especially shellfish), and eggs. If there is an allergy to eggs it is usually to the white portion. When in doubt either muscle test or use the sensitivity test. The B vitamins are in the yolk, so you can separate the yolk from the white. Eggs from goose or duck have almost five times the amount of B12 compared to chicken eggs. Egg yolks also have the added benefits of vitamins B2, D, and iron.

Vitamin B12 supplements come in two different forms. The most common form used is cyanocobalamin. Cobalamin is the actual B12 portion. Cyanide is added as a stabilizing agent to preserve the cobalamin in packaging. In order for the cobalamin to be activated, the cyanide must be removed by an enzyme. If the body is not able to remove the cyanide, not only will you not benefit from the cobalamin, but it will actually block the B12 component. When looking for vitamin B12, be sure to get *methyl*cobalamin and *not cyanoco*balamin. Methylcobalamin or methyl B12 is the natural form of B12. By using methyl B12 no conversion is needed, therefore, it is very absorbable.

Read your labels to be sure the ingredients are what you are looking for. For example, often the cyanocobalamin form of B12 vitamin is used as it is cheaper. This is not the best form of B12, but it is more stable when blended with other vitamins, especially liquid ones. Methylcobalamin has a rapid deterioration when blended this way, but it is stable on its own. If you give the blended form with the cyanocobalamin and you do not see the results you had hoped for, it may be due to the lack of conversion and absorption. Best results are seen when supplementing a pure form of methyl B12.

Due to improper digestion in those on the autism spectrum, a liquid or sublingual form is best. This is easily and quickly absorbed and enters the bloodstream more quickly. Noticeable differences in energy and behavior can often be seen almost immediately.

There are several good choices for liquid spray or sublingual droplet B12 vitamins in methyl form. The company Readisorb makes a liquid B12 spray of high quality but it has a slight taste to it. It can be found at www.ourasdkids.com for a good price. The company New Beginnings carries one called Methyl Mate that has a high potency (although you choose how much to put into the dropper), and it has no taste at all. It can be found at www.nbnus.net, 877-575-2467. New Beginnings also carries chemical-free products such as sunscreen, insect repellent, deodorant, and toothpaste.

MaxamRevitapop is a company that makes methyl B12 lollipops. Yes, they are lollipops made with methyl B12 so that it absorbs directly via your tongue for longer, better absorption. They taste good too. You can find them at www.revitaPOP.com, 888-MB12POP.

Vitamin B12 is often given as an injection to children on the autism spectrum. This method would be helpful in the beginning stages when his gut is not yet absorbing nutrients from his food, and his health and behavior are at their worst. Injections are in a mentholated form that helps build glutathione better. Parents are taught how to give the injections to their child, often while he sleeps. It is gently given in the buttocks where the muscles are large and there is little sensitivity to the shot.

Check with your doctor to see what degree of need your child has. As his gut heals, he will absorb this nutrient better from his foods and the need for supplementation will decline. When this occurs most children are completely fine with the sublingual drop form of this supplement.

In excess, B vitamins, especially synthetic ones can create hyperactivity. Natural forms will not do this. The foods you see in stores that read, "fortified with essential vitamins," are filled with synthetic vitamins. Watch your child for signs of behavioral changes after starting any new food or supplement.

Sea plankton is one of the best food sources of vitamin B12. A good, organic, non-GMO product can be found at www.newearthsuperfoods.com.

Remember, as your child's system begins to work more efficiently on its own, supplement dosages may need to be decreased or altered in different ways. Each individual is quite different. One child may do extremely well on B vitamins and another may get agitated or hyperactive.

Methylcobalamin has been helpful in dosages of 1,000ug per day for maintenance and 5,000 mcg per day for those with poor nutrient absorption or chronic illness. Check with your healthcare practitioner for your child's needs.

VITAMIN C

Vitamin C, which is water soluble, is one of the key vitamins to help the defenses of the immune system, and prevents anything harmful from entering the body. It is capable of killing viruses and bacteria. Vitamins C and E work best together because one will recharge the other. They both help to protect brain cells. There is a heavy demand for vitamin C by the brain, especially the hippocampus, which is deeply involved with memory and emotions.

Vitamin C reduces the stress hormone cortisol in the body after stress, therefore, it is needed in high concentrations by the adrenal glands.

Vitamin C in the form of ascorbic acid is often too acidic for the body. A buffered ascorbate form is best as it prevents heavy acidity. Between 500 mg and 2,000 mg per day, in divided doses, have been helpful for maintenance, but it can be taken to bowel tolerance when infection or illness are present, usually about 5,000 mg per day. Vitamin C is water soluble, so it will not become toxic in the body and any excess will be excreted. It may increase iron absorption, so if increased iron is problematic for a particular individual, it would be good to have iron levels checked with excessive use of this vitamin.

FAT SOLUBLE VITAMINS

The fat soluble vitamins are vitamins A, D, E and K. Omega-3 fatty acids are also oil based. They all need the proper digestion of fat for proper absorption. When the liver and gallbladder are congested, these fat soluble compounds are not able to be properly utilized by the body and we become deficient. They cannot be absorbed through either food or supplementation. The liver and gallbladder must be directly addressed (see the chapter on detoxification and organ support). While digestion is healing, and after, there are sublingual supplements available that absorb directly into the system via tissues under the tongue. Once digestion has healed and the body is able to absorb properly, these fat-soluble vitamins must be eaten with foods that contain some amount of fat to assist their absorption.

The body will not excrete what it does not need from fat soluble supplemental vitamins, so they can become toxic in excess. Do not be afraid of them, as they are incredibly important to have enough of in your system. Simply remember to have the intake of them monitored by your healthcare practitioner for your child's individual needs. When taken as natural food sources, such as cod liver oil for vitamins A and D, nature takes care of the balance, and no harmful excess should exist.

Oils and fat soluble vitamins will go rancid fairly quickly if not kept in the refrigerator, and always keep them away from heat and moisture.

VITAMIN A

Vitamin A is commonly low in children with autism. It is essential for the health of the digestive tract, the immune system, healthy vision, and cell communication, including brain cells.

Vitamin A can be difficult to absorb. By now you have begun to understand the importance of a healthy, non-congested liver and gallbladder in the absorption of these fat-soluble vitamins. Carotene from fruit and vegetables also need to be converted by the body into an absorbable form that can be utilized. Without proper absorption of vitamin A, the epithelial cells of the body become damaged. Epithelial cells are layers of cells that protect organs, blood vessels, lymph vessels, glands, and more.

The widespread use of processed foods has also contributed to the problem of vitamin A and D deficiency. Processed foods add synthetic vitamin A to their ingredients. When we eat these foods, more vitamin A is added to our system, but vitamin D is removed. Without a balance of the two, the one that is more deficient becomes further depleted and the one in excess can accumulate to toxic levels. Foods rich in vitamin A are egg yolks, fish, butter and liver. Luckily, cod liver oil carries this natural form of vitamin A along with vitamin D3. (See cod liver oil below.)

COD LIVER OIL

Most children on the autism spectrum or with any health issue are deficient in both vitamins A and D. Cod liver oil contains both. These two vitamins work synergistically. They complement each other and can do their jobs best when taken together. Most importantly, they will regulate each other and keep levels from getting out of balance and toxic.

Since cod liver oil provides more vitamin A than D, many began to have concern whether this could cause an imbalance of the two. Luckily, cod liver oil is a natural product, and offers both vitamins in their natural food form. When vitamins are natural, not synthetic, the body can utilize them correctly. This eliminates a toxic imbalance. Use caution with any synthetic vitamins and processed foods.

Cod liver oil is sold in liquid or softgel form. Three companies I trust to carry out the guarantee to be free of any fish oil contaminants, such as heavy metals and PCB toxins, are Nordic Naturals, Pharmax, and Carlson. They carry children's dosage of cod liver oil, but remember that most kids on the autism spectrum and with digestive disorders need more than the regular child's dosage. It may be best to purchase the adult formula. Nordic Naturals has their cod liver oil flavored in peach, strawberry, orange, lemon, or unflavored. Carlson has one in lemon, strawberry and unflavored. They all come in liquid or softgel form. Liquids are easy to disguise in a cup of juice. The company Pharmax makes a high quality cod liver oil. All are available in healthfood stores and at www.pureformulas.com.

VITAMIN D

Vitamin D is one of the most important vitamins and one that most people are deficient in. Many neurodevelopment conditions are associated with vitamin D deficiency such as depression, lack of motivation, dementia, Parkinson's disease, epilepsy, muscular sclerosis, and schizophrenia. Vitamin D helps neurons grow and survive, and is important in brain development and its protection. It also decreases heavy metal damage to the brain, and is anti-inflammatory.

Vitamin D is essential for fighting both viral and bacterial infections. It seems to be especially important in fighting viruses and is a far better choice in fighting the flu than mercury-based immunizations that only cover one strain of influenza. A 2009 pediatric research journal stated that children and infants deficient in vitamin D are more susceptible to viral infections.

Many problems for infants arise in utero. If a woman is deficient in vitamin D during her pregnancy, then the deficiency will be passed on to the baby. This can be especially common for babies born in the winter months, since we get much of our vitamin D from the sun. The kidneys must be working properly because they convert vitamin D to its active form. Vitamin D deficiency is also connected to inflammatory bowel disease and liver and gallbladder inefficiency.

There are many correlations between respiratory infections and low levels of vitamin D. Another 2009 study showed newborns with acute respiratory infection were born to mothers who were deficient in vitamin D, especially in the winter months. Vitamin D deficiency is also linked to asthma in children. If the mother is deficient in Vitamin D during pregnancy, it can affect the brain tissue of the fetus in early development.

Lack of this vitamin also has a connection to inflammatory bowel disease and asthma. Vitamin D deficiency may increase toxicity from fluoride. Those having seizures that are put on anticoagulant drugs may be deficient due to the drug lowering vitamin D levels.

Supplementation will assist the body's defenses against these issues. Sufficient amounts of magnesium are necessary in order to absorb vitamin D. The body actually makes vitamin D when the skin is exposed to sunlight. Overuse of sunscreen adds to the problem. More than 58 million children are vitamin D deficient. We need to get our children outside more. Instead of television or a video game go for a walk, sit in the backyard and play a game, go to the park, or go for a bike ride.

To increase your exposure to the sun, wear shorts and short sleeves if possible. A bathing suit is even better. I leave the sunscreen off for 10 to 20 minutes on hot days and much longer on cooler days. Use your own discretion on safety depending on the weather you are in.

The fear of skin cancer has resulted in vitamin D deficiency. Too much sunscreen and covering up completely eliminates our exposure. We don't want to burn, yet we need sun. Most commercial sunscreens contain cancer-forming chemicals. The skin is the largest organ of the body. It will absorb whatever we put on it. Be sure to buy non-toxic sunscreens. Local healthfood stores carry many brands, such as Jason, that make a natural, mineral-based, 45 SPF sunscreen specifically formulated for kids and their sensitive skin. Jason products are available at www.amazon.com. New Beginnings also carries a non-greasy, non-scented one that I like called Eco. You can find it at www.nbnus.com, 877-575-2467.

To test for vitamin D on your own from your home go to www.directlabs.com or call (800) 908-,0000. This vitamin D hydroxy test is only $59, instead of the usual $232 you would pay at a doctor's office, and comes without an expensive doctor appointment and wasted time. A phone consultation with a physician is available.

When supplementing with vitamin D, be sure to get vitamin D3, as it is the most absorbable form. Remember to take it with food, especially with good fats, for better absorption.

Sprays have far better absorption, especially for those with compromised digestive systems, and therefore, compromised absorption. Vitamin D is sold in any healthfood store in many forms such as sprays, drops, or pills. Get one with an oil base as vitamin D is a fat soluble vitamin and needs oil to absorb. Often vitamin E is taken with it. Remember to keep all oils in the refrigerator so they do not become rancid.

Mercola, www.mercola.com, carries a vitamin D3 spray. One spray from this product contains 1,000 IU of D3. The taste is slightly minty and pleasant.

The website, www.cpmedical.net, also carries a vitamin D3 spray but this one is 5,000 IU per spray. This is for those of you who have had blood work done and have been told by a professional that your child needs this amount. It is also the current recommended daily amount for most adults.

The company, Rainbow Light, makes a vitamin D supplement in gummy form called Sunny Gummies. Rainbow Light products are found in most quality healthfood stores and are available at www.pureformulas.com with no shipping fee.

Be sure you are giving your child the appropriate dosage for his age. Many supplements, especially for children, have very low doses. He may need to take several to get his needed daily requirement. This number has risen from 400 IU per day to as much as 2,000 IU for a child and up to between 5,000 and 10,000 IU per day for some adults. Vitamin D levels are easily tested in blood work.

VITAMIN D DOSAGE FORMULA

The amount of vitamin D we need each day in supplemental form depends on our level of current deficiency, how much of our body is exposed to sunlight every day, and how much time your skin is exposed. There is a formula for the breakdown regarding the varying requirements of vitamin D. This formula can be used for any person of any weight including pregnant women.

The formula is:

(basic daily vitamin D dosage) = (body mass in pounds) x 27

Twenty seven IU is the amount of daily vitamin D needed to keep blood levels at their optimum of 50ng/ml without getting any sunlight. For example, the basic daily vitamin D dosage for a 50-pound child would be 50 x 27 = 1,350 IU per day.

You must also take into consideration the amount of vitamin D gained by sun exposure. If your child wears long pants, a short-sleeved t-shirt, and a hat, he receives about 10% sunlight on his skin. To adjust for sun exposure, use this forumula:

(your daily need) x (% of your skin exposure) x 2

If the child in the example above needs 1,350 IU of vitamin D per day, you would multiply 1,350 x 10% x 2 = 270 IU of vitamin D gained from sun exposure. Now subtract that amount from your daily requirement: 1,350 – 270 = 1,080 IU vitamin D in supplemental form is needed per day. In the winter, we will obviously need more supplemental vitamin D than in the summer months when we are exposed to more sunlight.

If your child wears only shorts or swim trunks (lower legs, torso and arms fully exposed), he is receives over 50% exposure. If we get over 50% sun exposure for as little as an average of 15 minutes per day, we have our daily quota of vitamin D. For more information see www.vitamind-cholecalciferol.com/vitamin-d-dosage/.

Note: Be sure to keep vitamins A and D3 in balance (see vitamin A above).

VITAMIN E

A powerful antioxidant, vitamin E assists in many functions. It is brain protective, especially in neurons. Neurons are brain cells that are the messengers to the rest of the nervous system. In vitro tests show that vitamin E also blocks mercury toxicity.

Vitamin E as d-alpha tocopherol succinate is the most potent antioxidant form. It is also the form that enters the brain easily to combat free radical damage and lipid peroxidation. Acetate forms of vitamin E are cheaper, but are a waste of your time and money. Do not take the acetate form as it has low potency.

One of its favorite vitamins to assist is vitamin C, and visa versa. They are like the best friends who run to each other's aid when needed. The two work much more powerfully together than they do alone. Vitamin E also works with selenium and beta-carotene to protect cell membranes.

For proper absorption, be sure there is absorption from the liver and gallbladder working effectively. Generally, 400 to 800 IU per day is helpful. Discuss your child's needs with your healthcare practitioner.

VITAMIN K

Vitamin K is essential for the health of the brain, heart, bones, and blood clotting, and will even help regulate insulin and inflammation levels. When the gut lacks the necessary assimilation of fats, both absorption and production of vitamin K do not take place. This leaves the body deficient. The liver and the gut must be healed for proper assimilation.

My daughter was getting recurring nose bleeds. When people get nose bleeds, they are often deficient in vitamin K. Gut imbalance can cause this. When anticoagulants are taken for the bleeding, this only compounds the problem because anticoagulants thin the blood by blocking vitamin K.

The nose bleeds were a sign that my daughter's system had weakened and we needed to improve her diet and increase enzymes and probiotics to ensure better health in her GI tract. Supplements that assist the gallbladder may be helpful, such as A-F Betafood by Standard Process. This helped get her body back in balance. A-F Betafood can be found at most natural healthcare practitioners and at www.amazon.com.

True healing comes from the Candida protocol in this book and supporting the liver. In the meantime, you can supplement with vitamin K. Remember that if the digestive system is imbalanced, that the food and supplements may not be getting absorbed. Vitamin K comes from animal fats, liver, eggs, full fat cheese, and butter. Non-animal sources are leafy green vegetables, natto (fermented soy beans), and fermented foods such as yogurt, kefir, and sauerkraut. Fruit and juice are high in salicylates (aspirin-like substances) and block vitamin K.

AMINO ACIDS

Amino acids are essential nutrients required for a variety of processes in the human body. They are needed for many stages of healing, are the building blocks of proteins, and are essential when building neurotransmitters for the brain. We will go into detail on those that specifically support the brain and symptoms associated with their deficiencies in the chapter on supporting the brain.

Branched-chain amino acids refer to their specific chemical structure and include L-leucine, L-valine, and L-isoleucine. These are helpful with increasing muscle tone and performance, fatigue, concentration, and brain conditions, especially those associated with liver disease. (L-leucine should be limited due to its ability to cause hypoglycemia, especially in infants and small children.)

CREATINE

This amino acid is commonly low in children on the autism spectrum. Mercury can block its metabolism. This is often the cause of poor muscle tone and weakness in many of our kids. By supplementing with creatine, strength may be increased and poor muscle mass may be restored. Creatine is also important to brain cell communication and speech.

Blood and urine tests can offer information as to your child's creatine levels. Generally, one to three grams per day can be helpful, depending on weight, age, and need.

N-ACETYL CYSTEINE (NAC)

Sulfation is the process by which the body detoxifies. When sulfation levels are low, as is in most cases of autism, the amino acid N-acetyl cysteine can help to increase it. NAC will strengthen the detoxification system in the body and help during heavy metal detoxification. NAC also assists the methylation process by helping the body build glutathione, assists the liver during detoxification, helps replenish mitochondria, and benefits the respiratory system. NAC has been used for over three decades for bronchial congestion due to its strong ability to break up mucus. NAC will increase the GI mucosa, which will assist healing of the gut. NAC has been shown in studies to greatly reduce viral infections such as influenza. Due to its sulfur content, it may increase the growth of yeast in the digestive tract. For this reason, it is wise not to use it until yeast has been eradicated.

Amino acids may also help to chelate mercury before it enters the brain when mercury is attached to N-acetyl cysteine (NAC).

One study by The Pediatric Liver Center in London over a five-year period with 170 children, concluded that N-acetyl cysteine was safe for children. The results also showed higher incidences of recovery for these children with acute liver failure from non-acetaminophen-induced ALF.

Be sure to use N-acetyl cysteine because it has an acetyl group that will not allow it to become excitatory to the brain as cysteine alone can. NAC works so well that you want to limit your intake. With the increase in glutathione being built, there can be excessive release of toxins and the body may not be able to keep up. This could cause greater toxicity.

Dosages that have been known to be helpful are:

- 500 mg per day for adults
- 250 mg per day for age 14 to 18
- 100 mg twice a day from 8 to 13 years of age.

DMG (DI) AND TMG (TRI) METHYLGLYCINE

DMG and TMG are most important in the process of methylation. They are amino acids necessary for the production of glutathione and are extremely effective in detoxifying heavy metals from the body. Notable differences in autistic children are increased eye contact and speech.

Watch for possible increased irritability from DMG and aggression with TMG. The percentage of those with negative effects is generally less than 10%, but it is important to be aware of it. Always start with low dosages and work upward.

Helpful dosages have been: DMG 125: 1,000 mg per day and TMG: 175 to 2,000 mg per day. Dosages vary depending on age, size, and varying needs.

Various amino acid products are available at healthfood stores and online.

There is a product which has all of the important amino acids in it called My Aminoplex by Crayhon Research. The product was formulated by a man named Mark Schauss who has studied autism extensively. You can check out their websites for additional information at www.cpmedical.com and www.VRP.com. They are the same company. This product can be purchased at (888)401-1105, from CP Medical, and they offer 10% off of your first order. If you go to their website, you will need the PIN number (726645), to order, so they told me it is easier to call. If you are already placing an order here, you may want to also purchase your Lipoceutical Glutathione (Readisorb) from them to save shipping on separate purchases.

Limit intake of glycine and glutamine as they have been known to increase excitotoxicity.

ADDITIONAL ANTIOXIDANTS AND HELPFUL SUPPLEMENTS

We talked about antioxidants in detail in the chapter on nutritional supplementation. Antioxidants prevent the attack of free radicals on cells, or prevent cell damage and protect them. Antioxidants work synergistically. They work far better for us if taken with another because they regenerate each other. Note that many vitamins and minerals also contain antioxidants.

CHLORELLA

Chlorella is a concentrated source of chlorophyll. It is a freshwater algae, a natural food. It helps balance the immune system, reduce inflammation, and protect us from toxins. Chlorella binds to toxins such as PCBs, car exhaust fumes, pesticides, herbicides, bacteria, and viruses. It also detoxifies the heavy metals lead, mercury, and cadmium. Chlorella is anti-inflammatory and assists in tissue repair and cell regeneration. It contains vitamin B12, and due to its high levels of beta-carotene, it assists the health of the eyes and vision. It also has anti-tumor and anti-cancer properties. Lastly, it acts as a natural antibiotic without any negative effects such as those seen with prescription antibiotics.

Chlorella is a food, so it is completely safe and will not interfere with medications. It is helpful for breastfeeding mothers to take as it reduces toxins and increases IgA antibodies in breast milk for the baby.

Chlorella is 60% protein with 19 amino acids, including all 8 of the essential amino acids. Chlorella vulgaris, such as Yeayama chlorella from Jarrow Formulas, is a strain that is easier to digest and has higher chlorophyll. It comes in both capsule and powder form. It is available in healthfood stores and online at www.pureformulas.com.

Always start slowly with a gram or less per day and work your way up to more. Chlorella is safe, but as the body detoxifies, initial symptoms of rash, bloating, gas or nausea may result. This will dissipate after the first one to two weeks. When taken for general prevention, one to two grams per day with food and a glass of water is sufficient. For detoxification, higher doses are better for binding, and it is more efficient if taken on an empty stomach, 30 minutes before food or 1 hour after. Start with 1 gram, 2 to 3 times per day. Slowly work up to 6 to 12 grams per day in divided doses with up to 2 glasses of water. Muscle test along the way to check for dosage levels. Do this for several months before going back to the preventative doses.

Note: When chlorella is taken with omega-3 fish oil or krill oil, it is even more effective. To modulate an overactive immune system, 5 grams of chlorella, 4 times per day, 30 minutes before food with omega-3 has been known to be helpful.

LIPOCEUTICAL GLUTATHIONE

Glutathione is known as the body's master antioxidant.

Glutathione boosts our immune system. It is the best cellular detoxifier, and autism clearly improves with cellular detoxification. It also reduces viruses in cells, helps to chelate heavy metals (especially mercury), and protects our cells and our neurological system from free radical damage. Glutathione also regulates protein and the building blocks of DNA.

Glutathione is a naturally occurring protein that is found in every cell of the body including the brain. With the necessary three amino acids—cysteine, glutamic acid, and glycine—glutathione can be made by our cells.

In some people, glutathione can be difficult for the cells to make. Candida disrupts protein digestion, which reduces glutathione production. Pathogenic bacteria in the gut can destroy enzymes.

The gastrointestinal system must be working properly so it can make the necessary enzymes that break down the essential three amino acids that make up glutathione. Mercury is a commonly found preservative in vaccines. Mercury kills enzymes, therefore weakening the antioxidant system by binding with glutathione and rendering it useless. The depletion of glutathione makes it so the body cannot detoxify mercury. These enzymes need vitamins and minerals from the foods we eat, largely fruits, vegetables and meats, in order to be produced by the body. A healthy diet and proper absorption of its nutrients are necessary in order for this to happen.

There also needs to be enough energy in the cells to complete this process. Toxins also reduce the body's ability to produce these needed amino acids. The sulfur content in L-cysteine gives glutathione its antioxidant strength. For L-cysteine to build glutathione, it needs vitamin B12, folinic acid, and trimethylglycine or TMG. Diminished levels of these nutrients are also known to cause hyperactivity. Vitamin D is also necessary for glutathione to become engaged. Some call it flu season, I call it low vitamin D season. Glutathione cannot do its job if there is not enough vitamin D. Supplementing with CoQ10 also helps boost cellular energy.

We must have enough glutathione in our system for proper detoxification. Glutathione destroys and removes toxins from our bodies and protects the brain from heavy metal toxicity. If we don't have enough glutathione to do its job, we become loaded with toxins. These toxins enter the bloodstream, cross the blood-brain barrier, and cause neurological and physiological damage.

Toxic waste from pathogenic bacteria in the gut is one of the many reasons why children on the autism spectrum or those with intestinal imbalance have congested livers. The liver will attach an oxygen molecule to the toxin, creating a free radical. Glutathione is the "go to" antioxidant in the liver, so it attaches itself to the free radical. This renders the free radical harmless to us and it has done its job. The problem is that this also uses up the glutathione molecule that has attached itself to the toxin.

If the liver is overwhelmed by a toxic load, it cannot keep up and becomes depleted of glutathione. This crucial antioxidant is also leached out of the system due to environmental toxins such as heavy metals, polluted air, carbonated sodas, chemical household cleaners, processed foods, stress, alcohol, and prescription drugs.

THE RIGHT GLUTATHIONE PRODUCT

Not all glutathione products are absorbable. Enzymes must be working properly with enough cellular energy for the glutathione molecule to attach itself to the free radical and neutralize it. Most oral glutathione supplements are destroyed by our digestive system through oxidation.

There is one oral liquid glutathione known to have strong bioavailability. This product is called by two names. In your practitioners office, it is called lipoceutical glutathione. In your healthfood store, it is called Readisorb. They are made by the same company but had to be put under a different label for the general public.

When purchasing glutathione, it is important to get the lipoceutical or liposomal form. A liposome is like a little bubble that keeps the molecules inside it safe, stable, and active. Lipoceutical glutathione is in its reduced state, and antioxidants must be in their reduced state to be effective. This is one of the only absorbable forms of glutathione. It costs more, but it works. Other forms are a waste of your money.

Compared to glutathione given intravenously, the lipoceutical oral form can be a far better choice. With IVs, they are administered once every day, bi-weekly or less, but the body uses glutathione at all times. When taking liposomal glutathione orally, you can decide how often it is needed. Your practitioner can guide you too, but there is the choice of taking it one, two, or three times per day and changing the amounts as your child heals. It is also far less expensive than going for an appointment and far less traumatic than an IV can be for your child.

The dosage to begin with will be quite small, perhaps barely an eighth of a teaspoon. It does have a strong, bitter flavor, but it can easily be mixed into any beverage.

The best price I found for liquid liposomal glutathione was on www.amazon.com. The company Get Healthy Again, www.gethealthyagain.com, also carries a liquid liposomal glutathione product called glutathione specialist that also contains 1 mg of methyl B12 all in one spray.

Whatever we choose we never want to replace the body's own ability to build glutathione, so any glutathione supplement should be used as a temporary measure.

Breastfed babies have higher glutathione levels. Breast milk gives bonded cysteine, which helps build glutathione and deliver it to cells. With proper diet for a healthy, balanced gut, the goal is to get the body to a healthy state in which it is able to make enough glutathione again on its own.

Glutathione also helps maintain levels of other antioxidants. One antioxidant that has a strong symbiotic relationship with glutathione is alpha-lipoic acid. Of the many beneficial antioxidants it is my first choice when the intention is to build glutathione levels.

Supplements helpful in building glutathione are:

- Alpha-lipoic acid
- N-acetyl cysteine
- Vitamin E
- Vitamin C
- Carotenoids
- Flavonoids
- Riboflavin (B2)
- Magnesium
- Selenium
- Silymarin (from milk thistle)
- Sulfur

The supplement C0Q10 (Ubiquinol) helps increase glutathione in the cells. See below.

ALPHA-LIPOIC ACID

Alpha-lipoic acid is another powerful antioxidant. It easily penetrates the blood-brain barrier allowing it to powerfully assist in heavy metal detoxification. Overall it is used to stimulate detoxification pathways.

Alpha-lipoic acid supports the life of glutathione, and glutathione in return supports and strengthens alpha-lipoic acid. Adding the amino acid acetyl L-carnitine to alpha-lipoic acid also helps to build glutathione.

Alpha-lipoic acid assists the cells and the blood in detoxification, including heavy metal detoxification. It increases the energy of the cells, strengthens other antioxidants and brings them back to their reduced state so that they are functional again, is helpful with liver disorders and diabetes. Alpha-lipoic acid also helps to balance blood sugar. Generally 50 mg per day is enough. It is found in many food sources such as brewer's yeast, liver, and potatoes.

CAROTENOIDS

Carotenoids are a group of vitamins that are strong antioxidants. A diet that does not contain enough fruits and vegetables can leave the body deficient of these. There are roughly 40 different types. Among the more commonly known are lutein, lycopene, and beta-carotene. Beta-carotene is a precursor to vitamin A. It is like a shape-shifter when it comes to the needs of others, especially the needs of vitamin A.

Carotenoids are food, so they will make what your body needs from them and excrete any excess. They have the capability to help other vitamins and antioxidants in the body that are in need of assistance. They assist selenium and vitamin E to protect cell membranes.

There are over 600 different carotenoids in orange, yellow, and some red vegetables. And there are over 300 anthocyanins that we know about; they are in deep red, purple, and blue fruits and vegetables.

CoQ10 (Ubiquinol)

Coenzyme Q10 (CoQ10) is a naturally occurring chemical compound. It is made in the body and builds with the help of fish oils, organ meats, and whole grains. C0Q10 is cellular fuel. It builds the ultimate energy molecule, adenosine triphosphate or ATP. It is what gives cells their energy. Without it our cells cannot function properly and our energy level decreases rapidly.

Ubiquinol is the active converted form of CoQ10. For various reasons, the body can have difficulty converting CoQ10 to ubiquinol. The immune system builds CoQ10, so if the immune system is weak, it will affect cellular energy levels. Supplementing with CoQ10 or ubiquinol are helpful for increasing one's energy levels, especially when taken with B vitamins. As we age our body' ability to make this necessary element diminishes.

CoQ10 has additional benefits such as lowering blood glucose levels, improving metabolism, improving heart muscle contraction, stimulating energy production, acting as an antioxidant, having the capability to increase cellular glutathione levels, and it protects the brain from excitotoxicity. It also assists the ability of mitochondria (which helps the messages from the brain get sent) to function properly.

CoQ10 or Ubiquinol in supplemental form is a fat-soluble substance that it is best taken with food and oils such as omega 3 fatty acids.

TRANSFER FACTOR

Transfer factor is naturally found in breast milk, but is now available in supplement form. By increasing Th-1 immunity it helps to balance Th-2, which often imbalances the immune system. It is valuable to the immune system when chronic infections, allergies, or autoimmune disorders are present.

Transfer factor may be helpful for chronic viral infections, such as those residing in the gut. Dr. Andrew Wakefield found strains of the same measles virus in the digestive tracts of children with autism as the ones used in their measles vaccinations. Transfer factor could be a useful agent for this.

The supplement usually comes from eggs or cows, so be aware of cascin as an ingredient when purchased through healthfood stores. Look for purified transfer factor such as Wellness Transfer Factor by Source Naturals found at www.pureformulas.com. Dosages that have been helpful are 200 to 1,800 mg per day, depending on age and weight.

SUMMARY

Even when we are feeding our child healthy foods they may not be absorbing the nutrients efficiently. Most children with autism, if not all, have poor absorption due to an injured and poorly functioning digestive system. Our cells and organs, such as the brain, rely on nutrients to fight off toxins, and build the chemicals necessary for healthy function and behavior. Our immune system is mostly developed in the gut.

Some supplements in liquid and sublingual forms are very helpful, especially during the healing process of the digestive tract when the gut cannot properly absorb nutrients. Specific nutrients will help to heal the lining of the intestinal tract so that the body will eventually be able to absorb enough nutrients on its own. When the gut is still injured and absorption is limited oral supplementation is best during this time.

Several companies are available to help with specific needs of children with autism. Once the gut has been healed and absorption is going well, then you may want to look into supplements that are available to help with additional specific vitamin, mineral, and antioxidant needs.

The products found in this chapter can be found at http://naturallyhealingautism.com/a-healthy-home/

CHAPTER 11

REDUCING INFLAMMATION

Children with autism often have chronic inflammation. This is not only a problem in the digestive system but also in the brain. Inflammation impairs brain cells and it can also kill them. If the brain cells are weakened, they are even less capable of fending off toxins or excreting them once they have entered the cell.

Inflammation also damages the blood-brain barrier. This is the brain's protective shield against toxins. Without it, the brain is vulnerable to much damage, whether it is from undigested food particles in the bloodstream, or environmental toxins such as heavy metals, pesticides, household chemicals, and more. The most common disorders caused by inflammation are anxiety and obsessive compulsive disorder, but many more can exist. One more critical factor is inflammation's ability to alter neurotransmitters.

Neurotransmitters are the brain's messengers. They affect things like mood, sleep, and appetite. Particularly vulnerable to inflammation is the neurotransmitter dopamine. When there is a deficiency in dopamine, it causes fatigue, lack of focus, moodiness, and problems with fine motor coordination. The amino acid L-tyrosine is especially helpful for this deficiency and its consequences. (This is discussed in detail in the chapter on supporting the brain.)

The most common places to look for inflammation are in the gut and the mouth. Problems with teeth are a common indicator that the immune system is fighting on an ongoing basis which can also lead to autoimmune disorders. The inflammation in the gut leads directly via the blood to inflammation and chronic disorders of inflammation in the brain. These products can be purchased at www.naturallyhealingautism.com under "healthy home products."

TESTING FOR GUT INFLAMMATION

The laboratory, Diagnos-Techs, offer a panel used with your child's stool that can give their inflammation markers along with a lot of other valuable information. The test can also check for IgA antibodies (gluten allergens), parasites, fungus, and more. Most alternative practitioners use this laboratory and have these tests on hand, or they can order them at Diagnos-Techs, 425-251-0596.

The website, www.crohns.net, also sells a pathology test that you can do from home; they send you the results via email. The owner of the site is Pamela Nathan. She is a licensed acupuncturist with over 30 years of experience working with people who have gut and digestive issues. She is available to help you with the results, if needed.

The following supplements are some of the best sources available for reducing inflammation and helping to heal the gut, and therefore the brain.

PRODUCTS TO REDUCE GUT INFLAMMATION, PROMOTE HEALING, AND ASSIST DIGESTION

ZINC CARNOSINE

Zinc carnosine is one of the best supplements to heal and protect the gut. Scientific data shows improved intestinal cells and improved gut barrier integrity. It also assists in balancing intestinal microbes and does not interfere with normal digestion. Even a dosage as small as 75 milligrams per day is known to heal leaky gut. Zinc carnosine can be found in most health food stores. The company Integrative Therapeutics makes a good product that can be found at a good price with free shipping at www.pureformulas.com.

DEGLYCERIZED LICORICE ROOT (DGL)

Deglycerized licorice root (DGL) has long been known as a digestive aid. DGL protects the stomach and intestinal walls by stimulating the stomach to secrete mucosal cells. Licorice also assists the immune system and the liver. It is helpful with acid reflux or

GERD, and helps to heal the gut by providing nutrients it needs. It is also helpful with stomach aches, as it is very soothing to the digestive tract.

The word deglycerized means that the part of the licorice called glycyrrhizin has been removed because it causes many people intestinal discomfort. With this substance removed, higher doses can be taken with no intestinal distress.

There is a powder from of DGL available from Vital Nutrients. It is a pure form that is free of all allergens and contains no sugars. There is also a quality chewable form available from Enzymatic Therapy. Be sure to get their formula that is fructose and sugar free for those with Candida and blood sugar issues. This product also contains glycine, which is helpful in promoting bile production, therefore assisting in the digestion of fats. This is especially helpful for people with poor liver function. They have a good taste and the chewable form is easy to carry around with you to eat one or two before meals. This product is also free of any allergens, and their products are all organically grown.

Both Vital Nutrients powder DGL and Enzymatic Therapy chewable DGL are available at many healthfood stores and online stores such as www.pureformulas.com.

L-GLUTAMINE

L-glutamine is an amino acid. Physical and emotional stress can reduce the body's ability to make glutamine. It plays an important role in maintaining and repairing the gut. It has also been shown to reduce the number of endotoxins that pass through the intestinal lining.

L-glutamine can increase excitotoxicity with long term use, but its benefits to gut healing are well worth using it. For this reason it is wise to use it for initial gut healing, (usually two to four weeks). Once intestinal health is restored use on an as-needed basis, instead of daily. See Glutagenics below for supplemental use.

GLUTAGENICS, AN ALL-IN-ONE-PRODUCT

One product I personally found helpful in healing my own gut and my son's was a product called Glutagenics by the company Metagenics. Metagenics is well-known in the holistic health field and is used by many alternative practitioners because they are backed by science. This product contains multiple gut-healing agents in one product.

Glutagenics contains the amino acid, L-glutamine, a safe form of concentrated licorice extract, and aloe vera leaf. All three are essential in healing the mucosal lining of the digestive tract. They have taken out the laxative effect of the aloe leaf for those who are sensitive.

Glutagenics comes in gentle-tasting powder form, so it is easy to add to any food or beverage and easy for the body to absorb. It can be purchased at www.pureformulas.com, 800-383-6008, for a good price and free shipping.

ALOE VERA LEAF

The leaf of the aloe plant has the strongest properties. I occasionally take one made by Next To Nature. I purchase it through a practitioner, but www.pureformulas.com sells aloe leaf made from high quality companies. They have one by Nature's Way in liquid formula. Nature's Way is a good company, and the liquid formula would be better for non-pill takers.

Aloe leaf cleanses the blood of toxins that have entered the bloodstream via a damaged lining of the gut. It assists in removal of these toxins, and soothes the digestive tract. Aloe leaf can have a laxative affect, which is helpful if constipation is an issue, but it can cause bowels to become too loose in sensitive individuals. Start with a quarter to a half of the recommended dosage and work up to bowel tolerance.

ALOE VERA JUICE

Aloe Vera juice is soothing and healing to the mucosal lining in the intestinal tract, and it has regenerative properties. Depending on an individual's size and tolerance, one quarter to a half cup on an empty stomach can be helpful.

BOSWELLIA

A great inflammation fighter for inflammation anywhere in the body is boswellia. Boswellia is an herb that has been used in

Ayurvedic tradition for centuries. It has been shown in clinical studies to support healthy GI function, joint, and respiratory health. It is used to remove natural toxins from joint tissues and support healthy blood circulation. Boswellia promotes a healthy, normal inflammatory response, therefore it can assist with additional inflammation in the body such as the brain.

Boswellia is sold in most health food stores in capsules that can be opened up to give to children. It is also available in both capsule and powder form online at www.pureformulas.com. Generally, adults take about 200 mg per day, half that amount for children. As it is herbal, a standardized form will be most beneficial.ce or twice a day can be helpful.

QUERCETIN

Quercetin is an antioxidant flavonoid found in fruits and vegetables. It has both anti-inflammatory and antihistamine properties. It can be very effective for any inflammatory reaction or allergic reaction.

HYDROCHLORIC ACID (HCl)

Hydrochloric acid (HCl) is secreted by cells in the wall of the stomach. It gets food ready for digestion, especially proteins, so the enzymes can break food down thoroughly. If we do not have enough HCl in our stomach, the enzymes cannot do their job.

Although many people feeling the acidic burn in their chest or throat (heartburn or GERD) think this is due to too much acid backing up, it is actually a lack of enough stomach acid that causes this problem. When the gut is not in proper working order, the hydrochloric acid (HCl) production is minimized. It is the opposite of what you may think, but most adults and children with gut issues are deficient in hydrochloric acid and need supplemental assistance until the gut is healed.

When my gut was in poor health, I would find that I had a feeling of being extremely full or bloated after even a very small meal. Supplementing with HCl helped this immensely. There are several products that have proven helpful in building up the HCl and assisting with digestion; I have had personal success with two of them. One is Metagest by Metagenics. The other is Zypan from Standard Process. Both Metagenics and Standard Process products are practitioner grade and high quality. They can be found at many healthcare practitioners offices, but can also be found (usually at a better price) at www.pureformulas.com, 800-383-6008, and free shipping. They can also be found at www.amazon.com.

Muscle testing is a great way to help you know which product to give and at what dosage. Dosages vary due not only to one's size and weight, but also by individual need. This depends on the health of the gut. As you determine your starting dosage, remember to continue to muscle test about once per week to see if the need has changed. As the gut heals, the dosage should lessen, but this does take time.

High quality supplemental enzymes are already in their active form, so they do not need HCl to activate them. You may try taking quality enzymes before trying HCl to see if they do the job alone. The right dosage and product is essential for proper results. There are also products that contain both multiple enzymes and HCl, such as Digestive Enzymes Ultra with Betaine HCl by Pure Encapsulations. This can be found at www.pureformulas.com. See Enzymes below for more information.

ENZYMES

Enzymes can be extremely helpful with autism, ADHD, allergies, and more. From the use of enzymes, parents have documented better concentration, increased language abilities, and improved digestion and behavior.

Enzymes catalyze chemical reactions, meaning they cause things to happen, including breaking down food particles such as proteins, carbohydrates, and fats or assisting in detoxification. Also, they are not used up in the process. They continue on in the body as little garbage collectors cleaning up toxic materials in your body.

There is a significant amount of research and data that support enzymes as a viable alternative to gluten-free or casein-free diets. They are safe to use, and most of our bodies need them anyway. Enzymes help with a myriad of other ailments, including digestive difficulties, healing the gastrointestinal tract, allergies of all kinds, and viruses, to name a few.

Enzymes are produced in saliva, the stomach, the lining of the intestines, the pancreas, and the bile in the liver. When the GI tract is not working properly, including the liver, there is disruption in the ability to make enough enzymes for the digestion and absorption of nutrients. As we age, our body's ability to make enzymes decreases.

Enzyme supplements that are enteric coated purposely prevent digestion in the stomach, so they will not be released until they reach the small intestine. This way stomach acid won't destroy them. However, non-enteric-coated enzymes seem to outperform the enteric-coated ones if given before eating so that they will help with digestion of the food you eat.

It is valuable to take enzymes about 10 to 30 minutes prior to eating to give time for the capsule that encompasses them to dissolve so the enzymes can be released in the stomach at the same time the food enters it. I open my enzyme capsules into water and drink them just before I eat. This way I don't have to wait, and I know they are ready to do their job.

There are also enzymes that come in powder form such as Garden of Life's Omega-Zyme. This eliminates the waiting time and the need to open capsules. A good price for these is at www.crohns.net, and www.pureformulas.com. Another product I have have great success with is Digest Gold from Enzymedica. It is sold in healthfood stores and many online stores such as www.amazon.com, and www.pureformulas.com. It is important to switch your enzyme product about every month or so because the body will adapt to them. I go back and forth between Omega-Zyme and Digest Gold.

Gelatin capsules dissolve immediately once ingested, but vegetable capsules take about 30 minutes to dissolve. If you take an enzyme in a vegetable capsule and eat right away the enzymes may not be released in time and cannot work. I found out that my stomach did not like gelatin as much, and this can be another substance for which to check your child for sensitivities.

Enzymes work either metabolically or digestively. Metabolic enzymes work inside of cells. The cell wall protects them, which makes them hard to affect but not easy to replace once used up. Digestive enzymes are necessary to break down foods.

TWO TYPES OF DIGESTIVE ENZYMES:

1. Pancreatic enzymes are from the pancreas of cow or pig. These are often used when the pancreas is insufficient. The downside of this type of enzyme is that because it comes from an animal, it has a greater chance of creating an allergic reaction. Animals also come with diseases of their own, which can be transferred to those who ingest them. One company that makes high quality animal-based enzymes is Standard Process. They are used by many healthcare practitioners, especially chiropractors, and these practitioners will muscle test your child to know whether or not the product is right for him.
2. Plant-based enzymes are from fruits such as papaya and pineapple. Many come from fungal forms which are not harmful.

ENZYMES FOR GLUTEN AND CASEIN SENSITIVITY

There are many enzymes, and each has a specific job. The one that is most important to children with autism is a protein-digesting enzyme called dipeptidyl peptidase IV, or DPP-IV. This particular enzyme is able to break down the large protein particle in gluten and casein and transform it into a digestible form. Remember that meat and vegetables can also create exorphins. These are opiate-like chemicals that are created when certain foods are not broken down properly.

Trienza is a product from a company called Houston Enzymes that we mothers of children with ASD are most interested in. Trienza is a combination of three products that the company has blended together to cover the complete broad spectrum enzymes, plus the additional bonus of enzymes with DPP-IV activity. They come in both pill and chewable forms.

As far as enzyme companies go, Houston enzymes is one of the best anywhere. I cannot say enough good things about the quality and manufacturing practices of this company. Their customer service is equally as good. I have called them on many occasions to troubleshoot a problem, and they have always helped me find the answers I need.

They offer free samples, so you can try something new before buying anything.

They carry a wide variety of enzyme products to fit most individual needs. Look up their products at www.houston-enzymes.com, 866-757-8627.

SOME COMMON ENZYMES ARE:

- Dipeptidyl peptidase IV (DPP-IV) breaks down casomorphin (from casein) and gluteomorphins (from gluten)
- Proteases break down proteins
- Lactase breaks down lactose (found in dairy)
- Amylase for starch (carbohydrate) digestion
- Alpha-galactosidase breaks down beans and other fiber-rich foods
- Xylanase helps digest fruits and vegetables (phenolic foods)
- Beta-glucanase for fiber-rich vegetables and grains
- Lipase breaks down lipids or fats
- Bromelain and papain are enzymes derived from pineapple. They break down proteins. Note: Some people exhibit sensitivities to fruit or citrus, so watch for signs of this from your child.

Cellulase may interfere with some time-released, cellulose-based medications. Ask your doctor or check your labels for hydroxypropyl cellulose, or hypromellose.

ENZYMES FOR THERAPEUTIC USE

If given on an empty stomach, enzymes work therapeutically. This means they help with specific causes of problems like inflammation, viruses, or many other problems. If proteases are taken between meal,s they will reduce inflammation throughout the body, especially in the gut. Bromelain and papain, derived from pineapple and papaya have been deeply studied and are well known for reducing inflammation. Watch for phenol sensitivities with these two enzymes. See phenols below. Remember that when enzymes are used therapeutically, they must be taken one hour before eating or two hours after. There are several therapeutic enzyme products on the market. We will discuss just a few.

WOBENZYME N

Wobenzyme N is an enzyme product by Douglas laboratories that helps reduce inflammation in the body when taken on an empty stomach; otherwise, it helps food digestion. It is only sold in pill form. They are small pills, but if your child will not take a pill, you can crush it up and put into a small amount of beverage. Test for dosages and spread them out through the day. It is sold at most healthfood stores and online at many sites such as www.amazon.com and www.pureformulas.com.

SERRAPEPTASE

Serrapeptase is an enzyme product that has been studied extensively and is also shown to assist with inflammation. The inflammation can be anywhere in the body such as the gut or a joint injury. It can be found at www.crohns.net.

VIRASTOP

Virastop is an enzyme product made by Enzymedica. It is made with eight high-potency protease enzymes that are combined specifically to assist elimination of proteins in the bloodstream and aid the immune system. When used away from food, protease enzymes target the film covering of viruses that are made of protein. This breaks down the parasite and destroys it. Research has shown that these protease enzymes also break down other pathogens in the bloodstream, such as fungi from Candida, bacteria, and other parasites. Virastop is made from plant based enzymes with no fillers. It can be found in some healthfood stores and online at www.amazon.com and www.pureformulas.com.

CANDEX

Candex is an enzyme product used to break down the cell walls of yeast. Because the cell is destroyed, it does not have a slow death where it releases die-off toxins; therefore, there is no die-off reaction to the individual. I have found this product to be a helpful adjunct to the Candida cleanse products discussed in the chapter on pathogenic microbes; however, I have not found it to fully destroy Candida on its own. Candex is sold in many healthfood stores and at online stores such as www.brainchildnutritionals.com, www.amazon.com, and www.pureformulas.com.

MUCOSTOP

Mucostop, by Enzymedica, is extremely helpful anytime there is a problem with excessive mucus, especially during or after a head cold. It leaves you feeling naturally balanced, not dried up and uncomfortable as over-the-counter medications do.

PREBIOTICS AND PROBIOTICS

Probiotics are anything that increases the positive or "friendly" bacteria in the gastrointestinal tract. Probiotics will assist in replenishing the constantly-affected bacterial levels of the gut. They also help to crowd out the "bad" bacteria.

We all carry bacteria in our gastrointestinal tract, sometimes called intestinal flora. Some of the bacteria are "good" or "friendly" and some of it is "bad" or "unfriendly." When there is an imbalance in the intestinal system anywhere, there is usually an overgrowth of the bad bacteria, also known as Candida or yeast.

Stress, the use of antibiotics, vaccinations, and poor diet—especially one high in refined sugars and carbohydrates—will cause an overgrowth of bad bacteria. They become toxic to the entire body via the bloodstream and disrupt everything from internal organs to the brain. Often, behavioral issues stem from Candida overgrowth, along with intestinal problems.

GETTING RID OF THE BAD AND BUILDING THE GOOD

This is one of the most important steps in healing not only your child's gut but his overall being as well. Up to 80% of the immune system is built in the gastrointestinal tract. Without health here and with inflammation and malabsorption, it is the source of immune deficiencies, distorted detoxification pathways, improper brain function and development, behavioral and cognitive problems, inflammatory bowel disease, and more.

The first step in rebuilding the GI tract is through the use of prebiotics and probiotics. Prebiotics are a source of food for the good bacteria, the probiotics. They help the environment in the gut so that the probiotics can flourish.

My absolute top choice in probiotics is Dr. Ohhira's OMX sold by Essential Formulas. They contain both prebiotics and probiotics. Not many products contain both in one like Dr. Ohhira's does. While the probiotics were being fermented, they created their own food, the prebiotics, and they were encapsulated together. This enables the probiotics to be much more efficient in the gut after ingestion.

Dr. Lichiroh Ohhira, Ph.D. is an award-winning microbiologist and scientist from Okayama University in Japan. There are two different formulas: original and professional, and which one you choose is a personal choice depending on the individual. They both carry 12 carefully selected strains of bacterium, and both contain prebiotics and probiotics in each capsule with their own food supply of organic acids, enzymes, and bacteria. This includes micronutrient vitamins and minerals and amino acid byproducts.

Their "original" formula has a three-year natural fermentation process. Each capsule of the original formula has 900 million bacteria count or colony forming units (CFUs) per capsule.

The "professional" formula has a five-year fermentation process. Each capsule of the professional formula holds 600 million CFUs. It may seem odd that the professional formula has less CFUs, but the main value is in the organic acids. The professional formula has stronger organic acids which are better for chronic illnesses and have faster results.

Other probiotic products taken in the billions can create an autoimmune reaction in individuals who have an autoimmune disorder. The body may attribute too many organisms as an invasion and see it as a threat, and this could cause a negative immune reaction. The professional formula is great for those who need to stimulate their immune response without causing this autoimmune reaction. Since autism falls into the category of autoimmune disorders, the professional formula is often a better choice for our children. The lower CFUs in Dr. Ohhira's products will not cause this immune reponse to happen; this is why I feel safe with Dr. Ohhira's products.

Sometimes supplemental strains can worsen an imbalance in the gut. Scientific studies have shown that Dr. Ohhira's probiotics demonstrate the ability to cohere in the digestive tract. The five-year fermentation process maximizes its properties and allows only the strongest bacteria to survive.

Either the original or the professional formula will be beneficial in repopulating the good bacteria to crowd out the bad. They will also help create good digestion and pH. The company will send free samples, so that you can try each and see which seems to work best for your child.

Dr. Ohhira's probiotics also have a proprietary strain called TH10. This has the capability of breaking down the biofilm coating on the cells of yeast. Biofilm is a protective coating that surrounds many of the microorganisms in the gut that we are trying to eradicate. Not all probiotic supplements have TH10, and therefore, this capability. If the biofilm is not broken down, the yeast can hibernate and stay protected.

The fermentation process allows the bacteria to stabilize, so no refrigeration is required of these products. This makes them easy to take while traveling. They are 100% vegetarian, hypoallergenic, and contain no dairy or gluten. They are all natural and non-GMO.

Dr. Ohhira's probiotic package says that it contains fermented soy. I spoke with the company about any possibilities for allergic response. They explained that the soybeans used in fermentation are pre-digested and structurally modified to reduce or eliminate any reaction to soy. At the end of the fermentation process, the body does not recognize it as the same protein because the protein no longer has the same molecular structure. Therefore, the body does not see this as soy and will not have an allergic reaction to it.

Dr. Ohhira's probiotics come as a small softgel. If your child will not take any pill form, then just puncture the softgel and squeeze the product out into a small beverage. The taste is benign, so it easily mixes in without notice. These products can be found in most healthfood stores and for a good price at www.crohns.net.

HLC MINDLINX

HLC Mindlinx contains specific strains of lactobacillus crispatus and lactobacillus rhamnosus that have been proven in scientific trials to degrade wheat and dairy exorphins and to attach to and colonize intestinal epithelial cells. Mindlinx is made by a company called Pharmax that has an impeccable reputation.

Mindlinx is an essential product to assist in both gut healing and the breakdown of gluten and casein. It has been discussed in detail in the chapter on the gut and brain connection.

PROBIOTICS VS. ANTIBIOTICS

Antibiotics are non-specific to what they will kill, so the good is destroyed along with the bad. When taking them during antibiotic use, take the probiotic away from the medication to keep some good bacteria around.

With the use of antibiotics, it is important to regulate bowel movements. If diarrhea arises, then it is wise to begin probiotic use while taking the antibiotics. Probiotics should be taken throughout the course of antibiotic treatment anyway to insure growth of good bacteria along the way. Antibiotics will destroy and deplete your good flora weakening your gut, immune system, and more.

It is very important that you take probiotics at least two or more hours away from the antibiotic so they don't cancel each other out. The antibiotic will eventually kill most of the good bacteria in your gut, but at least you will be keeping some of the good numbers up for protection.

For children up to adult weight, one capsule of Dr. Ohhira's professional formula per day should maintain some balance. Teens and adults at adult weight may need two per day.

POST ANTIBIOTIC TREATMENT

Whether or not you have taken probiotics during the course of antibiotics, it is essential to rebuild the good flora. Probiotics should be used along with antibiotics. People hear to the contrary because the two can cancel each other out. This is true if they are taken too close to one another. To avoid conflict, take the probiotics at least three hours away from the antibiotics.

The importance of taking probiotics along with the antibiotics is to keep some balance in the gut along the way. The antibiotics will kill both the good and the bad. It is important to keep the numbers of the good flora up with the probiotics. This assists the immune system, prevents leaky gut, and more. Rebuilding the good bacteria as quickly as possible is important because our immune system begins there, as well as our ability to absorb nutrition from the foods we eat. When numbers of good bacteria get low, pathogenic microbes such as bacteria and viruses, and fungi such as Candida can get out of control. This not only ffects the body but the brain and behavior too.

Many people think that if they eat yogurt every day that it will do this for them. Yogurt will not build up the numbers of good bacteria to where they need to be. Besides, most commercial yogurt is pasteurized to the point where most of the good bacteria have been destroyed. It often contains sugars and often food dye as well.

After antibiotics are finished, it is a good idea to continue with a replenishing program. When rebuilding, take a higher, therapeutic dose and treat like you would for Candida cleansing. For children up to adult weight, one capsule of Dr. Ohhira's professional formula once per day may be enough. If you notice they are still yeasty after a week, increase the dosage by one more per day. Symptoms to look for are increased behavioral issues, any digestive issues including stomach ache, and a strong smelling, soft serve yogurt-looking stool. Too many probiotic capsules may cause diarrhea. If this happens at two per day, back off to one per day. Too much too soon may also cause a die-off reaction. See the chapter on the diet or Candida cleansing for more about die-off.

When I was rebuilding my own flora after antibiotic use and parasites, I was taking five professional formula capsules twice per day for two to three weeks before I backed off to two per day for a week, then one twice per day for maintenance. Always let symptoms be your guide. It usually takes a month or more to rebuild the good flora, so be patient.

Muscle testing is a great way to learn dosage needs. (Muscle testing is talked about at length another chapter.) After a month go back to the maintenance dose of one in the morning and one in the evening. If the child is young, they may only need one per day. This is the same protocol that is used for a Candida or yeast overgrowth. Watch for any signs that the professional formula is too much for them. Signs to look for are abnormal bowel movements (diarrhea) or energy levels, and immune system and behavioral changes. You can always switch to the original formula and see if it feels better.

An adult post-antibiotic dose or Candida cleanse dose is five capsules twice a day. Some people take them at this dosage for up to a month before going back to the maintenance dose. It is safe. I only suggest less if it is working well so you will save on expense.

Spray supplements are very absorbable since they go straight into the bloodstream. For spraying follow the directions on the bottle. Protein foods interfere with the product, so it is recommended not to eat them for 15 minutes before and 30 to 45 minutes after spraying. Slowly work up to 8 sprays, 2 times per day along with Dr. Ohhira's probiotics for an additional boost if you like. This is also great for non-pill takers.

If there is a particularly high amount of stress in your own life or your child's, or if a cold or flu are beginning, it is wise to increase the number of capsules taken daily from one or more, depending on their weight. If I feel like I am catching a cold or flu, I will take up to 5 twice a day for several days until all symptoms have disappeared before dropping back to the maintenance dose.

Candida imbalance will not go away and never return. This is where you learn to watch for the signs of irritability and digestive disturbances. Another time to increase dosages for a few days is after a birthday party or occasion where sugary and trigger foods have been eaten. One day can throw a sensitive person back off balance. Not to worry. Muscle test for dosage needs for Biogard spray or Dr. Ohhira's probiotics. Muscle test and use needed dosages every day until you are back to your maintenance dose, and symptoms have disappeared. You will learn along the way what is needed and when.

Note: Dr. Ohirra's probiotics are great for when you are traveling because they do not require refrigeration as most probiotic formulas do. There are many therapeutic uses of Dr. Ohhira's probiotics such as healing leaky gut, food allergies, parasites or Candida issues. Dr. Ohhirra's probiotics can be found in most quality healthfood stores or at www.crohns.net (877)240-7528, for a good price. This website also has additional educational information on these products. Essential Formulas is the company that distributes Dr. Ohhira's probiotics. They have been very helpful answering my questions over the years. They can be reached at (972)255-3918.

MAINTENANCE WITH PROBIOTICS

It is beneficial to take probiotic supplements every day to keep the good bacteria thriving. Our systems are constantly fighting against some sort of toxic stress. The probiotics will help keep the friendly bacteria plentiful, therefore strengthening the immune system.

Everyone in my family takes a maintenance dose of two Dr. Ohhira's probiotic supplements every day—once in the morning and once in the evening. The dosages are increased if the need arises, such as when someone has eaten higher sugar content foods, if anyone is not feeling well, or if there has been an increase in stress, etc.

Tip: probiotics are most helpful when taken away from food. Don't worry, if you need to hide them in food or in a beverage, they will still work.

I would also like to add that Pharmax, the company that makes the probiotic product HLC Mindlinx that we spoke of earlier, also has very high quality general probiotics.

NON-PILL TAKERS AND INFANTS

Probiotics rebuild the "good" bacteria that have been destroyed by toxic exposure, viruses, bacteria, improper diet, and stress. One company that has a specific probiotic for infants is Pharmax. They have a product called HLC neonate that has been used in extensive studies and n proven safe and effective. This is sold at quality healthfood stores or at www.pureformulas.com.

Dr. Ohhira's small capsules are easy to swallow if you have a pill taker, but for infants, just puncture a capsule and squeeze it onto your fingertip. The company recommends the original formula for infants. Most babies will suck it off of your finger easily. One capsule per day should be enough. It is likely that you may only need to do this from one to three days with an infant. It varies depending on their age and degree of symptoms.

If the baby is breastfeeding and the mother is taking the product, the baby will get the probiotics through mother's milk. Essential Formulas is the company that makes this product. They are very knowledgeable and friendly. It would be best to ask them for recommendations since every case is different. They can be reached at www.essentialformulas.com, or call (972)255-3918.

Most probiotics are capsulated powder forms that can be opened up or gel caps that can be easily punctured and squeezed into a food or beverages. They are fairly tasteless, like enzymes.

OMEGA-3 FATTY ACIDS

The essential fatty acids derived from omega-3 oils are DHA (docosahexaenoic acid) and EPA (eicosapentaenoic acid). They are called essential because the body cannot make them on its own. Whereas DHA helps to build and protect the brain, EPA helps with the functioning of the brain. We need both.

Omega-3 oils are necessary for proper function of the brain, nervous system, and visual function among others. They also help reduce inflammation in the brain and the body. This is helpful in healing the gut, thereby improving the immune system. Besides reducing inflammation, omega-3 fatty acids also down regulate cortisol and increase thyroid hormone transfer to the brain.

The American Psychiatric Association endorses fish oil for use in psychiatric illness.

Several studies show the improvement in intelligence and behavior from higher consumption of omega-3 fats. Growing evidence also shows that low levels of omega-3 fatty acids are associated with hyperactivity in children. Omega-3s are known to improve social engagement and eye contact.

A study done by Dr. Gordon bell at Stirling University in Scotland showed two-thirds of children with autism showed a deficiency in omega-3 fatty acids. When the diet is supplemented with omega-3 fats, parents report less aggression, irritability, and hyperactivity, and improved sleep.

The essential fatty acid, DHA, makes up over 60% of brain and nerve tissue in the body and constitutes roughly 40% of the brain. DHA is necessary for the wiring of the brain, its connections and for the stimulation of neurotransmitters (messengers responsible for connections to and from the brain).

Decreased levels of DHA have shown the decrease in cognitive ability and behavior. DHA has also been shown to decrease inflammation in a part of the brain called the hippocampus which effects memory and learning.

The neurotransmitters most effected by omega-3 fatty acids are dopamine, affecting motivation and drive, and serotonin, a neurotransmitter that is important in sleep, mood, and appetite. This is also why omega-3s are significant when used in treating depression, anxiety, violent and aggressive behavior, and even schizophrenia. Omega-3 fatty acids help these two important neurotransmitters bind to their needed receptors.

It has been found that vaccinations stimulate an ongoing immune system response in the body and in the brain. Immune activation of this sort can induce depression. Omega-3 fats have been found to reduce depression and support overall mood (Watanabe s, Kanada s, et al. Physiol. Behav. 2004; 81:605-13).

DHA protects the brain by strengthening the mitochondria that creates energy production in cells and improves the health of the cell membrane improving brain connections. They assist in bringing the supply of serotonin to the brain and directly prevent penetration of excitotoxins (chemicals that improperly excite the brain and make it toxic).

Another incredibly important aspect of DHA is that it can actually reduce damage to the brain. DHA is absolutely necessary in the development of the neurological system of the unborn child, the developing child, the adult, and the elderly. Unfortunately, we are not getting enough of DHA in our diets today. It is transferred to an infant through breast milk, so the mother must be sure that she is taking a high quality omega-3 supplement to increase levels in both herself and her child.

DHA also reverses insulin resistance, therefore reducing the risk of diabetes, and reduces stomach fat. It activates cell receptors called peroxisome proliferator-activated receptors (PPAR's), which are beneficial in the treatment and prevention of diabetes. PPAR's are also known to heal the gut.

Our main source of these important essential fatty acids comes from deep-sea fish and crustaceans called krill. We can get a small amount from flaxseed oil and walnuts, but these non-fish sources, called alpha linolenic acid, require a conversion to take place in the body. Only about 1% is actually converted to DHA; not nearly enough for our body's daily needs.

The American diet is all too plentiful in omega-6 fats which greatly limit the body's ability to convert the alpha linolenic acid to DHA by inhibiting the enzyme necessary to do so. Omega-6 fats are obtained from such foods as corn oil, safflower oil, sunflower oil, peanut oil, canola oil and soybeans. Not only do these oils promote inflammation and suppress the immune system, but the omega-6 fats come in and compete with the omega-3 fats. Unfortunately, the omega-6 fats win and the omega-3s get pushed out and are lost from the body, therefore leaving you even more depleted and creating a downward spiral.

We must be careful that the fish we eat is not contaminated with heavy metals such as mercury or other pollutants that will only make existing problems worse. The larger the fish, the higher it is on the food chain, and the more mercury and pollution it may have in its meat. As an example, swordfish is known to contain the highest amounts of mercury. Wild, non-farmed smaller fish such as sardines, mackerel, herring, and trout contain the least amount of toxins and higher levels of omega-3s.

Grass fed cattle and game will have greater concentrations of omega-3 fatty acids in their meat because they graze on grasses, berries, and plants that contain omega-3 fatty acids. Enhanced brands of omega-3 eggs can now also be purchased. American women have 40% less omega-3 fish oils in their diets than European women do. One possible reason may be that Europeans eat more organ meats than do Americans. Today, it is rare to find an American eating beef or chicken liver. Americans also eat more omega-6 fats than Europeans, which further depletes the system of omega-3 fats.

Sea plankton is another good source of omega 3 fatty acids from a plant source. A good organic, non-GMO product can be found at www.newearthsuperfoods.com.

An interesting additional note is that recent research has concluded that when supplementing with omega-3 fatty acids, there was twice as much improvement found in girls than in boys. It is likely that this comes from the female body's need to store omega-3 fats for their childbearing years, as well as for building their brains. Females also have higher levels of estrogen which protects the brain.

- Some physical signs of fatty acid deficiency are:
- Excessive thirst
- Frequent urination
- Dry skin
- Dry hair
- Brittle nails
- Dandruff
- Rough, dry or bumpy skin

KRILL OIL

A lesser known product that contains omega-3 fatty acids in a much more absorbable form than fish oil is krill. After researching what I offer you below, I tried the product for myself. I had been taking quality fish oil supplements for many years. When I first began taking krill oil, I noticed a huge jump in energy and alertness, and it also regulated my digestive system.

Krill are a shrimp-like crustacean found in ocean waters. You may recall that they are the main food source for whales. We are now learning that krill is superior to regular fish oil for humans due to its absorption ability.

Krill has all the benefits of fish oil and a lot more. It contains all the benefits of DHA and EPA but is more absorptive due to its phospholipid structure. The fats in our cells (including our brain) are in phospholipid structure, which means that the fatty acids have the same chemical make-up as the cells in our body, so the krill is more bioavailable. Due to this increased absorption, it means that you can take less to get the same benefits. Remember that the brain is 60% fat.

Krill contains phospholipids which are able to directly enter the body's cells. They are a "gatekeeper" that decides which chemicals get to enter the cells and which do not. Aluminum is a heavy metal commonly found in children on the autism spectrum, and it is known to weaken and destroy this phospholipid structure, therefore weakening our body's ability to protect the brain.

Krill also contains phosphotidyl choline, which is important in brain development. This is crucial for pregnant or nursing moms. Phosphotidyl choline is a precursor for the neurotransmitter acetylcholine, which assists in the transportation of messages to and from the brain. Acetylcholine also plays a strong role in memory, cognition, and mood, including depression.

Along with all of the original benefits of omega-3 fatty acids, krill is helpful with ADHD, lowering cholesterol, balancing blood sugar, autism, dyspraxia, aggression, depression, anxiety, dyslexia, cognition, and helpful in reducing inflammation and pain.

Krill is also full of antioxidants. Krill feed on a type of algae called phytoplankton that give them a vital source of nutrients. Krill contain vitamins A, E, and D, and a carotenoid compound called astaxanthin. Astaxanthin protects cell membranes from oxidative damage by penetrating the membrane or wall of the cell, so it is neuro-protective, which means it protects the brain. Astaxanthin also assists the cardiovascular system, increases immune function and immune response, increases insulin resistance, and indirectly assists the liver.

These antioxidants rate at 378 to 431 on the ORAC scale (oxygen radical absorption capacity). This measures how antioxidants really perform their job.

Fish oil rates at an 8 on the ORAC scale. These antioxidants help prevent the oils from getting rancid so they last longer and is the reason krill keeps its potency longer than fish oil, has no fishy taste, and does not leave us burping up the taste of fish.

WE ARE REALLY TAKING THEM FOR OMEGA-3s

In comparison, fish oils contain their omega-3s in a less stable triglyceride form that is different from the body's natural state. A conversion needs to take place during digestion so that the acids in fish oil can be absorbed by cells. In those with a less than optimal working GI tract this assimilation may not fully take place and many of the important ingredients are lost.

One study at The University of California at Berkeley showed that krill oil, with its phospholipid structure, markedly outperformed omega-3 fatty acids from fish oil in its triglyceride form.

Studies have found that krill oil is completely safe at any dose with no fishy after taste. It is more stable, so there is less possibility for it to go rancid like other oils. Krill are at the bottom of the food chain, so it has very little potential for contaminants such as mercury or PCB toxins.

CHECK FOR QUALITY AND DOSAGE

After researching and personal trial I would recommend the supplement Captain's Krill Oil oil over other krill oil supplements and over fish oil supplements for your omega-3 fatty acid requirements. Here's why:

Due to krill's incredible absorption rate, you can take less to get the same benefits of fish oil. The Oxygen Radical Absorptance Capacity (ORAC) shows krill oil's antioxidant value to be 48 times higher than fish oil. Only half the dosage of krill oil was needed to get the same results from the same amount of fish oil.

Whenever there is something new drawing the attention of the public eye—and wallet—we find many companies jumping on the band wagon to get a product on the market. This is happening with krill oil. It is crucial that our kids get the very best products available and not a cheaper, less potent substitute. This is especially true when it comes to omega-3 fatty acids, which have an incredible effect on their brain, their mood and their overall health and energy. Always check for artificial dyes and colors.

The best krill oil product is not by the company that was the first one to get a product on the market. Also, beware of the company that claims to be the best, or even have the best selling product. When you really research a product, the truth can be found. There is a website called www.aprovenyou.com. These people call themselves "the geeks" and research everything they look into at the deepest level. When researching krill, I found them extremely helpful. There are a lot of krill oil products coming out now, and all make strong claims, but I wanted the truth.

As I dug deeper, I found that the others had tested rancid or had lowered potency. Some of those companies advertise higher potency. If there is not an adequate amount of phospholipids in the product, it will not offer the needed results. Lower prices can also mean less active ingredients. For a full blown explanation from the geeks see their website. To save you the time, I will tell you that the only one I would choose is Captain's Krill oil. Captain's krill oil's freshness, purity, and price make it the best choice.

DOSAGES

We mentioned that krill oil is about 50% more potent than fish oil. This is when there is an adequate amount of phospholipids and astaxanthin. What this means is that you don't have to take as much krill oil to get the same benefits as fish oil. Absorptive factors vary per individual due to age and state of health. Some studies have found effectiveness at one-half to one-third that of fish oil.

Krill oil supplements should contain at least 40% phospholipids, a high enough amount of astaxanthin, and at least 150 mg EPA and 90 mg DHA in one pill.

The typical dose is one to three softgels per day. They can be punctured and squeezed into any food or beverage. Higher doses are recommended for the first 14 to 30 days, and then lower slightly. For example, if you are taking two pills initially, then lower to one pill after the initial time period. Most health professionals recommend one gram of krill up to ten years of age for the proper results. One capsule of Captain's Krill Oil contains 300 mg omega-3s, 150 mg EPA, 90 mg DHA, 420 mg phospholipids, and 2.5 mg astaxanthin. Remember, you do not need to refrigerate Captain's Krill Oil.

The best places to purchase are either www.amazon.com or www.stillsmilin.com. I buy mine from www.stillsmilin.com. They offered a reduced trial price that was significant. When you purchase, you become an autoship customer, which means that every 30 days they will automatically send you another bottle. This is how they keep their prices down. You can cancel at anytime with no questions asked.

Watch for changes in behavior, energy levels, and mood. Remember that natural supplements can take a few weeks for some people to notice differences.

There still seems to be uncertainty about the possible allergic reaction for those with shellfish allergies because krill is a type of crustacean. For now, it is advised not to take krill if you have this known allergy. If there is concern of a shellfish allergy, the next best choice is taking a fish oil supplement for your omega-3 needs.

For studies on krill oil, go to:

www.aprovenyou.com/wp/krill-oil/krill-oil-vs-fish-oil-what-the-science-says.

OMEGA-3 FATTY ACIDS FROM FISH OIL

The old days of taking fish oil supplements that taste awful and leave us burping them up all day are gone. Choosing the right essential fatty acid will make it easy to take. Some are even strawberry or orange flavored. If you find yourself burping up a fishy taste, then the oils are probably rancid.

DHA provides most of the developmental and protective benefits of omega-3 fatty acids. For this reason, children on the autism spectrum or those with behavioral or learning difficulties, benefit more from taking a supplement with higher DHA than EPA, but we do need both. EPA assists in the functioning of the brain.

One study done with 90 children ages 7 to 12 showed that children with ADHD have lower tissue levels of both EPA and DHA than children without ADHD. The study found that, "An increased red blood cell level of DHA was associated with improved reading and lowered parent ratings of oppositional behavior."

In a subgroup of 17 children with learning difficulties, "Increased DHA was associated with lower parent ratings of oppositional behavior, hyperactivity, restlessness, and other ADHD symptoms." (Milte CM, et al. "Eicosapentaenoic and docosahexaenoic acids, cognition, and behavior in children with attention-deficit/hyperactivity disorder: a randomized controlled trial." Nutrition, 2012; Jun; 28(6):670-7.)

EPA (not DHA) can act as a blood thinner, so if one is on blood-thinning medication, has issues with coagulation, or anticipates surgery, it is important to consult a physician before taking it. Many people take omega-3s to assist their cardiovascular system because of the blood thinning properties and the anti-inflammatory effects. Omega-3s also help with hypertension by lowering blood pressure. If you already take blood pressure medication, it is likely that it is a blood thinning agent. I like to take omega-3s before I get on an airplane to avoid any possible clotting effects from sitting for long periods of time.

QUALITY OMEGA-3 OILS ONLY

There are a few companies that make omega-3 supplements that have the highest quality and no after taste. They now come in many forms such as liquid, small soft gel capsules, or chewable. Most importantly, purchase from a company that follows the highest standards when it comes to removing any traces of toxins, such as heavy metals such as mercury, polychlorinated biphenyls (PCB), or other impurities from their sources.

If you want to choose an omega-3 in fish oil form instead of krill oil, there are a couple of companies that follow rigorous standards for purity and quality. Do not try and save yourself money when it comes to supplements, especially omega-3 fatty acids. Buy quality products and be sure to keep them refrigerated. Oils turn rancid if they are not refrigerated. Due to DHA being polyunsaturated, it is a good idea to take it with some vitamin E to add antioxidants. Always take them with food for best absorption.

Harvard University used Nordic Naturals Pro-Omega supplement for a study on bipolar disorder. They know how important omega-3s are in mental health and mood, and they must have also known of the high quality behind this company and their products.

Nordic Naturals has a product called Pro-DHA that has a greater concentration of DHA to EPA ratio, which is often best for children with additional needs. The Nordic Naturals Omega-3 Juniors smell like strawberries on the outside and are fine for those who will swallow small pills; however, when bitten into they taste like fish. I'm sure it was for this reason that another product was released by Nordic Naturals in a "gummy" form. These are called Nordic Omega-3 Fishies. They are the only ones I could get my daughter to eat before she would swallow pills (pills have higher dosages). You must give a high enough dosage to maintain benefits. Nordic Natural products are available for purchase in most healthfood stores or online for a good price at www.crohns.net, and www.pureformulas.com.

Pharmax is another company with the highest quality standards for their products. They have a liquid form, high DHA fish oil formula that comes in a base of essential oil of orange. It actually tastes like oranges. This makes it easy to add to juices, especially orange juice. Be sure to keep this and all oil-based supplements in the refrigerator. Pharmax is sold in most quality healthfood stores and at many online stores such as www.pureformulas.com.

DOSAGES

Check with your healthcare provider regarding your child's needs. Due to the nature of an individual's biology and size, dosages will vary. Most studies conclude needing 500 to 1,000 mg per day of omega-3 fatty acids (combined DHA and EPA) to improve symptoms. These are often adult dosages, which usually refers to anyone over the age of 12.

Children with special needs often require more than the general sugested dosage used for a child. I was told by a pediatric neurologist at the Amen Clinic (see the chapter, "Supporting the Brain"), that my son needed to take up to 2,000 mg per day to gain the results we were looking for. Jacob was an average-sized 15-year-old at the time. When in doubt, check with your health practitioner for individual needs.

Be sure to check the label to know how many milligrams are in one pill or one teaspoon. Sometimes they will give a dosage, but it will be for two or three pills. You may have to give more of them to get the required amount ingested. If chewable are easiest, but the dosage of each is extremely low, you can give your child as many as needed to provide the desired amount. In this case, it may prove more cost effective to try a liquid form.

It is important to be sure that your child is getting enough of these essential fatty acids. It's easier to use a supplement that carries the complete amount needed in one pill rather than having to give your child five of something unless you need the doses split up over the course of the day. It is best to avoid giving omega-3s in the evening, as they are known to increase energy (not hyperactive energy) and may effect sleeping.

The following recommendations are the minimal daily dosages established by the International Society for the Study of Fatty Acids and Lipids (ISSFAL).

- Infants (1 to 18 months, 0 to 15 lbs): 32 mg per pound.
- Children (1.5 to 15 years): 15 mg per pound
- Adults: 500 mg (With a minimum of 220 mg EPA and 220 mg DHA)
- Pregnant and lactating women: 300 mg DHA per day.

VEGETARIAN OMEGA-3S

For vegetarians looking for an omega-3 supplement, there is one made by the same Dr. Ohhira who makes the quality probiotics I talk about. This omega-3 supplement is called Essential Formulas Ohhira Vegetarian Living Oils. It is made from seed and plants, all non-GMO. These contain EPA, DHA, vitamin E, antioxidants, and micronutrients. They are a balance of omega oils 3, 6, and 9, with a ratio of 4:1:1. They are available at healthfood stores and at www.crohns.net. More information is available at this website.

Chia seeds are another source of omega 3 fatty acids with about eight times more omega 3's than salmon. They are also loaded with antioxidants and fiber.

Note: If you are not vegetarian, it would be best to take the fish oil or krill oil supplements. In order for flaxseed oil to be converted to EPA and DHA, you need an enzyme called delta-desaturase. Many children with ASD lack enzymes already, so it is likely that this commonly decreased enzyme will not be available in their system. If insulin levels are high, this enzyme may also be inhibited. Also, as mentioned above, the conversion is limited.

ADDITIONAL INFLAMMATION FIGHTERS TO KNOW ABOUT

It is more than likely that your child's gut is inflamed. This inflammation can spread in the body to areas such as the brain. Hormonal imbalances also create inflammation in the body. Some of the many safe and effective drug-free supplements that can help with inflammation are:

BIOPURE PROPOLIS VAPORIZERS

Propolis is a resin-like substance made by bees. It contains flavonoids that are strong anti-inflammatory agents. They can be taken as a supplement, but when the vapors are inhaled, they quickly enter cells via the bloodstream. Due to the different regions bees travel, propolis can vary in its constitution. The company, Bee Family Farms, www.beefamilyfarms.com, is certified to contain the necessary active flavonoids in their propolis. They also carry a variety of portable vaporizer to choose from.

INTESTIMEND

Intestimend is a liquid product that contains sulfur to help strengthen the intestines and the immune system. This can assist in reducing inflammation. It is sold at online stores, including www.brainchildnutritionals.com and www.pureformulas.com.

WOBENZYME N

Wobenzyme N is one of the best supplements available for the reduction of inflammation. It is enteric-coated so that it makes its way through the stomach to the small intestine for better absorption. Developed over 30 years ago, it is now distributed by Garden of Life for Douglas Labs. It is available to purchase at most healthfood stores and many online sites such as www.crohns.net, www.pureformulas.com, and www.amazon.com. It comes in a small tablet form. If crushed, it will loose the enteric coating but will still be beneficial.

SERRAPEPTASE

Serrapeptase is a proteolytic enzyme that aids digestion and is used for all types of inflammation.

CURCUMIN (TURMERIC)

Turmeric contains curcumin. It is an herbal antioxidant that is a strong natural anti-inflammatory and it is good for your brain. Dosages of 500 to 1500 mg per day have been known to be helpful.

QUERCETIN

Quercetin is natural anti-histamine and is excellent for allergic reactions. I have had personal success with it many times. I have used it for poison oak and a jellyfish sting, too. It is also helpful with asthma and general inflammation reduction.

VITAMIN D

Vitamin D is anti-inflammatory, among its many other benefits. Take this fat-soluble vitamin with food, especially other good fats. Dinner is a good meal to include vitamin D.

GAMMA GLOBULIN

Gamma globulin is used in cases of extreme immune dysfunction and those with digestive and intestinal issues. It is known to be especially helpful for those with recurrent or ongoing infection in the gut.

Processed from IgG antibodies, these large molecules cannot be absorbed so they stay in the gastrointestinal tract. An oral powder form is now available. Check with you healthcare practitioner.

SUMMARY

Children with autism often have chronic inflammation. This breaks down multiple systems of the body including the immune system, and it impacts the brain's ability to function normally. Inflammation breaks down the brain's main protective system known as the blood-brain barrier. Inflammation can kill brain cells.

Children with autism often have gut inflammation. It is the common source to many of their neurological issues. If you choose, testing can be done to know the degree of gut inflammation, but many moms already know this to be apparent. There are many natural products that assist in reducing inflammation in the body, and healing the gut. The digestive system must be healed in order to prevent further inflammation to the brain. Enzymes have many beneficial uses when healing the body, assisting with digestion, and reducing inflammation. Probiotics rebuild the good bacteria in the digestive tract, therefore building the immune system and reducing inflammation. Omega 3 fatty acids help with proper function of the nervous system, the brain and help to reduce inflammation. Additional supplements that are helpful are vitamin D3, vitamin E, milk thistle seed, curcumin (turmeric), quercetin, bromelain, and licorice root. Licorice root is also helpful for the adrenal glands.

The products found in this chapter can be found at http://naturallyhealingautism.com/a-healthy-home/

CHAPTER 12

DANGEROUS FOOD ADDITIVES

Read your labels, and know what to look for. Our foods today are poisoned routinely by large manufacturing companies that choose to add ingredients that are chemical in nature. Many of these foods actually make us crave more food. They also contain sugars and toxins that will invade the central nervous system. This means your child's brain! We are exposed to many more chemicals in our foods than our parents and grandparents were.

EXCITOTOXINS

Excitotoxins are toxins that will excite the neurons in your brain. They can also be referred to as neurotoxins because they damage and destroy the brain and spinal cord. What most people do not realize is that these toxins are in the foods they commonly eaten every day. The problem with these toxins is that they will excite brain cells to death. They literally die. This causes the brain to secrete glutamate and aspartate (excitotoxins), which cause negative behavioral changes. This can cause faulty wiring of the brain, especially during its developmental stage.

Children on the autism spectrum and with ADHD are particularly sensitive to these chemicals because their detoxification systems are not as capable as others to handle them. It is also vital to protect their brains from any further harm.

Those who are particularly sensitive and should not consume these products are children, babies, and pregnant women, and also those with depression, migraine headaches, heart issues, any nervous system disorder, kidney problems, or vascular disease. Remember that all of us are susceptible to harm by these toxins, not just those with an existing neurological condition or a compromised immune system. The elderly are also quite susceptible to these dangers.

WHAT IS GLUTAMATE?

Glutamate is an amino acid and a neurotransmitter for the brain. It helps stimulate brain cells, which help neurons to communicate. It all sounds good until it is too much of a good thing. When these neurons get over-excited, it can cause seizures and even kill brain cells.

The brain has a normal control system that regulates the amount of glutamate released in the brain. Protein carrier molecules bind with the glutamate in the brain and help keep it safely stored until it is needed. This system is delicate and susceptible to breaking down. Even microscopic amounts of glutamate can trigger excitotoxicity or death of brain cells. In large quantities, glutamate increases the production of free radicals, causing greater injury to the brain, blood vessels, and the blood-brain barrier. It can also cause oxygen deficiency in the brain.

When other forces, such as foods with added excitotoxins, or hypoglycemia (low blood sugar) come into play, the glutamate system can become overwhelmed. Infants and children are extremely susceptible to this system becoming impaired because their brain is still developing and their protective blood-brain barrier is not yet intact. Glutamate can easily pass through the placenta and enter the bloodstream of the fetus during pregnancy.

Mercury is a heavy metal known to inhibit the protective protein carrier molecules, therefore, causing excitotoxicity. Mercury interferes with this system as long as it is in the brain, and this destructive process can go on for many years. Glutamate is intricately involved in the formation of brain circuitry so the accumulation of glutamate causes mis-wiring of the brain.

The results of mis-wiring can be subtle and include poor cognitive abilities, memory trouble, or an inability to control anger. Sensory-processing disorders increase when glutamate activates certain genes. These genes affect the nervous system's ability to adapt to changes in stimuli. Learning, absorbing, and analyzing information can become difficult or impossible. The effects on the brain vary per individual based on biology. In more extreme cases, the child ends up with Asperger's syndrome or autism.

Excitotoxins can be found in ingredients of monosodium glutamate (MSG), aspartate or aspartame (artificial sweeteners such as Nutrasweet), hydrolyzed vegetable protein (cysteine), and aspartic acid. Two common foods that increase glutamate levels in the body are tomato's, and soy products, especially soy milk. Soy milk is hydrolyzed, therefore increasing the level of free glutamate.

MONOSODIUM GLUTAMATE (MSG)

Used as a flavor enhancer or artificial flavor, the most commonly used excitotoxin in our food is monosodium glutamate, also known as MSG. It is cheap to use and it will fool your brain into thinking that the food tastes better than it does. Food manufacturers and restaurants know and like this.

The USDA has defined MSG as "naturally occurring," so it is allowed in our food and is regarded by them as safe. Do not be fooled by this. MSG is known to cause behavioral problems, and worse yet, MSG excites neurotransmitters (the brain's messengers). As I mentioned before, these nerve cells become so excited that they are excited to death, and the effects begin in as little as 15 minutes after ingestion.

MSG also negatively affects neurotransmitter levels. There can be up to an 80% drop in acetylcholine, which is involved in learning and memory. It is also known to greatly reduce norepinephrine, which is involved in attention and focus.

Children are four times more susceptible to the dangers of MSG and aspartame than adults are (Neurotoxicology 2 (1980), Olney, Excitatory Neurotoxins as Food Additives.) There is a fine tuned pruning process that occurs in the brain during development. Glutamate and aspartate affect this process and can cause faulty wiring of the brain and its functioning. Low blood sugar, or hypoglycemia, can trigger glutamate levels to rise and cause negative behavioral changes. Aggressive behavior, loss of emotional control, and hyperactivity are common symptoms. One study done using glutamate and aspartate on mice showed extreme damage to the cells of the retina, affecting vision. The younger the animal, the worse the damage is.

We have mentioned that the part of the brain called the hypothalamus has no blood-brain barrier. It also has the highest number of glutamate receptors. This is especially important during puberty because the hypothalamus controls the endocrine system throughout the body. Through this system, the brain regulates growth, metabolism, and the onset of puberty. Damage from MSG to this part of the brain in a newborn causes an extreme deficiency of the immune system that can last their entire lifetime. Glutamate will bind with aluminum and increase its absorption in both the bloodstream and the brain.

The hypothalamus uses glutamate as a neurotransmitter. Excess glutamate causes excitotoxicity destroying brain cells. MSG can also affect the adrenal glands. The hypothalamus is involved in emotion, learning, and memory.

Biological changes from glutamate levels may include problems with the endocrine system, leading to reproductive problems, hypothyroidism, and weak adrenal glands.

Damage to the hypothalamus via excitotoxins can lead to:

- The lack of growth hormone excreted by the hypothalamus causing stunted growth
- Early onset puberty
- Reproductive problems
- Trouble producing breast milk following birth
- Thyroid trouble
- Weak adrenal glands
- Obesity
- Anger
- Cognitive problems
- Poor memory
- Asperger's syndrome
- Autism

ANGER, LEARNING PROBLEMS, AND OBESITY

It is noticeable in today's society how much more aggressive people have become. We already stated that MSG affects the hypothalamus, which affects hormones. Due to the rise in hormonal activity during puberty, the effects of MSG are heightened, and can increase episodes of anger and rage.

The combination of heavy metal toxicity, processed foods, and excitotoxins all play an integral role. Federal data and research concluded in a 2013 report from the Center for Disease Control (CDC), "Mental Health Surveillance Among Children," that up to 1 in 5 American youth, an estimated 7 million to 12 million, experience a mental health disorder each year. The CDC reports that this rate is increasing. The ability to learn, maintain proper behavior, and cope with emotions affects 13% to 20% of youths under the age of 18. The estimated cost to families and society is $247 billion a year in treatment, special education, juvenile justice, and decreased productivity.

According to The American Academy of Child and Adolescent Psychiatry, only 21% of these children receive treatment due to a shortage in pediatric subspecialists and child and adolescent psychiatrists.

A boy about the age of eight was seated near me on an airplane once. I heard the parents telling the stewardess that he had just been diagnosed with autism. The boy seemed to be doing fine. After take-off his parents asked the stewardess to open up a can of food they had brought for him. He began eating his can of spaghetti with "o" shaped pasta and within minutes he started rocking back and forth convulsively. To please him, the parents opened up a green lollipop and handed it to him. His symptoms now were almost uncontrollable. The difference in this boy from his food intake was shockingly obvious to me, but I do not think his parents even made the connection. Read your labels and know what to look for. The more education you have regarding nutrition do's and do not's, the better off your child will be in both health and behavior.

Obesity is also on the rise. Glutamate affects the hypothalamus, which affects the endocrine system. In studies done on mice, those exposed to MSG were consistently extremely obese. They also had stunted growth, and all had trouble with sexual reproduction. Obesity from excitotoxins is not food driven, this is why so many people have trouble losing weight. It is actually a problem with brain function, largely the hypothalamus.

MSG contributes to metabolic syndrome. This occurs when the metabolism and insulin levels become imbalanced. This can lead to type II diabetes, especially in young people. It is one more reason why MSG contributes to obesity.

Some food establishments will advertise in their window or on the menu that they do not use MSG. Other places use it all the time without giving this knowledge to the general public. Unfortunately, the majority of the general public has little to no awareness of the dangers of using MSG. Now that you do, remember to ask. Be aware that they may also tell you that they do not add MSG, but it may be contained in the sauces and other products that they purchase.

It is also possible that they do not *add* MSG to their preparation, but their purchased ingredients do contain it. If you notice that your child shows symptoms such as hyperactivity, fatigue, headache, stomach ache, or anything else after eating at a particular restaurant, it is best to avoid the establishment in the future.

Restaurants routinely add MSG as a flavor enhancer. Ask your server if MSG is used in their food. If they do not know, ask them to find the manager for you. Some places will remove it if you ask, but if you don't they think it's just fine to give it to you. It is also used in most of the foods sold in grocery stores. I myself was surprised when I looked at the label of my son's favorite ranch salad dressing and found it contained MSG.

Remember that the health of the consumer is not the main interest of food manufacturers. What they want is for you to like their product and buy more so they can make more money.

See Leptin resistance in Chapter 11 for more information regarding obesity.

FOOD LABELING

Due to the growth of public knowledge regarding the dangers of MSG food manufacturers have become quite clever when it comes to ingredient labels. The ingredient is often masked under a different name.

COMMON HIDDEN SOURCES OF MSG

The following may contain enough MSG to serve as common reaction triggers. Take this list with you to the grocery store.

Some of the hidden sources of MSG on ingredient labels to look for:

- Anything ending in "ate" is bad, such as glutamate
- Glutamic acid
- Yeast foods and extracts
- Autolyzed ingredients, such as autolyzed yeast extract
- Hydrolyzed ingredients
- Calcium caseinate
- Sodium caseinate
- Textured proteins, such as textured vegetable protein (TVP)
- Natrium glutamate (natrium is Latin/German for sodium)
- Gelatin

OTHER POSSIBLE SOURCES OF MSG:

These ingredients often contain MSG, but not always:

- Carageenan
- Malt extracts and flavorings
- Maltodextrin

Take this list with you to the grocery store. Ask if so called "fresh" products contain MSG or anything else they know of. Often fresh-cut deli meats from the grocery store will contain MSG. It is hidden in foods you may not have guessed it would be in, including salad dressings, condiments, and sauces.

The following may contain enough MSG to serve as common MSG reaction triggers and glutamate in general.

- Glutamate
- Glutamic acid
- Monosodium glutamate
- Monopotassium glutamate
- Yeast extract
- Yeast food
- Yeast nutrient
- Autolyzed yeast
- Autolyzed yeast extract
- Torula yeast
- Autolyzed soy protein (any protein that is autolyzed)
- Any protein that is hydrolyzed (such as whey, pea, or corn)
- Hydrolyzed vegetable proteins
- Calcium caseinate
- Protein isolate

Another interesting fact is that ovaries contain glutamate receptors, so the ingestion of glutamate or MSG may increase chances of ovarian cancer. This is due to MSG creating free radical damage to tissues.

SUPPLEMENTS THAT BLOCK OR REDUCE EXCITOTOXICITY

Supplements that are known to block excitotoxicity are vitamin B12, ginkgo biloba, grape seed extract, and pycnogenol. Supplements that reduce excitotoxicity are alpha lipoic acid, CoQ10, acetyl L-carnitine, creatine, and all of the B vitamins.

ASPARTAME/ASPARTATE

Aspartate is another neurotransmitter normally used by the brain. It can become a neurotoxin in the same way glutamate can, and it is the main component in the artificial sweetener aspartame. It is ironic that so many people trying to lose weight will drink diet sodas containing aspartame. Obesity caused by excitotoxins does not depend on food intake. Aspartate and glutamate cause the same damage to the hypothalamus that lead to obesity. That diet soda is actually contributing to your weight problem, and it's killing your brain.

Aspartame and aspartate cause the same excitotoxicity damage to the brain as glutamate. In addition, aspartame is known to raise levels of the neurotransmitter phenylalanine in the hypothalamus and other parts of the brain. This can contribute toward many behavioral disorders including schizophrenia and seizures. Aspartame can also cause depression.

Phenylalanine causes the release of norepinephrine and dopamine, which control the release of the pituitary hormones. Noted are:

- Growth hormone
- Thyroid stimulating hormone
- Luteinizing hormone: essential for reproduction in both males and females
- Vasopressin: affects the brain's response to stress, regulation of aggression, social behavior and sexual behavior
- Prolactin: stimulates the production of breast milk, strengthens the myelin for the central nervous system, regulates the immune system
- Oxytocin: regulates neurotransmitters in the central nervous system, is responsible for the ability to bond to another as in maternal bonding, trust, and empathy, also social recognition, and regulating anxiety

Note: The toxic affects of excitotoxins is multiplied when more than one exist in the diet. Often the ingredients glutamate, aspartate, aspartame, and hydrolyzed vegetable protein are used with two or more together.

BABY FOODS MAY CONTAIN THESE INGREDIENTS!

Infant formulas often contain high levels of free glutamate. Of special concern are soy-based formulas, and those that contain casein hydrosolates which come from cow's milk. Due to their effects on the hypothalamus, the emotional center, and the amygdala, where our brain senses fear, we see behavioral problems, especially anger. Soy is covered in more detail in chapter 17, allergies and the gut/brain connection.

WHAT PROTECTS THE BRAIN FROM EXCITOTOXICITY?

Beyond good nutrition the following assist in blocking excitotoxicity, therefore helping to prevent its damaging effects:

- Magnesium: an absolute necessity (as magnesium lactate or gluconate and foods rich in this such as broccoli and spinach)
- Calcium pyruvate
- Zinc
- L-leucine: a branched amino acid that promotes the glutamate inactivating enzyme, glutamate dehydrogenase (GDH).
- Antioxidants: especially vitamins C and E
- Glutathione or anything that increases it
- CoQ10/ubiquinol together with niacinamide protects the brain from excitotoxicity
- Pyridoxine (vitamin B6); reduces glutamate in both the blood and the brain
- All B vitamins, especially methylcobalamin (B12)
- Grape seed extract
- Alpha lipoic acid
- The essential fatty acid DHA directly blocks excitotoxicity
- PQQ (pyrroloquinoline quinine)

ARTIFICIAL FOOD COLORINGS

Although the Food and Drug Administration (FDA) would lead us to believe that the amounts of artificial food colorings in many of our foods are safe, they are wrong. FD&C dyes are not safe. They are allowed to have a certain percentage of lead, mercury, arsenic, benzidine, and more because they were too hard to remove, so they said it was acceptable to contain some. The FDA themselves have told us that lead damages the brain. As we have seen in the chapter on heavy metals, no amount of these toxins are safe.

Today, we have five times the exposure to food dyes as our grandparents did. In 2009, almost 20 million pounds of coloring were certified as acceptable by the FDA. Although natural food colorings such as beta-carotene could be used, it is cheaper to use the synthetic ingredients, even though they are dangerous. Once again, money comes before health. The money will be spent in the future on health issues created by these chemicals.

These artificial colors make food look more appealing to the eye. They also cover up spoilage issues such as poor flavor and color. They are used in everything from cosmetics to cereal and soda—and they come with a price.

- Blue #2: It has been known for years to cause brain tumors called gliomas. Glial tumors account for one third of all brain tumors.
- Red #2: The most commonly used dye, shows increased immune system tumors, hypersensitivity to allergic reactions and triggers hyperactivity. It is known to cause urinary bladder tumors.
- Red #3: In 1990, the FDA noted as a thyroid carcinogen and banned it from use in cosmetics and topical drugs, but it is still allowed in candy, baked goods, and oral medications.
- Green #3: known to cause urinary bladder tumors.
- Yellow #5 (tartrazine): a derivative of coal-tar. This yellow food coloring is associated with asthma, hyperactivity, and behavioral problems in children.

- Yellow #6: known to create adrenal tumors and hypersensitivity reactions. Hypersensitivity can be to external stimuli such as light and noise or internal moodiness such as irritability or depression.

FD&C colors in medications are allowed to contain double the amount of lead as food colorings. Sadly, these medications are being taken by people who are already sick, and therefore with weak immune systems.

Always read your labels. It is surprising what foods contain these toxic chemicals. They are often not where you would expect them to be. Eat only natural foods. There are many natural foods to choose from with color. Green vegetables, white cauliflower, green and red apples, yellow and red pears, red beets and strawberries, blueberries, and more. Shopping at your local farmers market is your safest and best bet.

For additional information on artificial food colorings, go to www.feingold.org.

SUMMARY

Many foods today contain dangerous chemicals, natural or added, that can create behavioral disorders, cause tumors, and even destroy brain cells. Children on the autism spectrum are more susceptible to the potential damage to the neurological system from these toxins due to weakened defenses in immunity and detoxification processes. It is important to educate yourself as to what these chemicals are so that you are able to find them on food labels. They are often well disguised by food manufacturers.

To increase your knowledge further there is also extensive information on some websites such as www.feingold.com.

It is best to avoid these toxins completely, but if ingestion occurs there are supplements that can help protect against their dangers.

The products found in this chapter can be found at http://naturallyhealingautism.com/a-healthy-home/

CHAPTER 13

ENVIRONMENTAL TOXINS

Our families are the most important thing in the worlds to us. We must educate ourselves in order to protect them. There are many environmental toxins that we live in and around. Studies are coming out regarding their safety, or lack thereof, but most people are either unaware of the dangers or disregard the warnings rather than give up conveniences. Autism has many contributors, but there are specific ones among them that most people use daily. These toxins affect the neurological systems of fetuses and children at an even greater rate than they do adults.

Allergies to food are more often thought about, but environmental allergies are just as common and as dangerous. Fatigue, headaches, anxiety, depression, and many more symptoms are linked to environmental toxins.

Remember that your SRT or N.A.E.T. practitioner (see the chapter on alternative therapies), can desensitize for an allergy to many of the below toxins. Strengthening detoxification in the system and heavy metal detoxification are all important. Each is covered in this book.

I found a homeopathic remedy called Enviroprotect that reduces the symptoms and addresses the causes of environmental toxins in the body. It is made by Apexenergetics. Most natural health practitioners carry this in their offices or are happy to order it for you. I have found this product to be immensely helpful. It comes in a liquid with a dropper for easy use, and can be carried in your purse for use as needed.

The liver is the detoxifying organ and is always in need of support. We have discussed this in its own chapter. Bioray makes a product called Liver Life that is very helpful for the health of the liver. It is sold at most healthfood stores and online at many sites such as www.pureformulas.com. These products can be purchased at www.naturallyhealingautism.com under "healthy home products."

Toxins are cumulative. Yes, small amounts over time build up and cause disease. Precautions can be made to detoxify the body or prevent them in the first place. Due to the nature of biology, each of us can tolerate different loads of toxins. These factors include our body's ability to detoxify, health of DNA, repair enzymes, amounts or toxins absorbed, strength of cellular enzymes, age, genetic inheritance, possible pre-existing diseases, the number of toxins we are exposed to at different or concurring times, and the overall strength of the immune system.

The list of the top ten chemicals in consumer products that are suspected to contribute to autism developed by The Children's Environmental Health Center are:

- lead
- methylmercury
- polychlorinated biphenyl (PCB's)
- organophosphate pesticides
- organochlorine pesticides
- endocrine disruptors
- automotive exhaust
- polycyclic aromatic hydrocarbons
- brominated flame retardants
- perfluorinated compounds

For information on environmental toxins in your food, air, and home go to, www.ewg.org.

PESTICIDES

There are over 3,000 chemical additives that can be found in our food. Many of these chemicals are known to be dangerous to our health.

It is important to know what our children are eating, since they are even more vulnerable than adults. A growing fetus is most susceptible.

Pesticides are found in most foods, so we do our best to eat organically. But what about the pesticides that are in the air we breathe? One study found that the closer pregnant mothers were to organophosphate pesticide applications, the greater the incidence of autism. (Eric Roberts "Maternal Residence Near Agricultural Pesticide Applications and Autism Spectrum Disorders Among Children in the California Central Valley", www.markschauss.com.)

The counties most implicated were Fresno, Imperial, Kings, and Tulare counties in California. The top three pesticides implicated were organochlorine pesticides, endosulfan used in tomato processing, lettuce, alfalfa and cotton, and dicofol used on cotton, oranges, beans, and walnuts. The pesticides become airborne and are inhaled. The closer the pregnant woman lives to the source, the more likely her child will be born with autism.

Beware of schools located near agricultural fields that are sprayed with pesticides. Contact your state governor and senator and any local figure of influence to, at least, not have any spraying done during school hours, although many pesticides are in the air for days after they are sprayed. If your child is in a school near a known agricultural field that uses pesticides, then the best solution is to change schools to one in a safer location.

ELECTROMAGNETIC FIELD POLLUTION (EMFs)

I looked into the effects of electromagnetic field radiation many years ago. I knew they had to be harmful. When I started writing this book, I spent more time behind a computer than I ever imagined I would. My son happens to be a tech head, too. I wanted to protect my family. We do not have to be on computers all day long to be bombarded by the negative effects of EMF. We can be out in a serene desert or in the mountains and we are still affected by satellites and cell phone tower radiation.

Pregnant women need to be especially careful since studies have shown that since the bones of a fetus and those of young children, including the cranial bones that surround the brain, are much thinner; this allows them to absorb twice as much radiation as an adult. (Wang and Fujiwara March 2003). Electromagnetic radiation (EMR) can easily penetrate their brain tissue.

There is no protective blood-brain barrier until six weeks after birth. When it has developed, EMR has the ability to damage it. Without the blood-brain barrier intact, toxins can easily enter the brain via the bloodstream causing damage to nerve tissue and neurotransmitters such as dopamine and serotonin. The cells of a fetus, and those of children, are also dividing at a rapid rate. This allows greater risk for damage from electromagnetic radiation (EMR).

Endotoxins are components of cell wall structure. They are broken down and released due to EMR. Endotoxins can cause both an immune system response and an inflammatory response, especially in the lungs. Related symptoms are fever, bacterial infections, increased blood pressure, and severe diarrhea.

Dr. Geronimo Rubio from the Rubio Cancer Center says, "Electromagnetic frequencies such as those from cell phones can alter genes and affect the DNA."

Studies from the Bioelectromagnetic Laboratory have shown EMF "increases the production of free radicals in animal brains which can lead to cancer, inflammation, heart disease, and other serious illnesses."

The voltage of a pregnant woman in her bedroom and of children in their bedrooms has been shown to be a predictor of autism and other neurological disorders. Molds are also known to increase the release of biotoxins by 600 times when in the presence of EMR pollution. For more studies and information go to www.klinghardtacademy.com.

The growth of beneficial bacteria is much slower when in the presence of electromagnetic field pollution. Metal dental fillings and orthodontic devices containing metal wires can act as antennae for EMF and lead to ADD, insomnia, aggressive behavior, problems with concentration, and even Parkinson's disease.

There are hundreds of studies on the negative effects of EMF pollution on the immune system, enzyme synthesis, nervous system, learning, mood, and behavioral patterns.

Years ago when I still had mercury amalgam fillings, I would notice that my teeth would hurt when I used a wireless phone. EMF pollution is likely the reason why. A new retainer for my teeth gave me headaches I had never experienced before. My allergy elimination practitioner told me to unplug the computer in the room I slept in because the wire in the retainer was acting as antennae. I unplugged all devices, including the modem. As soon as I did this, the headaches went away.

In her book, *Zapped*, Ann Louise Gittleman gives detailed information regarding the negative effects of electromagnetic field pollution. This common invasion to the system and can affect DNA.

WHAT CAN I DO TO PROTECT MY FAMILY?

Luckily, there are products to harmonize or neutralize EMF pollution. They will help to protect your family from the harmful effects of radiation. These are products that you can use ongoing on your phones, cars, household electrical appliances, and more.

Dr. Igor Smirnov, Ph.D. took many years of research and study to invent and design an electromagnetic radiation (EMR) shield that could neutralize the negative effects of EMR on the human body. The MRET-Shield (electromagnetic radiation optimum neutralizer) was patented in the US in April 2002.

Man-made EMF fields are structurally different than those found in nature. The electromagnetic fields our body's cells use to communicate are a subtle low frequency. The natural fields are random, noisy, and fluctuate in amplitude and waveform. The artificial EMF is regular and constant. These regular fields cause our cells to become stressed and create a series of biochemical reactions inside the cells.

Stress proteins harden the cell membrane and weaken its ability for active transport causing toxins and free radicals to build up inside the cells. Studies have shown that these free radicals cause leakage in the blood-brain barrier just after EMR exposure. This also interferes with the normal processes of DNA repair which leads to disease. Multiple experiments show these effects of EMR exposure are eliminated when EMR was removed.

The MRET-Shield creates an "optimal random field" or "noise field" that neutralizes the exposure on a biological level. This is able to happen without causing any disruption to your cell phone's transmittance.

In 2008, Dr. Smirnov developed the MRET-Shield into a nylon polymer material that can be easily applied to any electromagnetic field device such as cell phones, electronic appliances, fabrics, and even accessories that can be worn on the body such as jewelry.

When in the presence of electromagnetic radiation, it puts out low frequencies that resemble the same frequency of living cells in the body. This neutralizes the harmful effects of any electromagnetic field. The MRET-Shield needs no outside power source as it is activated by the electromagnetic field itself.

The company Gia Wellness has taken the technology of MRET one step further by combining an additional technology called ERT, a technology that is proprietary to Gia. The ERT has been added for dual action.

While MRET technology decreases the effects of electromagnetic pollution, ERT strengthens the body's ability to restore natural communication and resist stressors. It supports energetic body functions and communication of the biofield. It is an additional technology backed by studies from independent researchers and has been peer reviewed.

Distribution rights for the MRET-Shield Technology for many countries have been licensed to Gia Wellness. To save money, you can sign up as a distributor and get the products at the wholesale price, which is 30% off retail price. I wear the pendant on a necklace around my neck (it can also be put into a pocket). I use the cell guards on every family member's phone, and have the universal guards in our cars, on the microwave, refrigerator, TVs, toaster, hair dryer, and computers. I also have the home harmonizers plugged into certain outlets throughout our home.

Although they offer cell chips to put on your cell phones, they now recommend the universal guard for all smart phones because they are more like mini computers. There is also an air tube headset that allows you to talk on your phone hands free and does not allow the EMF radiation to transmit through the air tube as it does with most other hands-free devices. For more information on ERT or to purchase Gia products, go to www.giawellness.com/karenthomas.

Information and studies on Dr. Smirnov's MRET technology can be found at www.gqusa.com.

HELPFUL TIPS:

- Purchase a gauss meter to detect EMR fields. There are many sites available to purchase them including www.amazon.com. I was surprised to find that the microwave in our kitchen emitted radiation eight feet away.
- When talking on a cell phone in the car, crack the window to help dissipate the EMR radiation.
- Keep nightlights at least six feet from the bed.
- Move your bed 3 to 6 feet away from electrical outlets.
- Turn off electrical and wireless devices in the room when sleeping.
- Never use an electric blanket.
- Remember, EMR emissions come through walls. When an electrical device is on in another room, the EMR penetrates through the wall. Anyone on the other side will be getting that radiation.
- Computers give off the majority of their EMR from their back side. In a classroom or office, a person is affected more by the computer behind them.
- Texting is safer than calling because you do not hold the phone up to your head.
- Use a safe air tube headset (sold at Gia Wellness) with phones and always use a Gia cell chip.
- Never keep the phone directly against your body when turned on. People like to put them in their pockets over their heart or on top of their reproductive area on a belt loop or in a front pant pocket.
- Never use a Bluetooth headset that hangs on your ear next to your brain.
- Petition to have cell towers moved away from schools. To locate cell towers, go to www.antennasearch.com.

Paul J. Rosch, MD, Clinical Professor of Medicine and Psychiatry, New York Medical College; Honorary Vice President International Stress Management Association; Diplomat, National Board of Medical Examiners, Full Member Russian Academy of Medical Sciences; Fellow The Royal Society of Medicine; Emeritus Member, The Bioelectromagnetics Society says,

> "It is not generally appreciated that there is a cumulative effect and that talking on a cell phone for just an hour a day for ten years can add up to 1,0000 watts of radiation. That's ten times more than from putting your head in a microwave oven. Pregnant women may also be at increased risk based on a study showing that children born to mothers who used a cell phone just two or three times a day during pregnancy showed a dramatic increase in hyperactivity and other behavioral and emotional problems. And for the 30% of children who had also used a cell phone by age 7, the incidence of behavioral problems was 80% higher! Whether ontogeny (embryonic development) recapitulates phylogeny is debatable, but it is clear that lower forms of life are also much more sensitive."

Martin Blank, PhD, Associate Professor, Department of Physiology and Cellular Biophysics, Columbia University, College of Physicians and Surgeons; Researcher in Bioelectromagnetics; Author of the BioInitiative Report's section on Stress Proteins says,

> "Cells in the body react to EMF's as potentially harmful, just like to other environmental toxins, including heavy metals, and toxic chemicals. The DNA in living cells recognizes electromagnetic fields at very low levels of exposure; and produces a biochemical stress response. The scientific evidence tells us that our safety standards are inadequate and that we must protect ourselves from exposure to EMF due to power lines, cell phones and the like, or risk the known consequences. The science is very strong and we should sit up and pay attention."

For more information from experts go to:
www.electromagnetichealth.org.

Let's admit that we all use devices daily that can harm ourselves and our children such as cell phones, wired and wireless devices, automobiles, TV, refrigerators, hair dryers, and microwaves. We spend an average of 540 hours in our cars each year. We put hair dryers directly up to our heads and we talk on phones, and whether wired or not, they are hazardous to our health. Also, be particularly aware of radiation exposure on airplanes. The scary part is that all of this is far more dangerous for our children and unborn babies.

WATER SOURCES

Research has detected at least 11 chemical compounds from prescription drugs, antibiotics, hormones, heavy metals, and chlorine in drinking water. There are chemicals that are not filtered through our "trusty" municipal water sources, and they end up in the faucets in our homes. Along with these chemicals, there are disease-causing bacteria, some of which comes from your own household pipes. These drugs, antibiotics, and other toxic chemicals enter our bodies every time we drink unfiltered water or bathe in it.

We know the dangers of drugs and other chemicals, especially on a compromised immune system, but most do not realize the dangers of chlorine. Chlorine (bleach) is one of the chemicals added by your city's water company that is used to "clean" our water. Currently, many cities have begun adding ammonia to the water to make the chlorine "stretch" further. This way they do not have to use as much chlorine because it is more expensive. The downside is that ammonia is another poison to the human body.

Chlorine kills good bacteria in the gut. While we are trying our best to build up the good flora in our kids, we do not want to unknowingly killing them on a daily basis. In addition to drinking water, the water that we bathe and shower in can be just as dangerous, if not more. In a hot bath or shower, the vapors can directly enter the respiratory system, carrying harmful bacteria and toxins. The skin is also the body's largest organ. When the skin heats up, the pores open and allow greater absorption of anything it comes in contact with, including harmful chemicals.

Heavy metals often remain in our water sources or are added to them. Aluminum sulfate is used to treat public water, and is extremely toxic to the brain. Lead is another commonly found heavy metal in drinking water that affects DNA cell function, muscle control, and memory. If you have old lead pipes, you can be sure you are ingesting lead from that water. If you have newer PVC pipes, they may still have joints made from lead. Lead easily crosses the blood-brain barrier, especially in children, and is associated with aggressive behavior, anxiety, and poor learning and memory.

In most cities, the American Dental Association has convinced them to put the neurotoxin fluoride into your drinking water. They will tell you how lucky you are to have it and most people believe that, unless they have been educated to the dangers of this heavy metal (see the chapter on heavy metals). Fluoride increases the absorption of lead. The water passes through pipes, pulling lead along with it, and then once in your body it helps the lead absorb into your tissues, including your brain tissue. A child with autism is even more susceptible to the damaging neurological effects of lead.

There is controversy regarding the removal of minerals during reverse osmosis and distillation. To avoid concern, add quality minerals to it. One product to help with this is liquid Vital Minerals from www.herbprod.com, 831-688-8706. It is a concentrate of Inland Marine Minerals containing approximately 84 ionic minerals, most as essential trace minerals found in human blood and plasma.

Another choice for quality water without the dangers of contaminants is to purchase a high quality water filter. Many products do not properly remove all of the drugs, heavy metals, chlorine, or dangerous bacteria from the water. Sante For Health is a company that makes some of the best water filters available. Their filters are in multiple layers, including carbon. Carbon is needed to filter drugs and further purify the water. Unlike some of the other companies that claim their products work and charge a fortune for them, Sante's filters actually do what they say they will and are very reasonably priced.

Sante offer a large selection to fit your needs. There are filters commonly used by those on well water, filters for city water, above counter and under the counter alkalizing filters, radiation removing filters, and more. Sante's filters can be used at the point of entry on the main house water system or can be individually placed on shower heads, bath nozzles, or faucets. They won't change your water pressure and are easy to install. For more information, go to www.santeforhealth.com, or call 800-398-6735.

DIBILITATING DISEASE BLAMED ON BACTERIA-INFESTED SHOWER HEADS

There is an under-diagnosed, but increasingly common pulmonary disease called non-tuberculous mycobacterium complex. Common symptoms include excessive coughing that will not go away. The primary means of infection comes from shower heads. In one study, over 30% of shower heads harbored disease-causing bacteria. We are more susceptible to ingestion in the shower because harmful bacteria can directly enter our respiratory system. This disease commonly affects healthy individuals, so those with compromised immune systems beware.

RADIATION

The earthquake in Fukushima, Japan in April of 2011 released radiation into the oceans that is traveling the globe. It is estimated that the United States will have that radiation in their groundwater by the year 2015. It will make its way into food, public water sources, and wells. There are often other radioactive contaminants in our environment that we are not aware of.

WATER BOTTLES, TOYS, CARPET, AND MORE

Ken Cook, President of the Environmental Working Group, spoke to a senate subcommittee in January, 2013, regarding ten American newborns that had been found to have more than 200 synthetic chemicals in their blood. Among these chemicals were flame retardants, lead, stain removers, and pesticides.

Fetuses, infants, and young children are most susceptible to harm because their immune systems are not yet fully developed, and they are unable to detoxify properly. Once we saw birth defects and cancer, today we see reproductive development and disorders, diabetes, heart problems, asthma, autism, multiple learning disorders, and obesity. These toxins are endocrine disruptors which imbalance hormones, but they also are disruptors of the digestive system. They are known to increase bad bacteria in the gut. The number of chemicals has risen to over 84,000, but the EPA has only required testing on about 200. Some of the most harmful are:

Bisphenol A (BPA) is a chemical found in plastics, such as drinking bottles, baby bottles, toys, dental sealants, and the linings of food cans. Receipts are often coated in plastic which is absorbed into the skin as a toxin.

BPA is one of the most dangerous chemicals. Most diseases are linked to BPA's and phthalates (see below). They disrupt the health of the GI tract, cause asthma and autoimmune disorders. Note: probiotics lower blood levels of BPA. See chapter 11, for more information on probiotics.

Polyvinylchloride (PVC) is another potentially harmful compound that may also contain **polychlorinated biphenyl (PCBs)** which are synthetic, organic chemicals. PVC is commonly found in toys, vinyl flooring, countertops, and shower curtains. You can now purchase a shower curtain that says "Contains no PVC." They both also contain a toxic compound called phthalates.

Research shows the nursing child ingests about fifty times the daily amount of the synthetic, organic compound polychlorinated biphenyl (PCB) of adults. Both PCB and PVC are known to disrupt the hormonal system, and are linked to premature puberty, asthma, allergies, irregular menstrual cycles, breast cancer, and prostate cancer. One study done in 2009 found that those who lived in homes with vinyl floors were twice as likely to have a child with autism.

Endocrine disrupting chemicals (EDCs) are especially dangerous to a growing fetus. Mothers exposed to EDCs produce more testosterone, which can result in over-masculinity of the male brain. In the developing brain of a fetus, estrogen has the opposite effect and is non-feminizing or masculinizing. The best cellular detoxifier is glutathione. See more on glutathione in the chapter on basic nutrition.

The recycle numbers found on water bottles are an indicator of the compounds of which they are made. In general, #1, #3, #6, and

#7 are all products we do not want to use because they are potentially toxic. When these plastics heat up, as a water bottle may do in the car on a hot day, or when the cases are awaiting distribution in a lot or warehouse, the toxins are quickly released into the water or beverage. PCBs, #7, are the worst when heated. (Remember, unlucky number 7.) It is the one used to make plastic baby bottles. These are the same bottles most people put warm formula or warm breast milk into and feed to their infants and small children.

Do not store food in plastic containers. It is uncertain if the newer BPA free plastics still contain harmful chemicals. There are plenty of glass options that come with air-tight lids. Never heat food in plastic containers or on plastic plates, especially in the microwave. Beware of microwavable paper plates that have a thin plastic coating.

Drink from either stainless steel or glass. Glass is best, but there is the potential danger of an infant breaking a glass baby bottle. The company, Lifefactory now makes a glass bottle that has an outer encasing of plastic for better gripping and protection from breakage. These bottles can be found in most healthfood stores today and at www.amazon.com. "Kanteen" baby bottles made by Klean canteen are a nice option for stainless steel. They are available at many stores and online sites, including www.amazon.com.

PFCs (polyfluorinated chemicals) are known to be toxic and are used in the coatings of nonstick cookware, stain repellants in carpeting and clothing, and grease-proof paper used in the linings of packaging for certain food items such as popcorn bags.

Flame retardants, including PBDEs are found in mattresses (including crib mattresses), automobiles, carpeting, textiles, plastics and electronics. PBDEs are easily released from their product due to a lack of chemical bonding. The hands of babies who crawl on floors pick up the dust, which they then put into their mouths causing them to ingest the toxins. Mattresses emit chemicals inhaled. Newer items may not contain as much but beware of old foam or old carpeting.

PBDEs interfere with thyroid function, disrupt neurological development, cause reproductive problems, and cause cancer. There is a proposal to revise the 1975 flammability law in 2014 due to the increased knowledge of the dangers involved.

Although studies have shown that the chemicals do little to alter fires, the global flame retardant market is a financial powerhouse. In 2008, it was worth $4.1 billion with a growth expectation of $6.1 billion in 2014. Millions are spent lobbying and research distorted to keep these chemicals in use. If the proposal is met, the manufacturers would carry a "TB-117-2013" tag on July 1, 2014.

The dust and fiber from these products is easily separated from them, and they are easy to inhale. To help avoid contamination, wipe floors and countertops clean with a damp cloth to adhere to the dust and use a HEPA filter in your vacuum.

Nonylphenols, including nonylphenol ethoxylates

These chemicals are used in laundry detergents, shampoos, household cleaners, and latex paints. NPs have been detected in human breast milk, blood, and urine. They have been shown to adversely affect reproductive and developmental health in rodents. Safe alternative choices can be found at most health food stores.

Phthalates

These chemicals are extremely dangerous to the neurological system, thyroid function and are even known to cause cancer. Testosterone is needed for proper neurological development and is suppressed by phthalates. They are found in vinyl shower curtains, vinyl flooring, and toys, lotions, cosmetics, fragrances, nail polish, air fresheners and household cleaning products, and in recycled material #3.

Some products now will label themselves "phthalate free," although you are much safer purchasing your products at a health food store or via an search online at www.ewg.org. Manufacturers are not required to list phthalates on their labels. Often you will see the word "fragrance" listed. This is usually a mixture of chemicals that contain phthalates.

As a rule, I avoid anything that is scented. Laundry detergents contain strong perfumes, and after you wash your clothes, they touch your skin and are inhaled all day and night. If you really love scents, look for pure essential oils, and be sure to muscle test your child for them. Even though they are natural, they can cause allergies in ultra-sensitive kids. When in doubt, purchase from a quality health food store and have a conversation with the owner about the contents if necessary.

Phthalates have been implicated in lower sperm quality in men, fetal changes in males, and shorter pregnancies. Hauser, R., P. Williams, et al. (2005). "Evidence of Interaction between Polychlorinated Biphenyls and Phthalates in Relation to Human Sperm Motility." Environmental Health Perspectives 113(4): 425-430.

Frederiksen, H., N. Skakkebaek, et al. (2007). "Metabolism of phthalates in humans." Mol Nutr Food Res 51: 899-911.

Assay, SM. et al (2003) The Relationship between Environmental Exposures to Phthalates and DNA Damage in Human Sperm Using the Neutral Comet Environmental Health Perspectives

McIntyre BS, Barlow NJ and Foster PMD, (2002) Male Rats Exposed to Linuron in Utero Exhibit Permanent Changes in Anogenital Distance, Nipple Retention, and Epididymal Malformations That Result in Subsequent Testicular Atrophy., Reproductive and Developmental Toxicology.

Unfortunately, many products do not have to be labeled. Below is a site that offers the safe guidelines and allows a search on most products safety.

There are many companies that sell non-toxic cleaning supplies today. Grapefruit seed extract is a safe and excellent disinfecting cleaning agent. Just add a few drops to water and clean. Quality health food stores carry them as do many online sites. To search for healthy options or to search for the safety guide to any product go to: www.ewg.org.

To avoid searching through the maze of products, to assure you safety, quality, and affordability of non-toxic and phthalate-free products I have information offered on my website at www.naturallyhealingautism.com listed under "my healthy home." They are some of my favorites that I use in my own home for my family's protection and safety.

HEALTH AND BEAUTY AIDS

A study in England showed that the average woman puts on about 515 synthetic chemicals on her body every day. Shampoos, lotions, soaps, and make-up commonly contain harmful chemicals, gluten, perfume, and FD&C colorings. Phthalates, sodium laurel sulfate, and propylene glycol are most common. It is always safer to purchase these products from a quality healthfood store, but I still recommend reading your labels to be on the safe side. These products are absorbed through skin or by inhalation. Those that use an alcohol-based hand sanitizer on a daily basis have been known to have higher levels of alcohol in their blood.

Remember that everything we put in and on our body during pregnancy and nursing is absorbed into both ourselves and our baby. The products we place on our skin absorbs and reaches our circulatory system within thirty seconds. There are many safe organic choices in shampoos, soaps, lotions, make-up and more at health food stores, but they tend to be expensive and hard to sift through to find ones we are assured to be safe. There are high quality, non-toxic, and affordable products for adults and children that can be found on my website at www.naturallyhealingautism.com under "my healthy home."

PHENOLICS

Phenolics are petroleum-based products that are found in plastics, and the dyes in leather goods such as clothing and furniture. They are contained in many health and hygiene products such as toothpastes, hair dyes, disinfectants, and medicines. Phenols are also naturally occurring in many foods. They are very common allergens, especially for a child with autism or one who is sensitive. Phenols sensitivity is common in people with poor methylation. We discuss these foods and their effect on behavior in chapter 10, "reducing inflammation."

It is possible to be desensitized to phenol compounds through natural allergy desensitization, (see the chapter on alternative therapies).

AIR POLLUTION

The Clean Air Task Force released a study in 2002 on air pollution affecting Americas' children that told us that due to their size, children absorb 50% more air pollution than adults do. Those who live next to freeways or in areas where crops are sprayed with pesticides are more likely to have a child born with developmental disorders.

Know where the crops are grown from the food you eat. If the crop stands next to a highway, it is likely to have far more toxins in it. The best way to assure yourself is to know your sources. Local farmers markets are your best bet. Get to know the growers, and ask a lot of questions. You will learn who you can trust.

Environmental Protection Agency (EPA) studies indicate indoor levels of pollutants are up to 10 times higher than outdoor levels. A 2013 EPA study found that 30 million homes in the US have significant indoor air quality issues.

A Biopure propolis vaporizer can be essential for removing pollutants from the air. Propolis is a resin-like composite derived from bees. When vaporized, propolis destroys pathogenic microbes and air pollutants. When inhaled, propolis quickly enters the cells via the bloodstream. One study showed a reduction in indoor air pollution from 15% to 70%.

The Biopure propolis vaporizer is all natural, free of chemicals, and eliminates mold, bacteria, and viruses. It is known to be anti-inflammatory, anti-bacterial, and anti-fungal. The vaporizer is small and can travel with you. There is even a car model that plugs into the 12-volt power source in your vehicle. More information can be found at www.beehealthyfarms.com. Also, see more information under "mold" in the chapter, Pathogenic Microbes.

RADON

Radon is a radioactive gas from the natural decay of uranium found in most soils. It is the second leading cause of lung cancer after cigarette smoking. It commonly builds up in homes, rising up through cracks in the foundation or other crevices. Any home is susceptible to radon build up. It is estimated that 1 in every 15 homes in the United

States have elevated levels of radon. For an EPA map of radon zones in the United States go to www.epa.gov/radon/zonemap.html.

Regardless of your zone, all homes should be tested. For a list of devices, professionals, and laboratories that are approved, see the website of the National Radon Safety Board, www.nrsb.org, (866)329-3474. Test kits for radon are available starting as low as $26.

Contact your state radon program http://www.epa.gov/radon/whereyoulive.html

HEAVY METALS

There are several heavy metal toxins, and all adversely affect the neurological system. For more detailed information, see the chapter on heavy metals. The following are five of the most common heavy metals and some common sources.

- Mercury: vaccines, old thermometers, cosmetic products, chemical plants, mercury amalgam dental fillings, large seafood such as swordfish, tuna, and shark.
- Aluminum: vaccines, cosmetic products, lotions, aluminum bakeware, cans, public water supplies, some fruit, processed cheese, processed tea, herbs, spices, aluminum utensils, and concrete.
- Lead: soil, cans, FD&C dyes, old paint, newsprint, ceramic glaze, and herbal products.
- Cadmium: cigarettes, PVC pipes, clear plastic wrap (never heat products in this), foods, especially leafy foods, fertilizers, dry cement, organ meats, and shellfish.
- Fluoride: in public water sources and dental hygiene products, tea, decaffeinated coffee, infant cereals, grape juice, and wine. Fluoride-free toothpaste can be found at most healthfood stores. I purchase Xyliwhite, a xylitol toothpaste made by the company NOW. It is sold in most healthfood stores and can be purchased online from www.pureformulas.com and www.swansonvitamins.com. They carry both cinnamon and strawberry flavors.

SUMMARY

There is an abundance of environmental toxins that we are all exposed to in our daily life. A growing fetus and children are most vulnerable to the health dangers of these compounds, especially their neurological damage.

Safer alternative choices can be made to reduce toxins in the home. Keeping the body's natural detoxification defenses strong helps to protect it from additional damage. Supplements and therapies can also assist in protecting us. Education about environmental toxins is necessary in order to protect our children as best we can.

The products found in this chapter can be found at http://naturallyhealingautism.com/a-healthy-home/

CHAPTER 14

HEAVY METALS

Heavy metals are simply toxic metals. They can damage and even destroy the brain, the central nervous system, weaken the GI tract and our antioxidant system, rendering us incapable of detoxification. They also reduce levels of neurotransmitters (the brain's messengers) in the brain.

Many conditions, including autism, have been shown to be the result of an undeveloped or damaged blood-brain barrier prior to the age of six months. The blood-brain barrier is just what it sounds like: a barrier that protects the brain from harmful material in the blood. A newborn is up to 55% more susceptible to the dangers of heavy metal toxicity than an adult. Heavy metals can also be passed from mom in utero to the baby via the placenta.

Each heavy metal affects specific areas of the brain but also overlap on some. For this reason, it is important to test for all of them when neurological toxicity is in question. Heavy metal toxins, like any toxin, affect every individual at a different level. Due to the nature of biology, we are all able to detoxify various amounts.

There are 100,000 new cases of autism every year in the United States, and the number is rising. One in every 50 families in America has a child with autism.

Many conditions affect the level of neurological damage. Most commonly noted for increased risk are the individual's nutritional status, age, and the dosage he received. Results can range from poor memory and trouble with focus to severe autism.

HOW DO HEAVY METALS GET INTO OUR BODIES?

Heavy metal toxins are found in the foods we eat, the air we breathe, the soil we play in, inside household cleaning products, shampoo, soap, lotion, toothpaste, water sources, food colorings and preservatives, the pots and pans we use to cook our food, the coffee and tea we enjoy with breakfast, chalk and paints, medications, toothpaste, mercury amalgam dental fillings, vaccines, and more.

The most common heavy metals are mercury, cadmium, lead, aluminum, and fluoride.

MERCURY

The extent of mercury damage to the brain and heart depends on age, sex, and genetic factors. Infants, children, and the elderly are the most at risk. Males are also higher risk due to testosterone increasing mercury's neurotoxicity.

For more than 80 years, medical doctors have observed symptoms for those exposed to even very low levels of mercury.

Symptoms of mercury toxicity are:

- Excessive irritability/anger
- Timid behavior
- Depression
- Weakness
- Delirium
- Insomnia
- Apathy
- Impaired concentration
- Poor memory
- Abnormal motor coordination
- Suicidal tendencies
- Personality changes
- Obsessive compulsive disorder

The symptoms of mercury toxicity mimic many of the symptoms of autism. Higher levels of mercury have been shown to create symptoms that last up to 30 years! It aggravates every other medical condition.

The World Health Organization (WHO) admits that there are no safe levels of mercury exposure. Common exposure comes from vaccines, medications, coal emissions, dental amalgam fillings, and contaminated fish. Even in small amounts, mercury is dangerous.

Toxicologists consider mercury to be one of the most poisonous elements in existence. Mercury destroys the brain, and is completely destructive to all aspects of the nervous system. It inhibits the brain's ability to uptake and store the neurotransmitters dopamine, serotonin, and norepinephrine.

Mercury can affect any organ and is poisonous to all cells. The building of proteins for the cells is called protein synthesis. Mercury not only damages cells, but interferes with protein synthesis, a common problem among children on the autism spectrum. Mercury has a powerful effect on the immune system [See: Pollard KM. et al Met. IonsBiolSys.34:421(1997)). Research shows that the vapors from mercury amalgam fillings in the mouth can degrade the strength of the immune system by half.

Mercury also binds with Candida to resist its removal from the system. Mercury prevents the body from killing Candida. It prevents a natural type of white blood cell called neutrophils from destroying Candida and other foreign matter in the blood. It can even act as antennae in the body for electromagnetic field radiation (Klinghardt).

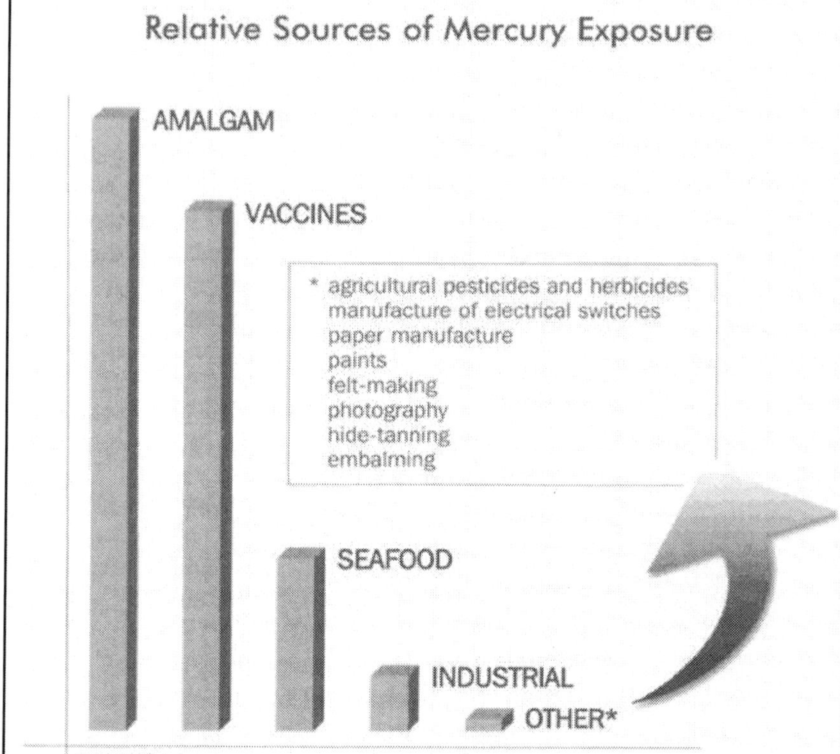

FIGURE 3.1

The greatest exposure to mercury toxicity currently comes from mercury amalgam dental fillings and vaccines. There is a tremendous amount of medical documentation regarding its dangers, even at low levels. The Centers for Disease Control (CDC) and the Food and Drug Administration (FDA) have chosen to ignore this knowledge. When mercury toxicity is found in people, it is usually blamed on the consumption of contaminated fish.

Even worse, the number of childhood vaccinations has increased to as many as thirty eight on the CDC's routine schedule. Thirty six of these are given by the age of two. Many contain unsafe levels of ethyl-mercury. Ethyl mercury (thimerosal) is added to vaccines to prevent bacterial contamination. When injected, it goes into the cells of the heart and the brain and greatly affects the immune system. Some of these vaccinations are given at birth, such as the hepatitis B vaccine. The most critical part of brain development is between the third trimester of pregnancy and the age of two.

Mercury is measured in Micrograms per Cubic Meter, or ug/m3. The Environmental Protection Agency (EPA) has documented an infant toxic at a poisonous levels at 2 ug/m3. Their current level of safety is 0.3 ug/m3. Mercury is detrimental to the brain at levels below 0.5 microgram. Mercury is also cumulative!

A LOOK AT STATISTICS

There is a direct link between increased doses of mercury and the increase in cases of autism. The listed number of vaccines below is recommended by the CDC, and usually administered to the child, before the age of two. This is the time period of the fastest brain development.

year	#vaccines	mercury	autism cases
1985	10	135 mcgs	1 in 2,500
1996	12	246 mcgs	1 in 350
2014	36	?	1 in 68

In 1996, the Hepatitis B vaccine and the Varicella (chicken pox) vaccines were added to the Center for Disease Control's routine schedule. Some vaccines, including the hepatitis B vaccine, contained as much as 12.5 micrograms of mercury per dose. This is more than 100 times the EPA's "safe" limit guideline when administered to infants.

My son was born in 1996. Over the past several years, I have talked to many parents and grandparents who had children born in that year who have been affected by autism. Until I found this research, I had continually asked the question, "What happened in 1996 to cause such an increase?" See the chapter on vaccines for more information.

In 1999, studies showed that multi-dose vaccines, such as the MMR and hepatits B vaccines, contained 62.5 ug of mercury in one individual appointment with the pediatrician. This, again, is over 100 times the Environmental Protection Agency's "safe" limit guideline for infants.

Autism affects four times as many boys as girls. Hormones play a part in this. The neurotoxicity of mercury is enhanced by testosterone, which is predominant in boys. Autism is sometimes labeled as an "extreme male brain." Higher levels of estrogen in females protects the brain, especially the hippocampus.

Mercury amalgam fillings are an extremely common source of mercury exposure. Although they have been known for years to be harmful, in the past they were cheaper to use than other materials. As it seems to always happen, money comes before health. As a result, many of us were given fillings of mercury amalgams that we have had contaminating our systems for years.

Chewing releases mercury vapors that we then inhale. Up to 80% of mercury is absorbed into the lungs and stays in the body. Hot items release the toxic vapors as well. Think about this the next time you drink coffee or hot tea. Due to the vibration of the amalgam fillings, brushing teeth, the use of water picks and dental work of any kind, also releases the toxic vapors. A dental drilling can release as much as 4,000 ug/m3. The safe limit set by the Environmental Protection Agency is 50 ug/m3, and this is not really safe at all! Do not have dental work done while you are pregnant!

Large fish carry high amounts of mercury than smaller fish. As a rule, the larger the fish, the higher it is on the food chain, and the higher the mercury content. Sharks, swordfish, and large tuna are among the highest because they are top predators. They have a highly absorbable type of mercury called methylmercury. The fats in the fish absorb the mercury. When we eat the fish, the mercury becomes extremely absorbable by the GI tract. As absorbable as the methylmercury is from fish, mercury amalgam fillings are almost ten times more so.

One study showed up to 30% of those tested had toxic levels of mercury. With the increase in coal-powered plants around the globe, these numbers are in the millions. Mercury emissions from coal-fired power plants, natural gas, and petroleum products emit as much as 5,000 tons of mercury into the atmosphere every year. Harmful toxins get into the jet stream and carry it thousands of miles into the air we breathe.

Due to the mother's elevated mercury blood levels, federal scientists estimate that 410,000 children are born every year at an increased risk to the harmful effects of this transference in-utero. Mercury amalgam fillings from the mother pass through the blood-brain barrier and into the fetus via the placenta and later through lactation. Breast milk has been found to have much higher levels of mercury, up to 80% higher, than the mother's blood mercury levels. This largely comes from mercury amalgam fillings in the mother. I would also use caution when choosing the type of fish you consume.

Those at highest risk of mercury toxicity are those with developing brains such as fetuses, infants, and children. Males are also at higher risk because testosterone enhances its neurotoxicity. Those with the lowered ability to fight toxins, such as the elderly and women of child-bearing ages, between 20 and 39, are also at high risk. Remember that when we are pregnant, our immune systems are depressed, so we have less capability of combating toxic exposure.

Have all mercury amalgam fillings removed by a bio-dentist, *before* conception and use the natural detoxification method discussed in the chapter, Natural Heavy Metal Detoxification. A bio-dentist is trained in the safe removal of the amalgams. During removal, vapors released are inhaled and ingested into your system if not removed properly. To find a bio-dentist, see the chapter on alternative therapies. We will talk about detoxification in the next chapter.

See the video on the vapors from a 25-year-old mercury amalgam filling at Dr. Klinghardt's site under heavy metal detoxification, www.klinghardtacademy.com. Also see Dr. Andrew Cutler's website, www.noamalgam.com.

SIGNS OF MERCURY TOXICITY

- Poor immune system
- Extreme irritability or anger
- Lack of impulse control
- Shy and withdrawn behavior
- Insomnia
- Fatigue

- Lack of ability to concentrate
- Depression (even suicidal)
- Poor memory
- Poor motor control
- Do any of these symptoms sound familiar to you?

SOME OF THE BIOLOGICAL AFFECTS OF MERCURY

- Can cause lifelong immune deficiency.
- Causes a loss of glutathione
- Resists removal of the pathogenic yeast Candida albicans
- Inactivates contacted molecules of glutathione two-fold.
- Reduces antioxidant levels
- Disrupts metabolism of creatine, causing poor muscle tone and weakness
- Renders the body defenseless against free radicals
- Interrupts protein synthesis
- Retards brain development by interfering with DNA and RNA function
- Depletes protein-bound sulfhydryl groups and lower the body's immunity
- Destroys glutamate transport proteins responsible for removing glutamate from neurons causing mis-wiring of the brain (often causing dementia and problems with motor control)
- Destroys enzyme functioning creating faulty wiring of the brain
- Promotes the production of inflammatory cytokines, which are essential in fighting viruses
- Disrupts protein digestion
- Can enter the area of the brain called the hypothalamus, which is responsible for metabolic function, hormonal

balance—including neuro-hormones—hunger, thirst, body temperature, and the circadian rhythm affecting the sleep-wake cycle. An injured hypothalamus can cause lifelong suppression of the immune system, and weaken the adrenals and thyroid.

- Can inhibit neurotransmitters (the brain's messengers) such as serotonin, dopamine, and norepinephrine.
- Increases your body's lipid peroxidation. This is when the fatty membranes in our body are oxidized by free radical damage. This, first and foremost, affects organs with a high fat content, such as the brain. It weakens the cell membranes and proteins within the cells. When this happens, enzymes are lost and cells cannot function.
- Increases susceptibility to seizures
- Renders the brain vulnerable to damage from excitotoxins

Phew, that's a lot!

Mercury damages the brain. It allows for the accumulation of glutamate in the brain, and disrupts normal enzyme function. These actions cause mis-wiring of the brain. The results of mis-wiring can be subtle, with poor cognitive abilities, memory loss, or an inability to control anger. In more extreme cases, the child ends up with Asperger's syndrome or autism.

The brain and the kidneys retain the most mercury. Mercury primarily attacks the cerebellar region of the brain. Long-term exposure affects:

- The amygdala, the center for fight or flight (fear)
- The neocortex, affecting sensory integration, motor control, spatial awareness, language and conscious thought
- Damage to the temporal lobes which are responsible for visual memory, emotion, and language comprehension

In my craniosacral work, I always find the temporal bones are jammed in children on the autism spectrum, and in those with ADD, ADHD, or learning disorders.

Mercury accumulates over time in the nervous system, and the results from exposure may not be seen for several years. The brain can hold mercury for more than ten years. It is crucial to detoxify mercury and other heavy metals from the system.

Proper nutrition and increased antioxidant levels help protect us from mercury exposure. Foods with high antioxidant content have deep colors such as blueberries and green leafy vegetables. Taking antioxidant supplements, such as vitamins E and C, selenium, magnesium, zinc, carotenoids, and alpha lipoic acid can all assist the body in removing mercury and other heavy metals. Selenium protects against mercury toxicity in an unborn fetus at about 200 mcg per day for adults.

During pregnancy, cysteine (also needed to build glutathione) is used to transport through the placenta. Supplementing with N-acetyl cysteine (NAC) and other amino acids that build glutathione can be helpful in blocking mercury from reaching the baby. NAC also helps chelate mercury from the body, so adults should not exceed 500 mg per day. See more information in the chapter "Basic Nutrition and Supplementation".

Many studies on vaccinations and mercury can be found at www.pubmed.com.

ALUMINUM

Aluminum is extremely toxic to the brain. Like mercury, there are no known safe levels. It is one of those heavy metals that is difficult to stay away from, and it is very easily absorbed in all forms such as injections, inhalation, or ingestion from food.

Aluminum is contained in vaccines, medications, pots and pans we cook our food in, food and beverage containers, acidic foods such as tomatoes, processed cheese, skin lotions, aluminum foil, utensils, and steam released from industrial paper plants and concrete. Aluminum is also put into water supplies in the form of aluminum sulfate, a toxic form of aluminum used in treatment of public water. Areas with higher levels of aluminum in water have been found to have higher incidences of Alzheimer's disease. There is consistent evidence of the connection between aluminum toxicity and Alzheimer's dementia.

Acidic foods tend to pull aluminum into them. Citrus juices in aluminum cans, soda and beer, and canned goods such as tomato sauce increase your intake of aluminum. The kidneys help to excrete aluminum, so those with weak kidneys and poor detoxification (like our children) have a harder time getting rid of it.

Certain foods contribute to increased aluminum absorption. Food combining is important here. If you have any concern regarding aluminum toxicity, reduce the intake of pecans and berries because they contain gallic acid, and apples that contain chlorogenic acid, which assist aluminum into the tissues.

Aluminum reduces the phospholipids or fat structure of the myelin (the carrier of messages to and from the brain). Remember when we talked about krill oil and the importance of phospholipids? Unfortunately, the brain holds onto aluminum and has a hard time letting go. Once in the brain, it distributes itself, but primarily affects DNA synthesis controlling how the cells function.

Aluminum depletes mineral absorption. When calcium levels are low, aluminum will attach to its receptors and becomes even more toxic and further deplete calcium. Low magnesium levels have been shown to increase absorption of aluminum by the intestinal tract. Remember that the intestines have a direct connection to the brain. Aluminum also displaces zinc, iron, manganese, and magnesium. When these are not in place, their dependent enzymes cannot do their jobs. Critical cell functions and detoxification processes are hindered. Aluminum is also capable of destroying cells altogether. Along with iron and mercury, aluminum increases the production of free radicals in neurons. Neurons are the cells that affect the brain and the nerves.

Aluminum affects the following neurotransmitters:

- Acetylcholine and the enzyme that breaks down acetylcholine, involved in learning and memory.
- Norepinephrine, involved in attention and focus
- Dopamine, focus
- Serotonin, mood, appetite, sleep

The brain absorbs glutamate at a higher rate when aluminum is available. Keep blood sugar levels from diving by eating small amounts of protein every couple of hours. Nuts are an easy snack that fulfills this purpose. By all means, avoid excitotoxins like MSG and foods that contain glutamate, such as hydrolyzed vegetable proteins, soy protein extract, protein isolate, and others mentioned in the chapter on dangerous food additives. Beware of restaurants that routinely add these ingredients to their food.

Keep magnesium and calcium levels in balance. Low levels of these minerals increase aluminum absorption. Read further on the benefits of magnesium in the chapter on general supplementation. The usually noted antioxidants are helpful here, and include vitamins C and E, N-acetyl L-cysteine, alpha lipoic acid, magnesium, and calcium pyruvate, which prevents absorption from both fluoride and aluminum.

LEAD

Lead is a heavy metal most commonly found in buildings built in or prior to the 1960s, although lead-based paint was not banned until 1978. It is found both in lead-based paint and the dust in these buildings. Exposure is highest for those who have lived in or visited older structures that have not been properly cleaned up. This includes schools of all kinds that our children spend countless hours in. Chicago has been found to be one of the most contaminated cities in the US due to multiple old buildings and a high level of poverty that has prevented clean up measures from happening.

Breathing in the dust or getting it on hands that end up in the mouth, even in minute amounts, can cause lead poisoning. It can also enter the body through a cut in the skin, and a piece of lead as small as a grain of salt can poison you.

Lead poisoning can come from:

- The dust from old lead-based paints
- Soil
- Lead plumbing fixtures
- Newsprint
- Ceramic glaze
- Cosmetics

- Imported toys, such as those from China
- Jewelry

A study released in May of 2000 by economic consultant Rick Nevin demonstrated that 65% to 95% of violent crime in the US and other countries was due to lead exposure.

The Mayo Clinic states that children under the age of six are especially vulnerable to lead poisoning. Lead crosses the blood-brain barrier and severely affects the brain, kidneys, cardiovascular system, and the reproductive system. Lead easily passes through the placenta from mother to baby, directly affecting brain development. This may cause mental retardation, difficulty with visual-motor coordination, and cognitive learning disabilities that can last a lifetime. Lead is known to be a contributor to ADHD. It also reduces iron and zinc in the body. Iron is needed for the production of the neurotransmitter dopamine. Zinc, among other things, helps protect the brain.

It can go undetected, showing no obvious symptoms; however, a child with low levels of lead in his system is more likely to fail the third grade due to learning difficulties. The heavy metal toxicity may be overlooked.

- Symptoms of lead poisoning include:
- Neurological problems (learning disabilities)
- Depression
- Poor memory
- Problems with social engagement
- Aggressive and even violent behavior
- Gastrointestinal problems
- Constipation
- Diarrhea
- Nausea and/or vomiting
- Poor appetite
- Weight loss
- Insomnia

- Metal taste in the mouth
- Excessive fatigue
- Hyperactivity
- Headaches
- Seizures
- Anemia
- Kidney problems
- Reproductive problems
- Weakness in the muscles of the hand

Lead disrupts normal brain neurotransmitter function of:

- Acetylcholine, affecting memory and motor function
- Dopamine, affecting autonomic motor control in the brain, behavior, and emotions
- Serotonin levels in the brain, which helps to regulate violence
- The GABA system, which we rely on to keep our brain signals calm; when this system is disrupted, we commonly experience anxiety

Lead is held in the bones by hormones. As we age, our hormone levels drop and lead begins to leak out of the bones. This often affects the heart, which we see has greater complications in elder years. In addition, by increasing glutamate toxicity, lead produces free radicals, worsening degenerative diseases.

Magnesium has been shown to be far more effective than the commonly used drug EDTA in the removal of lead. See the chapter on heavy metal detoxification for more information.

CADMIUM

Cadmium is an extremely toxic metal found in industrial workplaces, shipyards, construction areas, and agriculture. It is also found in nickel-plated batteries, plastics, electronics, cement, cigarette smoke, and bright orange, yellow, and red chalk and paints.

Our water, food, and soil are easily contaminated with cadmium. It is contained in the phosphates in fertilizers and is easily transferred in the atmosphere from one place to another. Cadmium travels through the air and lands in our soil and on the plants we eat, and contaminates water supplies. It is also found in the liver and kidneys of animals, so their meat may be contaminated with it.

When coal and oil are burned, the toxins find their way to the jet stream and contaminate countries across the world. Exhaust fumes from automobiles releases cadmium. People who live close to highways and busy streets are more likely to consume cadmium. Food crops grown close to roadways are found to have higher levels of this toxin. It has no definitive taste or smell.

Fruits and vegetables, especially grains, potatoes, and leafy vegetables, commonly grow in soil with high levels of cadmium. Shellfish and organ meats also have a higher content of this heavy metal toxin.

Typical effects of cadmium exposure are flu-like symptoms, including chills, fever, and muscle ache. Inhalation of this heavy metal can cause respiratory tract infections, kidney weakness and failure, and liver damage. Cadmium and lead are often found in learning disabled children.

Some of the biological effects of cadmium are:

- Problems with motor coordination and behavior
- Damage to the brain's blood vessel supply
- It increases your body's lipid peroxidation. This is when the fatty membranes in our body are oxidized by free radical damage. This affects organs with high fat content, such as the brain. It weakens the cell membranes and proteins within the cells. When this happens, enzymes are lost and cells cannot function.
- Depletes glutathione
- Depletes protein-bound sulfhydryl groups which lowers the body's immunity and weakens enzyme function
- Promotes the production of inflammatory cytokines, which are essential in fighting viruses

- Cadmium increases deficiency in calcium zinc, iron, and vitamin C
- Disrupts the transfer of trace elements in utero needed by the fetus' developing brain
- Reduces acetylcholine receptors
- Increases dopamine
- Damages myelin
- Lowers superoxide dismutase (SOD)
- Increases free radicals

Poor nutrition allows cadmium to stay in your body and is mainly stored in the liver, kidneys, and bones. If you suspect exposure to cadmium, test for kidney and liver damage. Weak bones are another symptom.

To reduce exposure, eat organic, local, whole foods. Farmers markets are best because you can get to know the growers and ask them questions. Find out if the crop is close to any heavily traveled roads. If you grow your own food or your child plays in the dirt around your home, you should test soil samples in those areas. Be sure to drink pure water. See the chapter on environmental toxins and heavy metal detoxification for more information.

FLUORIDE

Most of us grew up being told how important and beneficial fluoride is. We were told that is was important for strong teeth. Because of this, it is much harder for most people to accept its downfall. There are over 25 human studies and 100 animal studies connecting fluoride to brain damage and lowered IQ. Several peer-reviewed studies have shown fluoridation to weaken bones. Dental fluorosis is when tooth enamel becomes discolored and is due to fluoride disrupting the enamel during development. However, dentists will often tell us it's because of poor hygiene. Please recognize that the dangers of fluoride are real. What they did not tell us is that fluoride damages a part of the brain called the hippocampus, which has no blood-brain barrier to protect it. The hippocampus is responsible for emotions, behavior, learning, memory, and spatial awareness. It is the primary part of the brain affected by those with Alzheimer's.

- Reduces acetylcholine receptors which affect motor control
- Reduces lipids which help make up brain matter
- Reduces antioxidant levels lowering immunity
- Increases the absorption of aluminum
- Damages DNA repair enzymes and causes genetic damage
- Increases osteoporosis (the irony: fragile bones and teeth) by greatly depleting calcium levels
- Causes abnormal brain development
- Reduces absorption of iodine contributing to hypothyroidism
- Reduces male fertility and lowers levels of testosterone
- May contribute to hypothyroidism (under active thyroid)

Note: In many studies, more problems arose in males than females.

We absorb fluoride from dental treatments, brushing or rinsing with fluoride, and drinking water with added fluoride. When aluminum and fluoride are combined, as in fluoridated water in an aluminum pan or using fluoride toothpaste from an aluminum container, the toxic affects are heightened.

Interestingly, studies have shown that cities with added fluoride in their drinking water have equal or higher levels of dental cavities than cities without fluoridated water. The added fluoride did not reduce the number of cavities for those populations. Unfortunately, the body accumulates this toxin and absorbs up to 50% of each exposure in its tissues.

There are two factors of fluoride toxicity that are of greatest concern. The first is genetic damage. Damage to DNA repair enzymes affects the reproductive cells and is inherited by our children. The second factor of great concern to us is fluoride's effect on the brain. Common signs are difficulty thinking, poor memory, and fatigue. For the developing brain in a fetus, fluoride crosses the blood-brain barrier, accumulates, and then spreads to all areas of the brain.

Assisting in the removal and protection from fluoride are the cited antioxidants vitamins C and E, alpha lipoic acid, N-acetyl L-cysteine, magnesium, and calcium pyruvate, which prevents absorption from both fluoride and aluminum. It is helpful that many of the same antioxidants, vitamins, and minerals are used to protect us from all heavy metals. To reduce and remove fluoride poisoning it is important to clean out the liver bile ducts. See chapter four for more information on liver decongestion.

SUMMARY

Heavy metals are toxic metals. They can do severe damage and even destroy the brain and central nervous system. They also weaken the body's immune system and detoxification abilities. Infants and children are far more susceptible to the dangers of heavy metal toxicity.

There are several different kinds of heavy metals. They are found in food, air, water, household goods, mercury amalgam fillings, vaccines, and more.

The products found in this chapter can be found at http://naturallyhealingautism.com/a-healthy-home/

CHAPTER 15

VACCINATIONS; FUELING THE FIRE

My son was my first-born child. The greatest concern a new mother has is for her child. I was told stories by doctors that created fear in me if I did not vaccinate. At the time, my fear to not vaccinate overrode my fear to vaccinate. I listened to people who I still believe gave me the information they believed to be true. The risks of that information were largely unknown to me at that time.

We do what we hope is best for our child. Here we need to take out the word "hope" and replace it with "know." This brings me back once again to the need for self-education. Unfortunately, I had to learn the hard way. I hope that you do not.

I doubt that if a mother knows that the risk factors for her child becoming autistic, having some form of neurological damage or learning disability, contracting Type 1 diabetes, asthma or a lifetime of digestive disturbance or death, that she would feel more confident to vaccinate against rare diseases than not.

An infant's developing brain does not yet have the blood-brain barrier fully intact to help protect it, and inflammation weakens the immune system leaving the body vulnerable to bacterial and viral attack. If pathogenic microbes reside in the body, especially in an infant or a child, toxins pose a much larger threat. The brain is rapidly developing in utero and in the first years of life. Without a developed, or a strong immune system, toxins easily create havoc in the body. The neurological system is most vulnerable.

Vaccines are among the highest concern in America with 89% of Americans having vaccine concerns. Research shows that there is a connection between heavy metal vaccines and autism. The Center for Disease Control (CDC) admits that vaccines contain mercury, aluminum, formaldehyde, and MSG. These ingredients are toxic and should never be injected into anyone, especially pregnant women, infants, and children. Multiple vaccines injected into a 2 month old infant is equal to 10 times that dosage in an average 130 pound adult.

There is huge pressure from doctors to get vaccinations but no information regarding their safety. If they tell you they are safe, they are wrong. I find it strange that a doctor must see studies to prove to them what we have to say, but when I ask if I can see the studies to prove the safety of vaccinations, they have none. Yet, they are very willing to inject chemicals and viruses into pregnant women, newborns, children, and the elderly.

NO SUCH STUDIES HAVE BEEN DONE

No one can assure you that vaccines are safe. In order to do so, there would need to be long-term randomized, controlled studies. None have been done. Proper long-term studies take years (not weeks, as has been the case in the past). Studies that are done in three or four weeks are not sufficient to call the vaccines safe.

In order to develop a truly scientific study, one group would not be vaccinated and another group would have been. These children would be followed over the course of many years since it can take a long time for negative side effects to show up. In the end, if we concluded that the number of children who developed any of the diseases, neurological difficulties, autoimmune disorders, Type 1 diabetes, asthma, digestive problems, seizures, etc, were the same in both groups, then our minds could be put at ease.

These studies would also need to be done by people who had absolutely no ties—financial or otherwise—to the vaccine industry. No studies of this kind have been done, yet they still tell us that vaccines are safe. If they were indeed safe, then I doubt that the U.S. government would have paid out more than $1.5 billion from its Vaccine Injury Compensation Program to families whose children were either damaged or killed by vaccines.

We now have enough evidence and newly found knowledge regarding the brain's own immune system to justify a healthier, less invasive, and less neurologically damaging vaccination schedule. Even though the brain has a protective filtering system, called the blood-brain-barrier, which is not yet developed in infants and it is not impermeable to every toxin once it is developed. Vaccinations are a toxic overload that can create a cumulative effect on genetic outcomes. This downward spiraling affect can ultimately damages the brain's cells and its vital connections. Researchers call this damage "bystander injury."

"Bystander injury" is what I see so prevalent in children with autism or Asperger's Syndrome. One example is the child who hears the words that have been said to him, but will not be able to "connect" the meaning of the words spoken, thus creating learning disabilities, social difficulty, anxiety, and more.

SEEKING THE TRUTH

When it comes to vaccinations, most studies and research are either well hidden or the research company is paid by or is part of the company doing the study. Much is covered up by large corporations who stand to lose profit by public knowledge. Throughout the world, those countries following the CDC guidelines for vaccinations have seen an increase in autism. All data, scientific or otherwise, is left to interpretation. Take precautions now. It is better to self-educate than to listen to others.

Physicians are also covered against the liability act of 1986 if your child develops an illness or dies due to a vaccination. They are not covered against liability if your child does not receive a vaccine and happens to contract that illness. Later in this book I will give statistics that show the infinitesimally low number of those individuals who do contract an illness by not vaccinating (usually due to an already compromised immune system). The greater risk is to those who develop autism, other neurological disorders, or die following injections.

It is so controversial to not vaccinate your child that most try to disclaim it. Family members will deem mothers irresponsible for even thinking about not vaccinating. However, most do this without having any of the real facts. Let's be the generation that changes the statistic that says, "1 in every 68 children today is diagnosed with autism, in America, over 4 million children have Attention Deficit Hyperactivity Disorder (ADHD), and now 1 out of every 6 is categorized as learning dis abled."

THE BRAIN DURING DEVELOPMENT

The greatest development of the human brain begins in the third trimester of pregnancy and continues rapid growth until the age of two years. When a child is two years old, his brain is 80% developed. Detoxification pathways are not set until a child is about the age of three.

Many neurological problems can result from vaccination, including death. Autopsies done on the brains of children with post-vaccinal encephalitis (inflammation of the brain) showed a loss of the myelin. The myelin sheath is a fatty covering over the neuron pathways. The myelin helps to make connections in the brain. If your child has trouble with motor skills or speech, auditory, or visual trouble, it could be an issue of damage to the myelin. Remember earlier in the book when we talked about the benefits of omega-3 fatty acids during pregnancy and forever after? Omega-3s help protect the myelin, even while in utero.

Possibly the biggest problem is that too many vaccines are given too close together. How does anyone, let alone a trained pediatrician, expect the immune system of an infant or a small child to react to six viruses and a mixture of toxic additives to be received by an undeveloped immune system all at once?

WHAT'S IN A VACCINE?

Many of the common toxic additives are, but not limited to:

- Viruses, one or more
- Formaldehyde, a cancer-causing agent used to inactivate the virus
- Mercury (thimerosal), a neurotoxin used as preservative

- Aluminum hydroxide, added to promote an antibody response, a neurotoxin that is has been found to play a part in Alzheimer's disease
- Animal tissues, pig blood, horse blood, rabbit brain, dog kidney, monkey kidney, chick embryo, human diploid cells (originating from human aborted fetal tissue)
- Monosodium glutamate (MSG)
- Phenoxyethanol or ethylene glycol (antifreeze)
- Sodium phosphate
- Sulfites
- Yeast protein
- Antibiotics
- RNA and DNA (from animal and human cell tissue)
- Sorbitol
- Sucrose

WHO MAY BE MORE VULNERABLE TO VACCINES?

Many vaccinations today are given at a very early age, even just after birth on day one. Others are often administered when the child is only two months old. Since the human detoxification pathways are not yet fully set until the age of three, then why are viruses and preservatives as harmful as mercury and aluminum being used in early childhood vaccines?

The developing child's brain is far more vulnerable than a mature adult brain. The greatest growth of a child's brain is from the third trimester of pregnancy until they are two years old. Most "basic" vaccines are continued through the age of five, and the number of vaccinations recommended by the CDC for children by the age of five years old has tripled in the last two decades.

THE MOST VULNERABLE ARE:

- Infants born to a mother who have had Candida while she was pregnant from stress, poor dietary habits, or current or past antibiotic use (even if it was long ago). Candida is passed on to baby in utero. Antibiotics are also passed through breast milk creating bacterial imbalances and weakened immunity in baby.
- Children born to mothers with mercury amalgam fillings. Mercury from mercury amalgam dental fillings can leach into the mother's system. Mercury can cross the blood-brain barrier and affect the unborn child's developing brain.
- Exposure before, during, or after pregnancy to toxic substances such as pesticides, refineries emitting toxins, or toxic water supplies
- Babies born with or showing signs of any form of weakened immunity or health issues
- Those with a family history of neurological conditions
- Infants and young children with no history or signs of neurological conditions whose brain and immune systems are not yet fully developed
- The elderly

AUTOIMMUNITY

Artificially stimulating the immune system of a newborn with live viruses and toxic preservatives is dangerous. Many viruses are harmful to the immune system, causing it to attack the cells and tissues of the person who has been injected or exposed. This is self-attacking is known as autoimmunity. What we see commonly with autoimmunity are diseases such as autism, multiple sclerosis, ALS (Lou Gehrig's disease), and Parkinson's disease.

HOW DO AUTOIMMUNE DISEASES OCCUR

Autism falls in the category of autoimmune illnesses such as Parkinson's, multiple sclerosis, and Alzheimer's. As I have noted before a gene lies dormant unless activated by something that makes it active. Autoimmune diseases occur when the immune system attacks its own body. Often triggered by inflammation, the immune system responds but does not stop, and this is when it becomes dangerous. The overactive immune system is the problem. All of these autoimmune diseases have similarities and similar triggers.

In order for an autoimmune illness to occur, the body must undergo an injury that causes the body to start attacking itself due to an overabundance of free radicals released into the system. Ongoing inflammation for too long can cause the body to generate a large number of free radicals within tissues. For example, aluminum, lead, mercury, and cadmium generate a huge number of free radicals in tissues, especially in brain tissue.

A lack of antioxidants weakens white blood cells so they cannot protect themselves. This further weakens the immune system and the infection worsens. Further, if your body is fighting a viral infection, the immune system can become overwhelmed. Ongoing infections are one of the key root sources to disease.

Alzheimer's, for example, is largely activated by aluminum in the brain tissue, as are people with chronic fatigue syndrome. There is also a demand on glutathione (the body's natural antioxidant) for similar symptoms, including physical, chemical, biological, and emotional.

METHYLATION CYCLE DISRUPTION

Methylation is a process of gene expression; it passes on genetic information to specific genes. There are hundreds of different methylation reactions in the body. Most commonly noted is its role in the body's ability to detoxify. Approximately 15% of the population has a methylation deficit and poor ability to detoxify, and this number goes up to 54% with vaccinations, (www.klinghardt.com). Of those with autism, 85% are known to have reduced methylation.

When a person who is genetically susceptible and has a strong demand for the body's master antioxidant glutathione, such as after a vaccine is given, and the glutathione level drops low enough, the sulfur metabolism becomes disrupted. The methylation cycle (part of the sulfur metabolism, or detoxification) can become partially blocked and deplete some or all of several important sulfur containing metabolites including S-Adenosyl Methionine (SAMe), cysteine, glutathione, taurine, and sulfate. This can create such a weakening in the system that it allows disease to develop. Sulfation and methylation are covered in more detail in chapter five.

In autism, the drop in the SAMe part of methylation appears to be a significant part of the problem with normal brain development. In the chapter on heavy metals, we explained that aluminum weakens the phospholipid protective structure, and mercury destabilizes glutathione.

"There appears to be substantial evidence that vaccinations containing either a mercury-based preservative or live viruses, many given within a short period of time, were responsible for triggering many of the cases in genetically susceptible children. (D. Geier & M.R. Geier, international Journal of Toxicology, 2004 Nov-Dec: 23 (6): 369-76: and A.J. Wakefield, several publications beginning in 1977).

Supplements that assist methylation are calcium, DMG, folic acid, vitamin B6, vitamin B12, magnesium, zinc, and SAMe.

WHY VACCINES DON'T ALWAYS WORK

Even the CDC tells us that vaccines are not 100% effective. Vaccines are temporary and often create an inferior type of immunity compared to what your body would create naturally.

Vaccinations are supposed to fool your body's immune system so that it will produce antibodies that resist viral and bacterial infection like it would if you actually contracted the disease. However, vaccines cannot replicate the exact same experience your body would have had, and contracting a disease naturally would affect the immune system differently.

The immune system has two different components. The Th1 portion is cellular. The Th2 portion that makes up the body's fluids such as blood, lymph, bile, and mucus, is called the humoral component. These are free antibodies in your blood.

When we contract diseases such as measles, mumps, and chickenpox, they actually strengthen both portions of the immune system (Th1 and Th2). Vaccinations largely stimulate the Th2 part of the system but not the Th1, unlike a naturally acquired disease, which stimulates both. Th1 is the cancer fighter. If Th1 is not built up in childhood by fighting certain diseases, a person may become more prone to getting cancer as an adult. If Th2 is over-stimulated, it causes autoimmune diseases. Autism is in the autoimmune category.

VACCINE SHEDDING

Vaccine shedding is when a virus is spread via a vaccinated individual of any age. For three days post vaccination the newly vaccinated individual releases vapors via exhalation and carries it in his feces. It is known that vaccine viruses (given as either a dead or live virus) such as polio, HIB, meningitis C, whooping cough (pertussis), and measles are contagious from vaccinated people. It is known now that we may be causing some of the very diseases in which we were vaccinating to prevent. These diseases can be spread through the air from breath, cough, or sneeze, through saliva, and from feces. Be aware of contamination from changing any diaper from a child who has recently been vaccinated. Bath tubs can easily become contaminated as are swimming pools through a leaky diaper. See the article, "US MMR Measles Vaccine Failing - Vaccinated New Yorker Causes Measles Outbreak In Other Vaccinated New Yorkers - Not Caused By Unvaccinated Children," posted on April 12, 2014 by ChildHealthSafety at www.childhealthsafety.wordpress.com/2014/04/26/more.

The CDC tells us that the MMR shot (measles, mumps, rubella), even with its booster is only somewhere between 76% to 95% effective. They only started the booster shot years after they realized that it was not working.

A mumps epidemic affecting more than 1,000 people broke out in New York and New Jersey in August of 2009. A boy who had visited the United Kingdom during an epidemic came home to the United States and went to summer camp before realizing that he had contracted the disease. The boy had been fully vaccinated against the mumps and so had 77% of the New Jersey patients that also contracted the disease.

In December of 2014, and January of 2015, there was a measles outbreak in California. The state was thrown into a flurry of angry parents blaming those who do not vaccinate and government officials clambering to find some sense of control. Of sixty cases in this measles outbreak twenty nine were completely vaccinated. In 1500 U.S. cases of measles in the last decade there has not been one death, but there are eighty known reports of deaths due to the vaccine. Statistics show that the vaccine does not always work. In 2010, after the whooping cough outbreak the numbers released told us that 81 percent of those that contracted the disease were completely up to date on their vaccinations. Only eight percent had never been vaccinated.

The government jumps to action at reports of diseases, yet they do nothing about the reports of injured or dead infants and children due to adverse reactions from vaccines. They say it is a coincidence. Mainstream media exaggerates and twists the story and often gives inaccurate release of information. With pharmaceutical companies such as Merck who fund and release most of the "chosen" reports and an annual profit of over $800 million a year, it's no wonder we lack reductions in the reported numbers of injuries and deaths from vaccinations.

THEY SAY THAT MERCURY HAS BEEN TAKEN OUT, SO ARE VACCINES SAFE NOW?

Thimerosal, a mercury compound, is a preservative used in many vaccines. Thimerosal is 49.6% ethyl mercury by weight. There is no safe level of any type of mercury. Mercury is used to prevent bacterial growth in vaccines, *especially in multi-dose containers*. Mercury is known to cause brain damage and is still in many vaccines.

They try to tell us that mercury has been removed from vaccines. Does this mean from all vaccines? It does not.

Joint official statement by Pediatricians and physicians desire elimination of thimerosal from all vaccines. DTP vaccine by Smith Klein Beecham contains no thimerosal. MMR, varicella and inactive polio do not contain any thimerosal. Merck's Hep B vaccine became thimerosal free as of 1999, *but what about the rest of them*?

From the website of the Center for Disease Control, www.cdc.gov, the following was written:

> "Influenza vaccination recommended for U.S. children ages 6 through 23 months old. Thimerosal is used as a preservative in multi-dose vials to prevent contamination of the vial when individual vaccine doses are drawn from it. Single-dose vials without thimerosal are available."

I do not know anyone who has been offered a single dose flu shot without thimerosal. They are widely known to still contain thimerosal (mercury).

Some vaccines contain levels of mercury (thimerosal). For more information see http://www.cdc.gov/nip.vacsafe/concerns/thimerosal/joint_statement_00.htm

Does this mean these vaccinations are safe? No, it does not.

By the time an infant has reached six months of age, most have received 15 doses of these toxic vaccines. Mercury is known to have a cumulative effect on the body. Please remember what is stated above regarding the multiple toxins in each vaccination as a causation for genetic mutation. It is not just one toxin, such as mercury, that is the whole problem, but the cumulative effect. Additionally, when vaccines are not stored at adequate temperatures it often causes them to become tainted, or more toxic. This is a common and lesser known fact.

Over-stimulation of the immune system, often of those at incredibly young ages whose immune systems and brains are not yet developed, are highly susceptible to viral invasion and toxic overload. All of this before the brain is mature, the blood-brain barrier has developed, and detoxification pathways are in place can have a devastating effect on the neurological system.

The other side of "no more mercury" is that there are other harmful substances in vaccines, such as aluminum. Aluminum is a known neurotoxin that has deep connections to Alzheimer's disease. If your child is given a vaccine dose with multiple viruses in it, which is often the case, it creates chaos and destruction of their undeveloped immune system and brain. This is also the connection to autoimmune diseases and neurological disorders.

Beware of listening to your pediatricians when they try to assure you that their vaccines are safe. You have the right to ask to be shown the "possible side effects and risks" pamphlet that accompany vaccines. Merck, one of the common vaccine makers, apparently has a list included with each vaccine batch; however, no one I know has ever been offered to read it.

Today, mercury is still in many vaccines. The problem is that now many more vaccines are given, and they are given too close together with multiple viruses and other toxic additives, at very young ages, even just after birth.

We have discussed the dangers of mercury at length in the chapter on heavy metals. There are also many studies available at www.pubmed.com.

WHAT ABOUT THE FLU SHOT?

There is limited evidence that the flu vaccine actually even works. The CDC knows that they are incapable of matching every possible strain that may or may not come through your town each year. It is merely a prediction.

Dr. Donald Miller, a cardiac surgeon and Professor of Surgery at The University of Washington, found a review of 51 studies involving 260,000 children from age 6 to 23 months, found no evidence that the flu shot is any more effective than a placebo. However there is a risk of harm from the flu vaccine itself, particularly from the mercury, aluminum, and formaldehyde it contains.

Mercury is often found in the flu vaccine. There were several lots or batches of vaccines that they wanted to "use up" instead of discarding, so they are using them up on our children. Some of the lots had greater levels of mercury in their batches. It's like Russian roulette at the doctor's office. If they grab a dose of serum for your child's shot and that vial happens to be one of those more concentrated with mercury, your child gets an even greater dose than perhaps the next child in the same office will get.

The flu shot commonly still contains mercury along with many other harmful toxins such as aluminum, formaldehyde, and ethylene glycol (antifreeze). The shot also contains various antibiotics such as neomycin, streptomycin, and gentamicin. Think back for a moment on the chapter that discusses the devastating effects of antibiotics on the good bacteria our bodies need, including Candida growth and inflammation. Do we have to wonder why so many of today's children have digestive disturbances and weakened immune systems?

The Modernization Act of 1997 made the Food and Drug Administration (FDA) assess the risks of mercury in all food and drugs. The levels in vaccinations are far higher than those said to be safe by the FDA.

In the 2008-2009 flu season, two-thirds of flu vaccines contained a full dose of thimerosal (mercury). Each shot contains 25 micrograms of mercury, a mercury content of 5,0000 parts per billion. This is 250 times more than what the EPA says is safe! What I would like to know is how the CDC allows this to happen. What do we have EPA guidelines for if no one is going to enforce them?

Those at greatest risk from harm due to the toxins in these vaccines are the young and the elderly. They are exactly who are first in line for the shot. Those who get the flu do not die from the flu itself, but from complications of pneumonia or cardiac trouble. If one has an extremely compromised immune system and pneumonia or cardiac problems are likely, then it is a matter to discuss with your trusted physician and it is time to begin your own research.

See the website www.drtenpenny.com, for more information on vaccines but specifically for flu shots.

Study finds those getting flu shots have higher chance of Alzheimer's

"If an individual has had 5 consecutive flu shots between 1970 and 1980 (the years of the study) his/her chance of developing Alzheimer's Disease is 10 times greater than if they had 1, 2, or no shots." When asked why, Dr. Fudenberg stated that, "It is due to the mercury and aluminum buildup that is in every flu shot (and in almost all other childhood shots). The gradual buildup of mercury and aluminum in the brain causes cognitive dysfunction."

Dr. Fudenberg's comments above were from his speech at the NVIC International Vaccine Conference, Arlington VA September, 1997. His bio and achievements can be found at: http://www.nitrf.org/fudenberg.html

Note: When I researched the Internet for the above quote, it only seemed to appear on chiropractic sites and alternative treatment sites, so I wrote to Dr Fudenberg to validate that this was what he stated and also asked for a citation or article. His answer to me was:

Statement is correct.

See my papers, Hazards of Vaccines 1 & 2 in Internat. J. Clin. Invest., 2000 & 2004

Dr. Hugh Fudenberg, MD

Keeping in mind both that flu shots are not effective most of the time and the number of recent epidemics of pertussis (whooping cough) among vaccinated children, it may be time to re-think our vaccination schedule.

PNEUMONIA VACCINES

In 2000, the pneumococcal vaccine was added to the list of childhood vaccines. The most we have seen from this is its ability to create virulent bacterial infections in children. It means that the infections your child gets may become stronger, and therefore, harder to fight off due to this. This is just like the flu shot in that the only few viral strains it can protect against are the ones in the vaccine, and there's no proof of that either.

SCIENTIFIC EVIDENCE FINALLY QUESTIONED

The CDC said they had decided to change its decision to continue administering the hepatitis B shot to mothers who tested negative until a later date than at birth. Perhaps the outcry from parents whose children were injured or died due to reactions from the hepatitis B vaccine was finally heard. Also, the scientific evidence that was used to license its use at birth was questioned. Questioning sooner would be another good choice. Where are *our* studies to question?

A friend of mine just had a baby and she told me that her baby was given the Hepatitis B shot at birth. They are still giving the shot even though they said they were going to stop.

Be sure that prior to giving birth that you have been very clear with every caretaker who will be present and involved on what you do and do not want for your child. Also be very sure that those who say they understand your needs will truly follow them.

THEY DON'T KNOW EVERYTHING

What many physicians are not taught in school is that the number of people who died from the measles between 1900 and 1960 dropped by 97.7%. The death toll in the U.S. went from 133 per million to 0.3 per million by 1960. However, before vaccines for diphtheria and pertussis were ever introduced, they too declined by over 90%.

The greatest factors in better health have come from better nutrition, higher quality transportation of fresh fruits and vegetables, adequate refrigeration, and proper sanitation, such as trash removal and the installation of sewage systems. It is not due to vaccines.

The World Health Organization (WHO) states, "The best vaccine against common infectious diseases is an adequate diet," even though they continue to promote vaccinations.

Only four vaccines were routinely given 54 years ago; they were for diphtheria, tetanus, pertussis, and smallpox. At that time, autism was unknown. When first discovered in 1943, less than 1 in 10,000 children were affected by these developmental disorders.

WHAT'S HAPPENING NOW?

Until 1989, children were still only receiving three vaccinations. In 1991, the increase in infant vaccinations tripled their exposure to mercury. In 2012, children receive 36 vaccinations before entering kindergarten. More than 20 of these are given by the age of 6 months. In many areas 32 vaccinations are given before the age of 2. This correlates with the rise in autism spectrum disorders and learning disabilities. Over 4,000,000 American children have ADHD, and 1 in every 6 is classified as learning disabled.

Today, 1 in 68 children are diagnosed with autism, and by the time you read this book, the number will probably have risen again. Of normally developing children who receive their MMR shot (measles, mumps rubella), 30% become diagnosed with autism. The leading causes of death in children today, along with accidents, are genetic abnormalities, developmental disorders, and sudden infant death syndrome. Many believe vaccinations to be the cause. Autoimmune disorders such as Type 1 diabetes, rheumatoid arthritis, asthma, and bowel disease are rising in epidemic proportions.

In the 1950s, 1 in 7,100 children had Type 1 diabetes. Today it is 1 in 400. Though almost unheard of 25 years ago, today 300,000 American children have juvenile rheumatoid arthritis. In the past 50 years, 4 times the number of children have developed asthma and bowel disorders. In 1980 one in twenty seven children was diagnosed with asthma. In 2013 this number rose to one in nine. Common triggers for these are overreaction of the immune system and chronic inflammation or fungal overload. What has changed so dramatically?

CDC Vaccination Schedule Birth to Six Years (recommended months)

1983
DTP (2)
OPV (20)
DTP (4)
OPV (4)
DTP (6)
MMR (15)
DTP (18)
OPV (18)
DTP (48)
OPV (48)
Total= 10

2014
Hep B (1)
DTap (2)
Hib (2)
IPV (2)
PCV (2)
Rotovirus (2)
DTap (4)
Hib (4)
IPV (4)
PCV (4)
Rotovirus (4)

Hep B (6)
DTap (6)
Hib (6)
IPV (6)
PCV (6)
Influenza (6)
Rotovirus (6)
Hib (12)
MMR (12)
Viricella (12)
PCV (12)
Hep A (12)
DTap (15)
Hep A (18)
Influenza (18)
PPSV (24 if high risk)
Influenza (30)
Influenza (42)
MMR (48)
DTaP (48)
Varicella (48)
IPV (48)
Influenza (54)
Influenza (66)
Total= 36-38

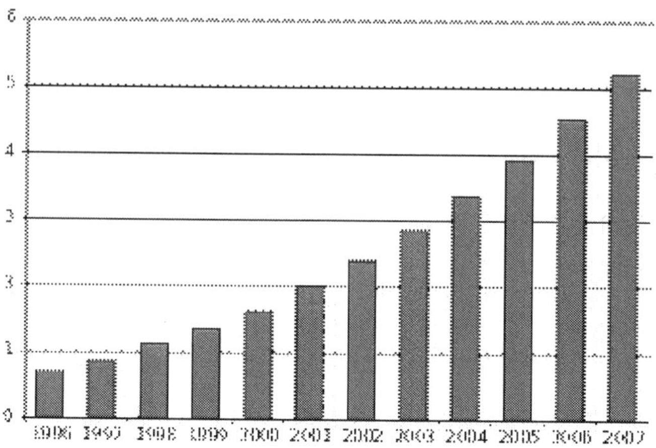

Reports of autism cases per 1,000 children grew dramatically in the U.S. from 1996 to 2007.

- 1985: 1 in 2,500
- 1995: 1 in 500
- 2001: 1 in 250
- 2007: 1 in 150
- 2014: 1 in 68

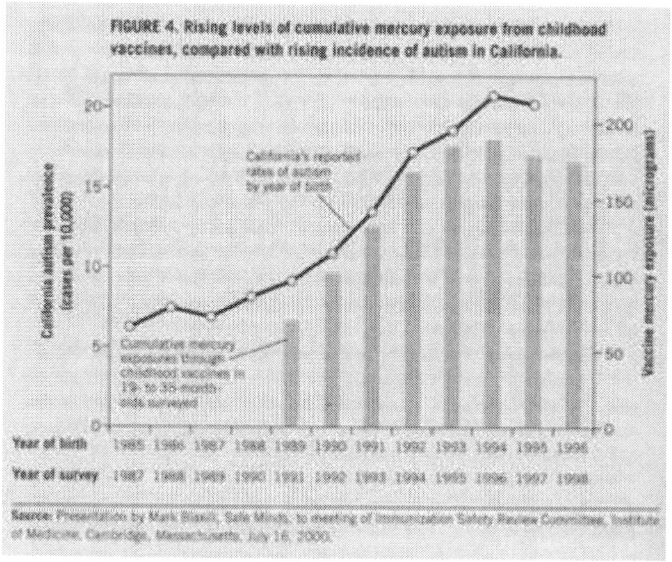

THE SCHEDULE MADE FOR THE MASSES

It seems far more sensible to consider a schedule that takes into consideration the best interest of the individual rather than what the government deems necessary.

The CDC, along with the 15-member Advisory Committee on Immunization Practices, has decided for the rest of us that all babies will receive the Hepatitis B vaccine the day of birth.

By the age of two, the infant has received 32 vaccinations on the committee's schedule. Dr. Donald Miller, a cardiac surgeon and Professor of Surgery at the University of Washington points out that, "7 vaccines injected into a 13-pound, 2-month old infant are equivalent to 70 doses in a 130-pound adult."

Family history and genetic testing for neurological weaknesses or disorders must be given before any vaccination is administered or it could result in a lifelong disorder or death for the child.

WHAT'S HAPPENING TO AMERICA'S CHILDREN?

How could the children of a well-developed, wealthy, and supposedly educated country like the U.S. be getting unhealthier by the year? Is it possible that it is because the most highly vaccinated children in the world are American? The U.S. ranks 31 in infant mortality!

AWARENESS OF THE DANGERS IN THE CDC's THREE MOST DANGEROUS VACCINES: Hepatitis B (Hep B), Diptheria, Measles, Mumps, Rubella (MMR), Pertussis Tetanus (DPT or DTaP)

THE HEPATITIS B VACCINE

The hepatitis B vaccine is known to be one of the most dangerous vaccines given with the highest rate of fatality. In 1994, the CDC decided for all of our children that they would add the hepatitis B (Hep B) vaccination to the routine schedule. After that, they began giving it to newborns in the hospital just after birth. The only way a newborn infant would be at risk for hepatitis B would be if their mother tested positive for it. This number is exceptionally low. A hepatitis B study conducted in June 1999, in North Carolina, showed the rate of positive testing new mothers to be only 0.2%. Interestingly, in order to justify the use of this vaccine for mass population, this rate needed to be at least 5% of the US population. The hepatitis B vaccine would also be inactive by the time the child was old enough to have sexual relations or begin recreational drug use to possibly contract the disease on their own. Why then would the medical establishments take it upon themselves to give the vaccine to all infants, including those born to mothers who test negative? Could it possibly be a financial decision more than a health-related decision?

The Canadian physician, Byron Hyde, M.D., has collected data from hundreds of cases of severe immunological and neurological dysfunction after receiving the hepatitis B vaccination. Symptoms included demyelinating disease, lowered IQ, pain, fatigue, loss of vision, and skin lesions.

Statistics from the National Health Interview Survey found that newborn infants in the U.S. that were vaccinated with Hepatitis B had three times the risk of autism spectrum disorders. In 1996, alone, there were 47 deaths reported among children from birth to age one from the Hepatitis B vaccination. In that same year in children under age fourteen there were 872 adverse reactions reported. Between 1992 and 2005, there were 36,788 officially reported adverse reactions to Hepatitis B vaccinations. Of these 14,800 were serious enough to cause hospitalization, permanent disabilities, or were life-threatening, (www.mercola.com).

We noticed the biggest difference in our own son after his hepatitis B vaccination at age two. Our happy, outgoing child became withdrawn, and hyper-fixated on everything to the point that he would not hear us if we called his name or stood next to him trying to get his attention.

THE MEASLES, MUMPS, RUBELLA VACCINE (MMR)

One report of two cases with young children who developed symptoms of Parkinson's disease, rarely seen in children, arose just after being vaccinated with the MMR vaccine. The measles virus is known to penetrate organs, including the brain.

When my son was ten years old I took him to a N.E.A.T. acupuncturist. If you'll remember from the chapter on alternative therapies, they are among the practitioners who will muscle test their client from a complete panel of serums to see what is keeping the body from healing itself. What she found astounded me. He had a remaining allergic reaction to the measles virus. The only exposure he had to measles previously was in his MMR vaccine over a decade before! His body was still trying to fight measles from the injection he received almost ten years earlier!

In 2012, Italy was the first country to admit that the measles, mumps, and rubella (MMR) vaccine was responsible for a child developing autism. A perfectly developing child received the MMR vaccine and immediately developed irritable bowel syndrome, loss of speech, and loss of interaction. He was then diagnosed with autism.

There has been an assault on doctors and scientists who stand up against vaccine safety claims. Dr. Andrew Wakefield is one of the doctors who has come out with scientific data against vaccines. Andrew Wakefield is a gastrointestinal surgeon from the United Kingdom. He is a man who had an impeccable reputation as a doctor, researcher, and surgeon. While working at the royal Free Hospital in London as senior lecturer and honorary consultant in gastroenterology he was approached by a mother of a child with autism who asked him for his help.

In 1995 he found that normally developing children who received their MMR vaccine began developing autistic type symptoms of diarrhea up to twelve times per day, inflammatory bowel disease, failure to thrive, withdrawal and loss of speech.

The highly reputable medical journal known as *The Lancet* released Dr. Wakefield's first MMR study in 1998. This publication offered the results of a case series showing the connection between the MMR vaccine and autism. Through testing Andrew Wakefield found that autistic children who suffer from ongoing stomach pain often had the cells that line their intestines growing live measles viruses. When these viruses were tested Dr. Wakefield found the viruses to be a genetic match to the virus in the vaccine. How did they know it was from the vaccine virus?

Vaccine viruses are made up of genetic material. These viruses become genetically altered when introduced to cell cultures. The measles virus is incubated in a culture of chick embryo. The genetics of a cultured vaccine virus are different from that of a wild measles virus.

When Dr. Wakefield released information in the Lancet in 1998 regarding his research findings on the connection between autism and the MMR vaccine the medical association, (and likely Big Pharma) did everything to destroy his reputation and tell the public that he was wrong. Later Dr. Wakefield tried to release 19 other studies showing the same type of findings *but they were never mentioned.* He was silenced and asked to leave his hospital residency. Over the years he has been well scrutinized by those who wish to disclaim his findings. It is difficult for the powerful medical associations to admit fault, and financial ties are abundant. Due to his findings Dr. Wakefield suggested that the measles vaccine be given as a single shot without mumps, rubella or any other virus included. This was denied.

The British Medical Journal made slanderous statements against Dr. Wakefield and his research. The statements of him being fraudulent, receiving funds, and more, ended in his credentials and license being removed. They continue this threat today. To see the interview with Dr. Wakefield from January 20, 2013 on the Alex Jones show, go to www.autismone.com.

Dr. Wakefield has, however, found many connections between autism and the MMR vaccine. He has finally been able to speak publicly about it. If you wish to hear the entire story straight from Dr. Wakefield himself then I highly suggest going to www.mercola.com. Search for the article entitled, Why Medical Authorities Went to Such Extremes to Silence Dr. Andrew Wakefield, April 10, 2010. There are also many additional ongoing studies and their findings available.

It is important to note that Dr. Wakefield found the greatest results in treating these children came from a gluten free/casein free diet. When he treated the inflammatory bowel disease he found their behavior improved, sleep improved and there was an increase in communication.

Researchers like to boast that since use of the measles vaccination has become widespread it has prevented many deaths. The decline in measles actually came pre-vaccine with the help of better sanitation, trash removal, sewage systems, improved hygiene practices, and better nutrition.

Now, instead of measles, thousands of previously normally developing children are developing autism after being vaccinated with the MMR shot. That's one family out of every 68 in the U.S. Is this really better? Most well-nourished children will recover from the measles without further complications. Studies that are published regarding the safety of vaccines or that discount findings like the one above almost always come from a scientist or author that have financial ties to the company involved. They do not disclose this information.

In support of this I will offer you information on a study done in Denmark, NEJM, 2002. Evidence against these findings was reported. There is often a twist in the format of the study. See Carol Scott's "MMR and Autism in Perspective: The Denmark Story," in the Fall 2004 Journal of American Physicians and Surgeons, posted online.

More interesting facts on the MMR vaccine noted by Dr. Mercola's article, "A User Friendly Vaccination Schedule," www.mercola.com:

- Live measles virus are found in the cerebral spinal fluid (the protective fluid in your brain) in children who become autistic after MMR vaccines.
- Antibodies to measles virus are elevated in children with autism but not in normal kids, suggesting that virus induced autoimmunity may play a causal role.
- A study published in Neurology this year implicates hepatitis B vaccine as a causative factor in multiple sclerosis.

A team of doctors, scientists, and lawyers have come together with Dr. Wakefield to bring the truth to public awareness. They are personally risking a lot for our health to go against the pharmaceutical companies and all of their power and control, especially monetarily. They are standing up for what is right and for our protection. If you would like to gather more information on this or assist in any way, go to www.academicintegrityfund.com.

MMR AND HEPATITIS B EXCEL THE RATE OF AUTISM

When the Hepatitis B vaccine was added to the CDC's schedule along with the MMR shot already in place it seems that the rate of autism accelerated far beyond what anyone had imagined. The rate of autism increasing correlates with the same timing that the number of vaccines increased on the standard CDC schedule. This is not due to the age of the mother at conception or the external environmental factors alone or anything else they try to blame it on.

The measles, mumps, rubella vaccine was introduced in 1988 in England. One possibility for the exponential increase in autism is that many current mothers were once inoculated with the MMR vaccine. Today's children are second generation vaccinated potentially causing greater susceptibility to its dangers. Additionally, in 1988 the United States added the second dose of MMR to the CDC's routine vaccine schedule.

DIPTHERIA, PERTUSSIS, TETANUS (DPT or DTaP)

Diphtheria is a respiratory bacterium. Pertussis or whooping cough is a contagious bacterial disease indicated by a hacking cough. Tetanus is an infection causing muscle spasms due to an open cut or wound. The vaccine for these three bacteria is called DPT or DTaP.

Due to high fever, encephalitis or brain swelling and other related health complications from this vaccine researchers thought that changing the bacteria used from a "whole" or all of its parts, to only those components of the bacteria said to be needed for the body to develop immunity, would be a safer idea. A DTP vaccine contains the whole bacteria, the DTaP vaccine contains only the said needed parts. The "a" means it is acellular, otherwise stating that it does not contain any cells. The DTaP vaccine is supposed to create fewer complications.

Although the DTaP shot may not have as many complications arise from its use it does still offer many potential risks. Pertussis, the whooping cough portion, is extremely toxic and damaging to the brain, and the vaccine is known now to offer little to no protection.

The 2010, whooping cough outbreak in California offered data from Kaiser Permanente Medical Center in San Rafael showed that out of 132 patients:

- Eighty-one percent were completely up to date on their whooping cough vaccination.

- Eleven percent had received at least one shot but had not had the full series.
- Only eight percent had never been vaccinated.

For more information see the article, "The cough spreads mainly through vaccinated populations," at www.mercola.com.

Many are quick to accuse any new outbreak on those not vaccinated. The truth is that whooping cough is naturally cyclical every four to five years regardless of vaccinations. Vaccines also create virulent strains making the bacteria and viruses stronger and harder to eradicate. One can be an immunized carrier of whooping cough but have no symptoms.

Either way there are potential risks. The best answer for you in the decision-making process is to be as educated as possible. There is an excellent book on the DTP vaccine called, A Shot In The Dark, by Coulter and Fisher. More studies can be found at www.pubmed.com.

There is also information regarding the statistics in Sweden whose sudden infant death, or SIDS, rate disappeared after eliminating the pertussis vaccination. After Japan decided that children needed to be at least the age of two before being allowed to be given this vaccination their SIDS rate also disappeared.

ADVERSE REACTIONS TO VACCINATIONS: (these are the recorded reactions).

Anaphylaxis, is a serious and rapid allergic reaction with symptoms ranging from itching, rashes, throat swelling, to death. It is always a concern with immunizations.

- DTP: fever (especially due to pertussis component), drowsiness, fatigue, persistent inconsolable screaming or crying, vomiting, anorexia, encephalopathy, convulsions, skin rashes, fever, diarrhea, cough, runny nose, ear infections, shock, seizures, loss of muscle control, hypoglycemia or diabetes, death, sudden infant death syndrome.
- MMR: Measles: mild non-communicable form of illness, measles, fever, rash, seizures, sudden infant death syndrome, and SSPE (Subacute sclerosing panencephalitis). SSPE is an abnormal immune response to the measles virus in children

and adolescence causing brain inflammation and swelling. SSPE can appear many years after the virus invades the body. It is progressive and often fatal. There is no known cure.

- Mumps: pruritus or chronic itching due to irritated sensory nerve endings, rash, deafness, seizures
- Rubella: Most common joint pain, stiffness, rash, and swollen lymph nodes.
- Polio: Polio induced paralysis with oral form, possibly contagious without getting disease with oral form.
- Varivax: local reaction: pain, rash, fever, some people seen with shingles down the road.
- HBV: Pain and fever, Guillain Barré syndrome
- HiB: Local reaction, fever.
- Hepatitis B: sudden infant death syndrome, death, damage to the central nervous system, blindness, seizures, multiple sclerosis (MS), Guillain-Barre syndrome, Bell's Palsy, Diabetes, Rheumatoid arthritis, Lupus, Idiopathic Thrombocytopenia Purpura (bleeding disorders due to low platelets in the blood from injured blood vessels causing purple spots on the skin), convulsions, and brain disorders such as encephalitis (brain swelling) and brain demyelination, immune dysfunction, visual and hearing impairments, including optic neuritis, and pancreatitis.

Please see "healing the genetic defect," and "what can I do if my child has an adverse reaction to vaccines" in chapter 16. For further information on homeopathy, see chapter two.

VACCINES AND THE FUNGUS CONNECTION

Our chapter on Candida/yeast/fungus showed a large amount of disorder in the gut that then found its way to other organs, including the brain. This can account for many behavioral problems, immune disorders, and even asthma. What many do not realize is the connection between mercury and Candida. Mercury prevents a natural type of white blood cells called neutrophils from killing Candida and other foreign invaders. Candida engulfs mercury molecules. Mercury hurts all epithelial (gut lining) tissues.

CLEARING OLD VIRUSES LEFT BY VACCINES

As I mentioned already, my N.E.A.T. practitioner found that my son's body was fighting measles (he had never had the measles except in his MMR vaccine). I had the practitioner desensitize him to this ongoing reaction.

Parasites often invade when the liver is weak and the GI tract is permeable, as in leaky gut syndrome. Parasites bring with them bacteria, viruses, and fungi. Viruses in the nervous system often come from staphylococcus and lungworm, but they may also reside in your child's body from vaccinations. (See the chapter on pathogenic microbes for more information on parasites and viruses.) Whether you are looking to clear old viruses left over from vaccines, or are working with clearing a current illness, there are many options. Here are a few supplements helpful in clearing viruses:

1. A homeopathic doctor can find the right constitutional remedy that fits your child's specific needs. See chapter two for homeopathic doctors.
2. There are homeopathic remedies sold over-the-counter. Homeopathy has been very successful in removing the damage from vaccinations. Guna-INF liquid homeopathies are used for clearing viruses. They are available at www.pureformulas.com. See the chapter on alternative therapies to find a homeopathic doctor for constitutional remedies.
3. The homeopathic agent Acute Virotox is helpful for fighting general viruses. It is available at www.pureformulas.com.
4. For specific flu viruses the homeopathic product Oscillococcinum is very helpful. It is sold in most stores and online for a good price at www.pureformulas.com, or www.swansonvitamins.com.

5. Monolauren is commonly used to fight flu viruses and bacterial infections. Lauric acid is commonly used to treat Candida. It fights only the bad bacteria, not the good. It has also been used against shingles, hepatitis C, herpes, and measles. It is available at www.inspirednutrition.com. They have descriptive usage information on their website. Muscle test for dosage.
6. Selenium is effective against chronic viral infections. There is a liquid selenium product from Pharmax available at www.pureformulas.com.
7. Immune force from www.gethealthyagain.com.
8. Virastop is an enzyme product made by Enzymedica. It is made with eight high potency protease enzymes that are specifically together to assist elimination of proteins in the bloodstream and aid the immune system. When used away from food, protease enzymes target the film covering of viruses that are made of protein. This breaks down the parasite and destroys it. Research has shown that these protease enzymes also break down other pathogens in the bloodstream such as fungi from Candida, bacteria, and other parasites. Virastop is made from plant-based enzymes with no fillers. Capsules may be opened up into food. It can be found in some healthfood stores and online at www.amazon.com and www.pureformulas.com. Opening up capsules and trying to hide things in food can be inconvenient with children, so a better choice might be homeopathics.

Muscle test with the thought of each product in mind, individually. The body will give the answers you need.

BIOPURE PROPOLIS VAPORIZERS

Biopure propolis vaporizers are essential for killing indoor airborne microbes, but they also help eliminate mold, bacteria, and viruses. Propolis is known to be anti-fungal. Research has shown propolis to defend against the negative effects of vaccines.

Propolis is a resin-like composite derived from bees. When vaporized, propolis destroys pathogenic microbes and air pollutants. Inhaling the properties of propolis allows it to quickly reach the cellular level via the bloodstream. The flavonoids in propolis are strong anti-inflammatory and reduce type one allergy. It is all natural and free of chemicals. The active flavonoids in propolis vary due to the regions in which the bees travel. The propolis sold by the company Bee Healthy Farms, www.beehealthyfarms.com, is certified to contain the necessary active flavonoids. They also carry the vaporizers. The Biopure propolis vaporizer is small and can travel with you. They even make a car model that plugs into the cigarette lighter or 12v power source in your car.

SUMMARY

The immune system and the protective blood brain barrier are not fully developed in infants and very young children. If they also have pathogenic microbes weakening their digestive tract, then they also have a compromised immune system. Vaccines are filled with heavy metals and other toxins along with multiple live viruses. Research shows that there is a correlation between toxins such as heavy metals, and autism. Sometimes this research is made difficult to find. Disruption of the body's detoxification system and genetic expression are noted.

Self-education is crucial. We are often told that vaccines are safe, and that they are the sole reason why there has been a decline in many diseases. Better sanitation and nutrition are greatly responsible for this decline. Natural immunity is stronger and safer. The only way to be sure of what is truly safe for your child is to do your own personal research. Much has been given here with additional resources offered. Seek as much knowledge as you desire to make the best educated decisions for your child.

The products found in this chapter can be found at http://naturallyhealingautism.com/a-healthy-home/

CHAPTER 16

HEALING VACCINE DAMAGE AND KNOWING YOUR LEGAL RIGHTS

YOU DO HAVE CHOICES

One of the greatest controversies today surrounds vaccines. The best way to make a decision for your child or yourself is by being informed, a process you should take control of yourself. There is a lot more information to research than that released by the American Medical Association and pharmaceutical companies who stand to profit.

On the other hand, there are many doctors who simply have only listened to their professors and never questioned it. If I can so easily find information regarding the risks behind vaccinations, then why can't a trained professional. The answer is usually that they have not bothered to look very far or do not have the time to. It is their responsibility—and falls under the Hippocratic Oath—to learn as much as possible and disclose that information to their patients before any injections are given so that people are able to make informed decisions—and are kept safe.

Not all practitioners feel the same way about vaccines, so there is obviously more knowledge on this subject than one or two or three practitioners has. Not all of them have the time or are willing to dig deeper into controversial subjects, especially this one, therefore *you* need to know best. Going against the grain can cause damage to reputations, so many choose to follow suit with the system—often to the detriment of our children.

If you know anyone who is currently pregnant or planning on getting pregnant, please give them as much information as you can so that they will be able to make an *informed* decision for themselves and their child based on all of the facts.

PROPAGANDA AND HYPE

We can become so emotionally involved that we won't even listen to ourselves even though we may know better. If emotion overrides you and you are not in a dangerous or life-threatening situation, it is best to do nothing. Separate yourself from the situation even for a short time to clear your head. If you need to gather more information for yourself before you act, then do so.

Proof that people are finally educating themselves was shown when the vaccine came out for Gardasil, which was supposed to prevent cervical cancer in young girls. They tried to make it mandatory for teenage girls to receive this vaccine, but this was stopped when the public learned too much. Mothers learned that 65 girls had died from the vaccine and over 18,000 reported significant health issues. Self-education is how we, the public, say, "NO.'

A CONFLICT OF INTEREST

A member of the World Health Organization (WHO) who is the director of the vaccine program in Finland received over 9 million dollars in 2009 for his research center from vaccine manufacturer GlaxoSmithKline. This creates the number one income source for the vaccine program. GlaxoSmithKline produces the H1N1 vaccine, Pandemrix. The Finnish government, following the recommendations from this director and WHO, purchased enough for a pandemic (just in case there happened to be one).

Several other doctors on the powerful panel of WHO have been named and are receiving funding from many of the large pharmaceutical companies as well. One of them, not so surprisingly, is in charge of fighting influenza. An emergency investigation has been launched since it has been discovered that this doctor has been receiving a salary from several of the companies who manufacture the swine flu vaccine. This is an extreme conflict of interest. Of course, they would recommend the vaccine if it put millions of dollars in their pockets.

If you would like the complete story, including the names of those doctors involved, please see "WHO Advisor Secretly Pads Pockets with Big Pharma Money" at www.mercola.com.

The only people who had serious complications or died from the swine flu were those who already had severely compromised immune systems. If I had a severely compromised immune system, I sure wouldn't inject a barely-studied serum into my body that also contains toxic additives. What would an already weak immune system do with that? Would it possibly be more beneficial in the long term to wash our hands more, take a lot of antioxidants and probiotics, and include more vitamin D in our diet before getting a potentially dangerous vaccine? Only after you do careful research can you make an educated decision.

Throughout my lifetime, I've caught the flu and then recovered just fine. I have to ask, since when did catching the flu become life threatening for all of us? Could it be that we have fallen for their propaganda?

A study done in 2008 showed that pharmaceutical companies spent almost twice as much money on promotion compared to that of research and development. In 2004, $57.5 billion was spent on marketing and promotion by the industry itself. In comparison, $31.5 billion was spent on research and development. [Gagnon M.A., Lexchin J, "The cost of pushing pills: A new estimate of pharmaceutical promotion expenditures in the United States." PLoS Med 5(1)].

No one who receives any type of funding from or is an advisor to any of the pharmaceutical companies should be allowed to give recommendations to agencies like the World Health Organization or anyone else who is making recommendations for the rest for the world (that includes both you and me).

These companies hold more power than we can imagine. They are inside government agencies. It is not likely that this will end. What we have to do is educate ourselves. You are ultimately in charge of what choices are made for yourself and your child. **Please make**

your choice from information that you have gathered and not what the media or anyone else says you should do.

EDUCATION BEFORE VACCINATION

Educate yourself completely on all information regarding vaccinations. This book offers many websites for further education, and there is much more out there. Remember that the brain is growing the most rapidly during the third trimester of pregnancy through the age of three, but the brain is only 80% developed even at age four. Anything that invades the child's system will have a direct impact on his brain.

Males do not have as much brain protection as females. Girls have higher levels of the hormone estrogen, which helps protect the brain. Boys not only have less estrogen, but higher testosterone, which exacerbates the toxic effects of both mercury, found in many vaccines, and Candida.

Please take into account your child as an individual. Many children who suffer from vaccine damage had parents who were not informed of neurological disorders such as mitochondrial dysfunction before the vaccine was given. Family history going many generations back and testing for neurological issues are crucial factors if you choose to vaccine. The one size fits all does not work for many and can leave a lifelong debilitation.

8 QUESTIONS TO ASK BEFORE VACCINATION:

(From the National Vaccination Information Center, www.NVIC.org)

1. Am I or my child sick right now?
2. Have I or my child had a bad reaction to a vaccination before?
3. Do I or my child have a personal or family history of vaccine reactions, neurological disorders, severe allergies or immune system problems?
4. Do I know the disease and vaccine risks for myself or my child?
5. Do I have full information about the vaccine's side effects?
6. Do I know how to identify and report a vaccine reaction?

7. Do I know I need to keep a written record, including the vaccine manufacturer's name and lot number, for all vaccinations?
8. Do I know I have the right to make an informed choice?

IF VACCINATING: A FEW GUIDELINES TO FOLLOW:

The following includes what should be standard knowledge before any vaccination is given. We cannot follow a "one-size-fits-all" model.

If you would like to vaccinate, there are possible choices that still have risks but are less invasive. Be sure you are doing what is best for your family's well-being.

- Always test for neurological susceptibility, including mitochondrial and gastrointestinal disorders.
- Only use single viruses in one injection. Never use multiple viruses at one time; this can overload the immune system.
- Be given proof that the injection contains no thimerosal (made of 50% mercury).
- Avoid live viruses. Examples are the combined measles, mumps, and rubella (MMR) vaccine; chickenpox (varicella) vaccine; and the live-virus polio (Sabin) vaccine.
- Spread single shots out three to six months apart. This allows time for the immune system to recover and time for you to determine if there has been any kind of negative reaction to the previous vaccine.
- Wait until after the age of two years (three to five is better) to begin vaccinations. The brain is in its greatest growth between the third trimester of pregnancy and the age of two years. At the age of two, the brain is still only 80% developed. If you feel the need to wait longer, then do so.
- Breastfeed for at least one year or more to help your baby build his immune system and aid in protection by receiving mom's antibodies to diseases. Breast-feeding delivers omega-3 fatty

acids (important for brain development and protection from disease).

- If bottle feeding, add omega-3 fatty acids to your baby's formula, especially DHA (docosahexanoic acid), and always avoid formulas made with cow's milk or soy.
- Never give vaccinations if your child has any sign of weak immunity including a slight cold, runny nose, or allergies. (Nine out of ten children are vaccinated by doctors even if they are ill.)
- Take vitamin C for at least two days prior and two days following any vaccinations.
- Never vaccinate if you have a family history of autism or other neurological illnesses.
- Must wait one month to give any live vaccines in patients with blood, plasma, or antibody transplant.
- Never give live vaccine in immuno-deficient conditions, except MMR in HIV patients (wild virus followed by measles is fatal for HIV patients).
- Allergy to egg whites often contraindicates vaccination (usually the median vaccine is grown in)
- History of febrile seizures, CI (contraindicated)
- If a family member has had a reaction, CI

DO THE BENEFITS OUTWEIGH THE RISKS?

Although it can be contested that many lives have been saved due to vaccinations, a lesser known fact is that the vaccinations have caused far greater damage to far more people than they were supposed to protect. While attempting to protect our children from diseases, we are injecting them with toxic serums that have caused even greater problems, including death.

Is temporary immunity from a vaccine better than contracting an infection on your own that would give you permanent immunity? Do the complications that come from vaccines cause more chronic illness such as neurological damage, immunological damage, or death than infectious diseases do?

Even if it is only one in a thousand odds of debilitating neurological disease isn't that too many? The statistics may not seem so real to you unless you have had a child who has been afflicted. A parent with a child on the autism spectrum, or with a physical or behavioral disease is left with the challenges of watching their beloved child go through life with physical and emotional struggles, not to mention their own emotional and financial devastation and the future financial impact on the country after the parent is deceased. Many parents are taking second loans out on their homes in order to pay for all of the needed therapies and treatments. Some children cannot speak or go without diapers. Many have severe aggression and anger outbursts. The challenges are so great that there is an 80% divorce rate for parents of autistic children. Are these better alternatives?

Why does the government feel they can take the authority to administer a "one size fits all" program when it comes to vaccinations? The consideration of each individual needs to be assessed. We do not know what small percentage may or may not be susceptible to injury or death due to vaccines.

THEY TOLD ME I HAD TO

It seems that with the growing knowledge of vaccine dangers, the two biggest reasons people still do get them are because of fear or perceived force. "What if my child were in danger of contracting a disease?" or "They told me I had to."

On one hand, there are the dangers of vaccines. On the other hand, there is the fear of the possible dangers of not vaccinating at all.

If you hear that a doctor or scientist has been discredited for what they have said, then I urge you to dig deeper yourself rather than listen to those who seem to fear what has been said. What might be the basis for their fear? Is it possible that they have either not educated themselves further than what their professors have taught them in schools controlled by the American Medical Association or that they have something financial to lose from increased public knowledge of the truth. Many scientific reports that are released to the public are funded by the very agencies that have to lose financially if Americans start finding out the real truths, and their data is deceptive.

In February of 2010, a news release came out about a new study that had found that the information released in 1998 by Dr. Andrew Wakefield had been found to be wrong. The information given was that too many parents were deciding not to vaccinate their children based on the 1998 study that referred connections to autism from the MMR vaccine. The news neglected to say who it was that was funding any contradictory release of information and who was so concerned about it—12 years later! I believe their hope is that now the pediatricians will be able to tell their concerned parents that the study they heard about from Dr. Wakefield was "proved" wrong and that they can feel safe now about going through with the vaccination.

I applaud those physicians who are willing to continue to educate themselves outside of the box so that you can serve your patients in the most educated and honored way possible. It is you and those who trust you with their health for whom you once took the Hippocratic Oath, "do no harm," that serves so well. It is a legal and ethical obligation, but it is also a personal choice to follow it.

Dr. Andrew Wakefield and a few others have been willing to speak up to the public, regardless of criticism. There have been few doctors who have been willing to risk their reputations and the scrutiny of fellow peers who almost seem to force a sense of discrediting on them for speaking out.

WHAT CAN I DO IF MY CHILD DOES HAS AN ADVERSE REACTION TO VACCINES OR CONTRACTS A DISEASE?

In the chapter on alternative therapies we discussed many of the ways in which homeopathy can be of great help. Adverse vaccine reactions and disease contraction can often be healed with homeopathic remedies. A professional homeopathic doctor will be able to assist you. These remedies inspire the vital force of the individual's system. Every person varies in their own mental, physical, and emotional susceptibility, so there is not just one remedy for all. The mental, emotional and physical are all treated to heal the whole.

Many look to homeopathy for prevention but only symptoms can be treated. Homeopathy looks to recognize the weakness in the body which has already occurred, not from a possibility of one in the future. In trying to prevent a disease we may be instilling the fear of that disease which can increase susceptibility. Prevention would be better used to treat the fears.

For information on homeopathy, vaccines, and autism see www.tinussmits.com. To find a homeopathic doctor go to, www.homeopathicdirectory.com, or www.homeopathy-cures.com. Most of the doctors have websites of their own and you can learn more before you call and interview them. Don't be afraid to ask questions.

Good hygiene, good sanitation, and good nutrition are the best defenses.

Building the positive gut flora with probiotics should be done daily. Vitamins A, D and C are known to prevent and treat the symptoms of many viruses including measles, polio and meningitis C. Infants and children can be supplemented with sublingual drops. Always breastfeed. Breastfeeding offers one of the most powerful immune builders and viral fighters known. Anything you as a mother ingests will be ingested by your baby, so take your vitamins and eat organic, nutritious foods. Nutrition is known to be one of the best preventative measures. Along with vitamins eat plenty of foods rich in vitamin A such as carrots, sweet potatoes, pumpkin, spinach, butternut squash, turnip greens, mustard greens, lettuce, and free range eggs. Get plenty of sunshine to add to your vitamin D levels. Teach your children good hygiene and be sure to practice it yourself. Regular hand washing during the day is great prevention, and so making it a habit to cough or sneeze into the inside of your arm instead of your hand. Lastly, always stay hydrated with plenty of healthy, pure water.

WHICH VACCINES WOULD BE PUT ON A SAFER SCHEDULE?

Dr. Andrew Wakefield suggested a safer way to vaccinate for measles might be with a single virus vaccine instead of the present multiple dosage with mumps and rubella. This was denied. If they want people to vaccinate they must give better choices. The DTP or diphtheria, tetanus, pertussis vaccine is another contradiction. They have made it impossible to get a tetanus vaccine without diphtheria and the dangerous pertussis virus combined in one shot. I suppose it stands that they can make more money this way. There should also be vaccinations available without all of the potentially harmful added toxins.

Dr. Donald Miller, a cardiac surgeon and Professor of Surgery at the University of Washington released an article at [LewRockwell.com in 2004, "A User-Friendly Vaccination Schedule."] In this article Dr. Miller, answers the question, "Which vaccines would be put on a user-friendly schedule?"

Dr. Miller stated, "Which vaccines should be put on this schedule (among those that do not contain live viruses or thimerosal) is not entirely clear." Due to pertussis and diphtheria being more infectious, Dr. Miller had originally included them in his top four. However, in the newsletter New Developments: New Angles on Developmental Delays (Spring 2005, vol. 10, No.3), in the News and Comments section (p.3) there was an entry titled "Friendly Vaccine Schedule Encounters a Glitch."

Apparently the D and T of the DPT are no longer available separately without thimerosal, so they can no longer be added to the "user friendly" vaccination schedule as it was previously written. Miller believes that, "the risk of the combined DPT vaccine, even after age two, outweighs its benefits, so it is better to do without these shots."

While still following the above guidelines this would leave only the following polio vaccine; The Salk polio vaccine, with an inactivated (dead) virus, one that is cultured in human cells, not monkey kidney cells.

A good case can be made for avoiding the three other newer vaccines on the CDC's schedule: The hepatitis B, pneumococcal conjugate (PCV7), and hemophilus influenzae type B (Hib) vaccines."

Dr. Miller says, "The best discussion on avoiding most vaccines on the CDC's schedule is on Dr. Sherry Tenpenny's (3-hour) DVD titled Vaccines: The Risks the Benefits, the Choices, (sold on Amazon.com and other sites).

Dr. Miller feels that the two best books on this subject are, Saying No to Vaccines: A Resource Guide For All Ages, by Dr. Sherry Tenpenny and Vaccine Safety Manual for Concerned Families and Health Practitioners; Guide To Immunization Risks and Protection, by Neil Miller.

Dr. Miller's web site is www.donaldmiller.com and you can contact him at dwm@u.washington.edu (mailto:dwm@u.washington.edu).

HEALING THE GENETIC DEFECT

Genes lie dormant until a trigger signals its protein receptor and engages it causing either a positive or a negative reaction. If autism, ADHD, pervasive developmental disorder, seizures, juvenile rheumatoid arthritis, Type 1 diabetes, asthma, and bowel disorders were not occurring in epidemic proportions 50 years ago, then what has changed? There appears to be a correlation with an increased number of vaccines.

Genetic defects may be triggered by physical or emotional trauma, or toxins such as those induced by vaccination. Vaccinations carry a number of toxins, not just one or two. The cumulative effect of toxins is extremely dangerous and cause for negative signaling on genetic cell structures. These genetic defects caused by vaccines are known to continue for four generations. Genetic mutations are reversible with the use of homeopathic remedies. See the chapter, "Alternative Therapies" for more information on homeopathy. For more information on the genetic mutations caused by vaccinations, please listen to the audio at www.klinghardtacademy.com.

My son was given the constitutional homeopathic remedy Thuja by our homeopathic doctor. This assists with nervousness around strangers, is intended to help over-sensitive people, and addresses any residual susceptibility or symptoms that he carries or his body has adapted to or compensates for related to vaccinations. The remedy inspires the vital force to restore that back to health. A constitutional remedy addresses the needs of the entire person including the physical, mental, and emotional.

We have covered genetics in detail in chapter four, "Genetic Susceptibility."

YOU DO HAVE CHOICES

You, as a parent, can refuse vaccinations but they try to make it sticky for you when it comes time to enroll your child in school. Do not fear. If you know what your legal rights and exemptions are, then you will have that to back you up.

I know a mother in my own town that our school system tried to stop with their threats and fancy wording. She was informed and brought out paperwork with all of her facts and legal rights on it. They responded with, "Oh, well, I guess you're right." She was able to enroll her children and that was the end of it.

For a list of exemption requirements in your state, go to http// www.909shot.com/state-site/state-exemptions.htm, and be sure to read the following article.

Religion is one of the freedoms in America. This can still be valid to stop immunizations. Additionally, a letter written by you stating that if your child shows any signs of adverse reaction after the immunization that the doctor will take full responsibility, personally, professionally, and financially, forever. Tell him he and a witness must sign it. This will stop him from proceeding. Lastly, let him know that neurological disorders or autism run in your family and that your child is predisposed to the dangers of vaccinations. It would not be safe for your child.

KNOWING YOUR LEGAL RIGHTS

I have been told by many mothers that they were told their child could not enter school without vaccines. Some were bullied and told that child protective services would be called on them. The most important thing of all is to educate yourself and know your legal rights. Each state has their own laws; go to www.nvic.org for more information on your state's requirements. You are the parent and may write personal beliefs exemption. If they argue, let them know your family has autoimmune weaknesses and are too vulnerable to viruses and toxins in vaccinations. Ask if they can give you a 100% guarantee that there will be no negative responses, and ask them to sign a form from you stating so. This usually stops them.

No one can make you vaccinate your child. Laws protect the medical establishments, but they don't protect you or your child if something goes wrong. In fact, they will say it was your fault because you allowed the shot when you feared it might not be safe for your child. They turn the blame around onto you.

In 1986, the U.S. Congress passed a law protecting both doctors and vaccine manufacturers from lawsuits connected to vaccine injury.

In 1949, it was only required to show proof of one smallpox vaccination in order to enter school. By 2003, most states required 34 doses of vaccines with multiple viruses. In 2013, it is 36 vaccinations by the time a child enters kindergarten. When will they stop? They won't. It's up to you to decide what your child will receive and will not receive.

See the article "How to legally avoid unwanted immunizations of all kinds" at www.mercola.com. Note that article three will show you how to obtain the immunization laws for your state. By knowing these laws you will know what you can do.

The rights in your state protect your vaccine choice rights. Sign up for the National Advocacy Information Center at www.nvic.org, to make a difference.

For Exemption from vaccinations:

Go to your public health department, and ask for an immunization waver. Have a notary public sign, and then send it back to the public health department.

Dr. Shari Tenpenny is one of the country's most knowledgeable and outspoken physicians regarding vaccines and the right to refuse them. She has scientifically sound information regarding the dangers of vaccines. She also offers treatment for those injured by vaccines www.drtenpenny.com. Please listen to my very informative podcast interview with Dr. Tenpenny on vaccinations at www.naturallyhealingautism.com

REVIEWS FOR QUESTIONING PEDIATRICIANS

Neurosurgeon, Russell L. Blaylock, has written two reviews on the subject of questioning pediatricians: "Interaction of Cytokines, Excitotoxins, Reactive Nitrogen and Oxygen Species in Autism Spectrum Disorders," in the Journal of American Nutraceutical Association [JANA 2003;6(4):21—35], with 167 references. And "Chronic Microglial Activation and Excitoxicity Secondary to Excessive Immune Stimulation: Possible Factors in Gulf War Syndrome and Autism," in the Journal of American Physicians and Surgeons [JAPS 2004; 9(2):46—52], posted online, with 54 references.

SUMMARY

There are various alternatives to traditional vaccinations. You have choices and you can choose what you feel is best for your child. You can refuse what you do not wish for. Resources have been given to provide further education. The information provided is for your learning process. Seek the advice of a professional homeopathic doctor for more information on healing damage caused by vaccinations.

The products found in this chapter can be found at http://naturallyhealingautism.com/a-healthy-home/

CHAPTER 17

ALLERGIES AND THE GUT/ BRAIN CONNECTION

Autism, schizophrenia, anxiety, ADHD, and other labels are just that—a label. One of the reasons we hear the word "recovery" so much now is due to the detoxification of the body and the healing of the gut. Yes, healing the gut does have that much power over the brain; do not let anyone tell you otherwise.

Dr. Andrew Wakefield is a gastroenterologist who used to work in London at the Royal Free Hospital. In 1998, Dr. Wakefield published research he had discovered while working with autistic children. He found that a part of the small intestine called the ilium had inflamed lymph nodes, which only become inflamed when fighting infection. These immune system fighters will encapsulate a virus if they cannot destroy them.

Many accounts of autism have been first noticed after a child has received the measles, mumps, and rubella (MMR) vaccine, so Dr. Wakefield began to explore this coincidence. What he and his associates found was that the same virus used in the MMR vaccine was the identical one found within these lymph nodes in the intestinal walls of these children. He suggested that these three viruses be spread out into three different vaccines and given apart from one another in single doses to allow the immune system the possibility to fight the invasion.

Sadly, all Dr. Wakefield has received from this famous release in the *Lancet* was ridicule. Things became so bad for him in the UK that he had to leave his homeland and move to Austin, Texas in the U.S. to practice medicine. Articles assaulting him are still found today. The parent movement and concern was so great in his findings that the medical and pharmaceutical movements continue to work at destroying his reputation in order to keep the public under their desires instead of their own. For a full interview with Dr. Wakefield regarding this issue, go to www.mercola.com, and enter "Wakefield interview."

Dr. Andrew Wakefield found that if a person was jaundiced (in which the liver is unhealthy and bile backs up to create yellowing of the skin and eyes), that some patients went into encephalopathy—their brain became diseased. If he treated the gastrointestinal tract, he found that the encephalopathy went away. This is a clear connection between the GI tract, the liver, and their effect on the brain.

Children and adults with autism and ADHD have intestinal symptoms. Most parents and doctors who work with children on the autism spectrum have found that if the child is treated for inflammatory bowel disease, there is vast improvement in behavior, sleep, verbal communication, and more. Here lies a key issue that must be addressed seriously if you want to see your child's physical and emotional/behavioral health improve.

The digestive system makes up to 80% of the immune system. These two synergistically functioning systems are crucial to the overall health of your child. When there is inflammation, cells die. Not only do we have immune system problems, but also malabsorption of nutrients and developmental delays.

Serotonin is a neurotransmitter (messenger for the brain) that regulates the function of such things as sleep, mood, and appetite. It is also important in helping to regulate those cravings for sugar. There are serotonin receptors in the GI tract that, when weakened, reduce the ability of the neurological system to build serotonin.

Due to the nature of biology, one person can be unaffected by a food or toxin, whereas another is greatly affected by the same product. Some individuals are so sensitive that merely touching a substance with their hands can cause severe reactions through absorption from the skin.

The cause of sensitivities and allergens may be biological or due to a weakness caused by genetics that was triggered by an environmental agent. The delicate balance of the intestinal system can be easily disrupted by Candida/yeast, vaccines, heavy metals, viruses, air pollution, food chemicals, and a high sugar, high carbohydrate diet. Many children are born with Candida/yeast in their gut that was passed on in utero from their mothers, so their system is already weak and detoxification channels poor at birth.

Children with a weak GI tract often do not absorb the nutrients from the food they eat due to an improperly working digestive system. They may even be eating some healthy foods, but the nutrition may not be getting in. If their body is not absorbing the nutrients from the food properly, then their body becomes starved of vital nutrients which also feed the brain.

LEAKY GUT: THE MAIN CAUSE

Intestinal permeability is very common. The gut lining is only one cell layer thick so it is quite vulnerable to damage. Damage to the mucosal intestinal lining creates large spaces or openings that allow bacteria toxins and larger food particles to leak through and get into the bloodstream. This is largely caused by the spores of the Candida. These spores have legs that act as screws that bore their way into the intestinal lining, and create holes in which the undigested food particles pass through.

When the gut lining becomes inflamed, it is unable to fight off bacteria, viruses, parasites, and Candida or yeast. Bacteria in the gut also inhibits production of enzymes, so if the gut is damaged, the needed enzymes for digestion and vital chemical reactions in the body are not produced. A healthy gut regulates the release of up to twenty five hormones to create such actions as digesting and utilizing insulin resistance or blood sugar balance, appetite control, and balancing brain chemistry.

Leaky gut mimics a myriad of disease and their symptoms including asthma, fibromyalgia, and rheumatoid arthritis as it affects the joints. Once in the bloodstream, the newly released toxins find their way to organs and tissues as far away as the brain. This causes chaos in the brain as its chemistry is affected.

Symptoms can vary from behavioral outbursts and inability to concentrate to anxiety or depression. Many children complain of stomach aches or headaches. Headaches, dizziness and stomach aches after eating may indicate leaky gut. These children also tend to have extreme fatigue off and on, or they may look emaciated. They are not absorbing the nutrition from the foods they eat, and their bodies become extremely malnourished. This also means that their brain is not receiving the vital nutrients it needs for proper growth and functioning.

We have discussed supplements to heal the gut lining in chapter eleven. They are also included in the healing program in this book. The gut balancing diet also helps to heal leaky gut.

HOME TEST FOR DAMAGED GUT LINING

Add about a teaspoon of apple cider vinegar to an ounce of water and drink it. If this creates a burning sensation in the stomach, you can be pretty sure there is damage to the gut lining.

TESTING FOR GUT INFLAMMATION

There is no need to put your child through an uncomfortable procedure in order to check for gut inflammation. The laboratory Diagnos-Techs offer a panel used with your child's stool that can give their inflammation markers along with a lot of other valuable information. The test can also check for IgA antibodies (gluten allergens), parasites, fungus, and more. Most alternative practitioners use this laboratory and have these tests on hand, or they can order them at Diagnos-Techs, 425-251-0596.

The website www.crohns.net also sells a pathology test that you can do from home, and they will send you the results via e-mail. The owner of the site is Pamela Nathan. She is a licensed acupuncturist with over 30 years of experience working with people who have gut and digestive issues. She is available to help you with the results.

FOOD ALLERGIES OR INTOLERANCES

If the intestinal lining is damaged, particles of food seep through into the bloodstream and cause havoc in the organs and tissues of the body and brain. These undigested food particles reach the bloodstream where the body sees them as foreign agents to fight against. The body will create antibodies against these foods and create an allergic reaction when the food is eaten. This is how we develop allergies to foods that we previously were not allergic to.

The gut lining becomes damaged due to factors such as an intense inflammatory response that leads to persistent inflammation (often the case after vaccinations due to mercury or viral exposure), overgrowth of bad bacteria such as Candida (caused in-utero, by vaccines, poor diet, or antibiotic use), invasion of parasites, contaminated food and beverages, chemicals in processed food, dyes, preservatives, bad fats, enzyme deficiency, NSAIDs (non-steroidal anti-inflammatory drugs, such as ibuprofen), prescription corticosteroids (e.g. Prednisone or hydrocortisone), a diet of highly refined carbohydrates, such as cookies, candy, soda, white bread, molds, and fungus from stored grains, fruit, and refined carbohydrates, viruses, GI disease, chemotherapy, and radiation treatments due to the harmful impact on the immune system. All of these things are contributing factors to what is known as "leaky gut."

True food allergies are caused by a reaction the immune system has created due to a response to antibodies. When the body does not carry antibodies such as IgE and IgG, there can still be a chemical sensitivity to the food. This commonly occurs when a food is not able to be broken down properly by the digestive system. Food intolerances are not caused by a reaction from the immune system but to that of a chemical. Intolerances and sensitivities can cause symptoms as serious as those of true allergies.

There is a difference between a true allergy and a food for which the body has created an intolerance. The intolerance mimics that of a true allergy, and undigested particles must now be eliminated by the body's detoxifying organs, largely the kidneys and the liver. Children on the autism spectrum already have poor detoxification pathways and congested livers, and their systems have an even harder time removing this debris while the toxins cause havoc in their central nervous system.

SYMPTOMS OF FOOD ALLERGIES OR INTOLERANCES

Symptoms of food allergies or intolerances are mucus in the throat or nose, runny nose and watery eyes, headaches, gastrointestinal problems, such as abdominal bloating or cramping, diarrhea, constipation, burping, nausea, irritable bowel syndrome, fatigue, arthritis, migraines, asthma, eczema, hives, acne or other skin irritations, ulcers, excessive salivation including drooling, sinusitis, ear infections, chronic cough, poor memory or inability to focus, emotional problems including depression, anxiety, hyperactivity, anger, muscle aching or cramping, insomnia, allergies to pollens, molds, and other environmental pollutants.

Food allergies may also trigger any form of behavioral change such as hyperactivity or anxiety, and emotional outbursts such as anger, impulsivity, or depression.

When the lining of the gastrointestinal wall becomes damaged, it allows otherwise non-penetrable products, such as large protein molecules, to invade the bloodstream. Once undigested food particles enter the bloodstream, the immune system sees them as foreign agents to defend against. Antibodies can then be created toward that food type and the body develops an "allergy" or sensitivity toward it.

The body sees a food as an allergy when the immune system gets triggered to release histamine. When there is a true allergy, to a food the body will create antibodies toward it. Often a test will have negative results for different reasons. For example, gluten binds to tissue, such as in the colon, so a blood test could easily come up negative, or an antibody for another substance may not show up in that particular blood test. This also does not mean that your child does not have intolerance to that food.

Food intolerances can create the same symptoms as allergies. The best way to know whether or not your child has an allergy is to simply remove the food from their diet for a few weeks and see if you notice a difference in their behavior or in their physiology. Often a difference can be noticed in days or within a week or two, but clearing a substance from the body can take up to three months for symptoms to subside.

Depending on their level of sensitivity, once their gut gets back into balance through a healing program, your child can possibly eat some of the foods he has developed sensitivities toward, although not every day. Initially, it is wise to only have that particular food about every four days to be sure that the body does not regress.

HOW TO GET PICKY EATERS TO EAT

Generally, the reward game works best. Let them know that they can have one bite of something they want if they will take one bite of something you want them to eat. Be persistent in them only getting one small bite of a favorite food for a small bite of a healthy one. As their GI tract heals they will become less picky.

ALLERGY ELIMINATION

We discussed allergy elimination practitioners in the chapter "Alternative Therapies". Please refer to that section to assist in healing the gut, along with the acquired food intolerances and organ weaknesses that are associated with it.

FALSE NEGATIVE TEST RESULTS

Be aware of food and allergy testing. Often a test will come out negative for an allergy, but there is still a strong sensitivity; this is commonly seen in gluten and casein sensitivities. The danger for your child lies in the false belief given by the negative test result. If you receive a negative test result, you may think it is all right to give your child that food again. Hopefully, the child's reaction is strong enough to the food for you to figure out what is safe to give and what is not. Hair analysis for food allergies has also been found to have poor results. Let symptoms be your guide.

ALCAT BLOOD TEST

This is a blood test that can give you the answers on a scale from the most allergic foods to the least allergic foods. I have found that this test has two sides. On one side, it can determine that a food or foods that you are eating regularly, although healthy, are not healthy for you. On the other side, this test is expensive and many doctors are uncertain of its efficiency.

I found that natural allergy elimination practitioners were the most cost effective and helpful in finding *and eliminating* allergies. See the chapter on Alternative Therapies for more information.

LET SYMPTOMS BE YOUR GUIDE

Using the symptoms of a food can be a lot less expensive than tests and doctors' visits. Our children typically eat from about twelve foods. Eliminate them one by one, except for gluten and casein, which I recommend eliminating from the beginning since they are both known to be such a big problem for children with autism, along with those with ADHD, asthma, allergies, and more.

There can also be withdrawal symptoms that the food is creating. When the body has an allergic reaction or intolerance to a food, the system will often, oddly enough, crave that food. Withdrawal symptoms similar to those you would experience if you went off of caffeine or sugar may occur for the child. The alternate possibility is that if you are in the middle of a Candida cleanse there can be similar symptoms, but they may be coming from the Candida die-off.

THE GOOD NEWS

Once we heal the gut lining, strengthen the good bacteria in the digestive tract, and naturally desensitize the system to allergens, we are usually able to eat the problem foods once again without any trouble.

TESTING FOR SENSITIVITIES

There are a couple of ways to test for food allergies or sensitivities, and the body will tell you how it responds to them. At night, just before bedtime, take a drop of the food in question and place it on the inside of your child's wrist. If it is a solid food, mash it up with a drop or two of pure water. Let the solution dry on the wrist and sleep with it there all night. Upon waking, check the area. If there is irritation and redness, then there is an allergy. If the area is clear, it is okay to introduce that food into the diet.

Muscle testing is also a great way to test if a food is agreeable with your body or not. Have your child raise one arm directly in front of him with the elbow straight, not bent. Gently press down on his wrist. The muscle should be strong. Then place any food or product you choose to test in his other hand. Test the same original muscle's strength again. If it now tests weak then the product is not good for him. If it tests strong, it should be safe.

For more detailed information on muscle testing please see the chapter on alternative therapies.

PHENOLS

Phenols are the natural colorings in foods such as in fruits and vegetables. Phenols are also in the artificial colorings that are in yogurt, candy, and popsicles, etc. Used industrially, they help form and are contained in plastics. They can be an allergen, whether from food or plastic products. People with poor methylation are often phenol sensitive. It is very common for children on the autism spectrum to be allergic to phenols. This is often due to an ill digestive tract.

Normally the body could properly utilize and eliminate phenols. Phenols and salicylates are in most foods. Candida/yeast overgrowth and leaky gut contribute to phenol sensitivity. Leaky gut will allow these chemicals to enter the bloodstream in high concentrations. This alarms the body and triggers an immune response which creates an allergy to these chemicals.

Proteins contain sulfites which turn to sulfates in the body. Sulfates assist with detoxification and digestion. People on the autism spectrum often have trouble digesting proteins, thus causing a deficiency in sulfates. This along with a weakened liver can cause difficulty digesting and eliminating phenolic chemicals.

Phenols are a natural chemical. Salicylates are a type of phenol. They are chemically similar to aspirin. Many people who are phenol sensitive are also allergic to salicylates. These sensitivities create a multitude of physical and behavioral problems.

Phenols are also produced in plants, including fruits and vegetables. The fiber content of fruit, though healthy, may be hard for some to digest also. Spinach and citrus are known to alter the sulphate transport system. This may be the reason why citrus should be avoided within an hour of taking many medications and natural supplementation.

The Feingold diet was developed by a pediatrician of the same name. It is a total exclusion of food additives, colorings, and salicylates to assist the body in healing, www.feingold.com.

We don't want to eliminate healthy, antioxidant-rich foods (such as blueberries) from the diet. For this reason, there are enzymes that allow them to be eaten. One great way to allow your child to eat these healthy foods while his gut is healing is through the use of specific enzymes. They are called no-phenol enzymes from www.houston-enzymes.com. It turned out that my daughter was extremely phenol sensitive. If she even ate a strawberry or had a natural popsicle without taking a no-phenol enzyme, her stomach hurt and she became very tired and emotional. The coloring of the food, natural or not, greatly affects her system. My daughter needed more of the no-phenol enzymes added to her dosage of Trienza enzymes.

Once the gut is healed the allergies often remain. The body needs to learn to recognize these foods as safe and no longer start an immune reaction when they are ingested. Natural allergy desensitization is often necessary. We had my daughter desensitized to phenols through natural allergy desensitization (see the chapter on Alternative Therapies). This worked wonders for her, and she no longer has any issues with those foods or products.

If your child tends to be constipated, the no-phenol enzyme product will help to loosen the stool. If your child's stool tends to be on the looser side, then the product Zyme-Prime from Houston enzymes will help firm the stool. Zyme-prime and no-phenol are both in the Trienza product, but at half the dosage. If you find that you want to assist in either firming or loosening the stool, you can purchase either of these products individually and increase their dosage. See if adding in one more each day helps the problem.

Prior to allergy desensitization, my daughter's stomach aches did not disappear with the regular dosage of Trienza. With the help of the staff at Houston Enzymes, I added in one no-phenol capsule along with the two Trienza, and she was better. She tends to be much more phenol sensitive than my son. Two Trienza helped his stomach right away. These products are available for purchase from many online sources such as www.houston-enzymes.com, www.pureformulas.com, and www.amazon.com.

Remember:

- No-phenol: This enzyme product will loosen the stool, so it is a good choice if your child has constipation. If taking Trienza and your child has constipation, add a no-phenol. Also, be sure they are drinking enough water. Constipation can come from dehydration. (Magnesium is also helpful with constipation. This is talked about in chapter 9, common nutritional deficiencies.)
- Zyme-Prime: This product firms the stool and is helpful with diarrhea. (Kefir is also very helpful in stopping diarrhea.

THE FEINGOLD ELIMINATION DIET

Dr. Benjamin Franklin Feingold, a pediatrician and. allergist, discovered that certain compounds in foods, natural or synthetic—caused an immunological response rather than an allergic reaction. He saw how diet can clearly create behavioral disorders. Those on the autism spectrum are particularly vulnerable, especially to food dyes.

One of the main components with the trigger foods is salicylates. Common in aspirin, salicylates are also in many foods, such as certain fruits, artificial flavors, preservatives, and food dyes. Many of the FDA-approved dyes also contain lead, mercury, arsenic, and other harmful toxins. These toxins attack blood cells, the nervous system, and the mitochondria (the cell's energy center).

LIST OF SYMPTOMS HELPED BY THE FEINGOLD DIET:

- Aggression, odd
- Asthma
- Autism
- Bedwetting
- Depression

- Dyslexia, learning disabilities
- Ear infections
- Eczema, hives
- Eye problems
- Headaches, migraines
- Irritable bowel syndrome
- Obsessive compulsive disorder
- Oppositional defiance disorder
- Seizures
- Sleep problems
- Speech problems
- Tourette syndrome
- Violence, aggression,

For more information go to; www.feingold.org.

Remember that muscle testing is an easy way to find sensitivities and that they can be desensitized. See the chapter on alternative therapies for more.

Since the symptoms for gluten and casein sensitivities are much like those of Candida/yeast overgrowth, it is best to remove potential allergens from your child's diet while on the Candida cleanse. The cleanse itself may cause symptoms of its own due to die-off reactions. This is covered in greater detail in the chapter on Candida.

I have had my N.E.A.T. practitioner (discussed in the chapter on practitioners), muscle test for several foods and other possible toxins and metals. When she finds one, we desensitize my child to that ingredient. In 25 hours, the body can be relieved of an issue. Let me note that this does not give you free reign to go out and eat as much of the problem food or foods that you had desensitized. It is a delicate balance and best to always use moderation.

THE B.R.A.T. DIET FOR DIARRHEA

If diarrhea is an issue the body will become dehydrated and may have difficulty removing toxins. The B.R.A.T. diet; bananas, rice, apple sauce, and toast, can be helpful for this, (short term). These will help to slow things down when it is necessary.

THE DOWNSIDE OF SOY

Soy is a common food allergy, and soy lecithin is often used as an emulsifier. This is unknown to most consumers who are allergic to soy and its many uses. Soy-based baby formulas contain free glutamate, which causes damage to the part of the brain called the hypothalamus which is responsible for many behaviors including the fight or flight response, hormones, aggression, sleep and appetite. Soy also leads to behavioral disorders. Glutamate will bind with aluminum and increase its absorption in both the bloodstream and the brain. Soy also contains phytoestrogens, which build estrogen in the body. Too much estrogen will disrupt the body's natural balance of the endocrine or hormonal system. Nonorganic soy is also genetically modified.

Soy contains the protease trypsin, which inhibits the absorption of calcium and magnesium in the body. There are a few natural, organic baby formulas on the market, such as Earths Best, which do not contain soy or harmful toxins. Be sure that you get an organic product and not a soy-based formula. You may find that one has a small amount of soy in it, but it is not soy-based (meaning that soy is not the main ingredient). I feel it is best to avoid soy completely in infants.

Ingredients are labeled from the highest content as the first ingredient to the lowest content being the last listed. For the lactose intolerant, they make lactose-free versions. There should be no processed oils, and the omega-3 fatty acids (DHA) should not be hexane processed. Hexane is a neurotoxin and a carcinogen. Nonorganic soy protein isolates are often hexane extracted also. The product should say "hexane free." Another product to look at is Natures One, www.naturesone.com. You can do a web search for "organic baby formulas." There are other choices, just remember the rules stated above.

Another good alternative is goat milk. Goat milk does not carry the allergens that cow milk does, and it is also much healthier for the human body.

FEEDING AND HEALING YOUR BABY

The gut lining can become inflamed due to an inflammatory response. This is due to factors such as pathogenic bacteria being transferred in utero to the baby, and vaccines, due to mercury and/or viral exposure. This is known as "leaky gut" and it will allow larger food particles and toxins to penetrate this protective mucosal lining. From here, these toxins enter the bloodstream and can cross the blood-brain barrier and enter the brain.

THE PROBLEM IS NOT MOM'S MILK BUT WHAT MOM ATE THAT WENT INTO IT.

Remember that what you eat goes into your milk. Sometimes onions are disturbing or broccoli will give your child gas, but a very common problem is cow's milk. Many children are lactose intolerant, and this can be a big part of the problem with a baby's digestion.

Eliminate the foods you think could be problems and wait at least a few days. If things get better, than it is likely that one of those foods was a problem for him. When you add the foods back into your diet, do so one at a time. Add only one food every two or three days so you have a good chance to see which one may be the problem.

There are many great books for breastfeeding moms. There is a good book by Sally Fallon called *Nourishing Traditions*. This book has a lot of helpful information on how and what to feed your baby and includes recipes. *The Nursing Mother's Companion* by Kathrine Huggins is also very helpful.

SUMMARY

Children on the autism spectrum and those with other physical and behavioral disorders commonly have a weak immune system and poor intestinal health. An unhealthy and damaged digestive tract causes inflammation and creates allergic reactions to foods that lead to toxins in the bloodstream that enter the brain. Symptoms can range from stuffy nose or headache to severe behavioral disorders including anxiety, depression, anger, and even loss of verbal communication.

Weak digestion also leads to a lack of absorption of nutrients from the foods we eat.

The child can be treated naturally for inflammatory bowel disorders and desensitized to allergic reactions to food. When the gut is healed parents notice marked improvements in behavior, sleep, communication and more.

The products found in this chapter can be found at http://naturallyhealingautism.com/a-healthy-home/

CHAPTER 18

GLUTEN AND CASEIN

As I speak with parents everywhere, the one thing they seem to have heard of is the gluten/casein connection to autism. This is a very big piece of the pie, although it is only one piece.

Dr. Andrew Wakefield found when working with the parents of autistic children that the number one thing that brought improvement in their child was going on the gluten and casein-free diet. Roughly 60% of these children improve within a short period of time.

Grains today are nothing like they were when our grandparents were growing up. Now they are more processed and often genetically modified. Wheat today contains about 90% more gluten than it did a century ago. Bioengineers work at creating wheat that has more gluten so that it is stickier. Gluten is used as a binder and is contained in almost all processed foods, including anything packaged or boxed. As the demand for processed food has increased, so has the demand for gluten. When people with gluten sensitivities eat gluten, their immune system reacts. Wheat and dairy both create inflammation in the body.

Gluten is the protein in wheat and casein is the protein is dairy products. Wheat, barley, and rye all contain gluten. Spelt, durum, and semolina are also types of wheat. Contrary to popular belief, because they are a type of wheat, they contain gluten. Oats normally do not contain gluten on their own, but due to cross contamination in agricultural processes, they often do. It is best to buy oats that specifically say "gluten free" if you are on a gluten-restrictive diet. Some supergreen foods contain ingredients that may be seen by the body as a trigger called a gluten "tag." They should be avoided if gluten allergies are suspected.

ALLERGY, SENSITIVITY, OR CELIAC DISEASE

Depending upon the degree of sensitivity, symptoms vary. One can be sensitive, allergic, or have full-blown celiac disease, which is actually an autoimmune disorder triggered by gluten that begins in the digestive tract. The physical and emotional symptoms of celiac disease and autism are quite similar. Some children have been misdiagnosed with autism, when the real cause is celiac disease.

Those with type O blood are often more symptomatic because their bodies tend to not do well with grains. Ethnicity also plays a role in food sensitivities, but children with ASD are often deficient in enzymes because their bodies do not make them properly.

Many people are deficient in the enzyme, DPP-IV (dipeptidyl peptidase-IV). This enzyme breaks down the proteins in wheat and dairy. When the enzyme does not work efficiently, or is lacking in the body, proteins such as gluten (in wheat), and casein (in dairy), are only partially broken down. These partial proteins are called peptides.

DIABETES AND WHEAT/GLUTEN

Gluten sensitivity is strongly associated with Type 1 diabetes. Type 1 diabetes is up to 30 times more common in people with celiac disease. Harvard University released a study that showed one in three people with diabetes developed it from whole wheat.

There are over 18,000,000 people in the U.S. with diabetes. It is estimated that over 5,000,000 are undiagnosed. Celiac disease often goes undetected, and 1 in 20 people will not produce symptoms. Malnutrition is also commonly found in people with celiac disease.

Testing for gluten sensitivity and removing gluten from the diet can often prove to increase both growth and better overall health.

SOME ALLERGIC SYMPTOMS TO LOOK FOR WITH GLUTEN, CASEIN AND GUT DYSBIOSIS:

- Hyperactivity
- Lethargy
- Extreme irritability, depression, anxiety
- GI problems: constipation, diarrhea, heartburn, gas, bloating

- Congestion, coughing, sneezing, difficulty breathing
- Ear infections
- Dizziness or poor balance
- Headaches or neck tension
- Skin problems such as rashes and eczema
- Muscle aches
- Trouble with focus or memory
- Watery eyes, dark circles, or puffiness under the eyes
- Excessive salivation
- Perspiration
- Insomnia
- Thyroid disorders

EMOTIONAL EFFECTS OF GLUTEN AND CASEIN

Peptides create opiate properties called caseomorphins, from dairy, and gluteomorphins, from wheat. Exomorphins are not only created by gluten-containing and dairy foods. Meat and some vegetables are also capable of generating these chemicals.

Exomorphins are absorbed from the gut into the bloodstream and ultimately the brain. Once in the brain, they create symptoms associated with autism. Exomorphins also have the same effect on the body as opiate drugs. They create symptoms that make us feel euphoric and intoxicated. That "spaced out" look you often see in your child's face could likely be due to these chemicals in his system. It's no wonder that the very people who are most allergic or sensitive to gluten are often the most addicted. Going gluten-free or casein-free, in the beginning, can mimic a drug withdrawal. The child will crave gluten and casein-containing products. Don't worry, this won't last too long. Most people see major improvements in their children in a very short period, often in days.

PHYSICAL EFFECTS OF GLUTEN AND CASEIN

Often these opiate receptors have already caused damage to the protective lining of the gut. Therefore, we need to heal the lining so it can do its job of blocking out toxic materials and absorbing nutrients from the foods we eat.

In addition, when casein and gluten are not properly broken down, they damage the process of methylation. Protein metabolism can leave behind toxins known as homocysteins. Elevated levels of homocysteins are associated with increased risk of cancer, Alzheimer's, and other neurological diseases.

There are certain vitamin deficiencies associated with gluten allergies. Among those are vitamin D, K, folic acid, B12, and vitamin B6. Folic acid and these B vitamins play a key role in the methylation cycle. Methylation is how the homocysteins are detoxified in the body. Without enough of these vitamins, methylation is hindered and the levels of homocysteins in the blood will rise. Supplementing with these vitamins will drop levels of homocysteins and therefore, assist methylation. Methylation also assists in maintaining appropriate levels of neurotransmitters (the brain's messengers), especially dopamine. Dopamine is associated with focus and motivation.

THE GOAL

Our goal is to create more balance, strength, and overall health by reducing inflammation, increasing the good bacteria and crowding out the bad, and providing an environment in which the body can heal. When the good bacteria helps to form a protective coating of the mucosal cell lining, B vitamins and digestive enzymes are naturally produced which helps restore balance. As this lining is healed, toxic material can no longer be absorbed through the intestinal lining and nutrition can be absorbed properly.

Instead of focusing on the symptoms, we must work to heal the causes. Loading the system up with supplements that very likely will not be absorbed does absolutely no good.

My daughter suffered stomach pain for many years. When we found that the pain was caused by gluten, we had our N.E.A.T. practitioner (discussed in the chapter on alternative therapies) stimulate points on Carly's body while she held a glass container with gluten in it. We were then not to touch gluten and anything containing it for 25 hours. At the end of that time, she was able to eat it again.

In the beginning there was still a slight discomfort in my daughter's stomach. After a few weeks, she no longer had any discomfort. Now she can eat gluten and be completely fine, but if she eats too much in a short period of time, she gets a stomach ache and often becomes more emotional or lethargic. Whole grains from a reliable source or sprouted grain foods like Ezekiel can be more tolerated by some who have trouble with gluten. Sprouted grains still contain natural enzymes, which make them easier for the body to digest. Rice, corn, millet, and quinoa are gluten-free.

Wheat and dairy are common foods and commonly added to most food preparations. Avoiding them can be difficult in the beginning, but it becomes easier with time. Luckily, awareness of this common problem has become so widespread that there are now many options for gluten-free and dairy-free foods. Most grocery stores have entire sections dedicated to gluten-free products, and there are countless gluten-free websites available.

GLUTEN-FREE WEBSITES

- Easy-gluten-free-recipes.com
- Glutenfreemall.com
- Foodphilosopher.com
- Mygluten-freetable.com
- www.pamelasproducts.com

GF AND MORE RECIPE BOOKS:

- *Breaking the Vicious Cycle* by Elaine Gottschall
- *Recipes for the Specific Carbohydrate Diet* by Raman Prasad
- Ecology health center cookbook: a sugar free, yeast free, gluten free and dairy free cookbook

The above books can be purchased at www.crohns.net.

AT-HOME TESTING

It is wise to test your child for gluten sensitivities since some children are not completely affected by it. The best and simplest test for gluten and casein intolerance that I know of, other than going gluten and casein free, is from www.enterolab.com. Enterolab can also test for fat digestion, egg sensitivity, soy, and more.

There is no need for an expensive appointment or any blood draw. Order the test online, and they will send it to your doorstep. This is a stool sample test because gluten binds to tissue in the bowel and can be picked up best this way. Often blood tests will show negative results when your child could very likely be positive.

The company will mail or email the results back to you. The results will be very specific and are on a percentage scale to let you know just how allergic your child is. There is professional assistance available if you need it, and the tests are often covered by insurance.

Know that even if your child comes up negative on the test for gluten or casein antibodies, he may very possibly have intolerance to them. Again the intolerance can create the same symptoms as an allergy, and they should be avoided.

The adrenal saliva test from Diagnos-Techs is a fabulous way to accurately measure the strength or weakness of the adrenal glands and get your gliadin (gluten) sensitivity score all in one easy at-home test. Most natural practitioners carry these tests in their offices and will give them to you to take home. If they do not have them ask if they will order one for you.

ENZYME SUPPLEMENTS FOR GLUTEN AND CASEIN

DPP-IV (dipeptidyl peptidase IV), is the only enzyme known to break down casomorphin and gluteomorphin. Breaking down these proteins fully prevents them from forming into peptides. Another interesting fact is that meat and vegetables can also create exorphins, and DPP-IV will assist with this also.

There is an enzyme product called AFP Peptizyde from Houston Enzymes that has high DPP-IV activity. It breaks down proteins such as gluten, casein, and soy. The product Trienza from Houston Enzymes is a combination of DPP-IV with additional enzymes to break down carbohydrates, sugars, and fats. Houston Enzymes make many enzyme products that target specific needs. Often, many of us need help with more than just protein digestion, so they have combined a few of their enzymes together to create an all-in-one formula in Trienza.

When these products are taken prior to eating gluten, it can assist the body in its digestion. Some people are able to eat gluten with DPP-IV enzymes, and their sensitivities are gone. If symptoms persist, they may have a strong enough sensitivity or an actual allergy to gluten that is severe enough that no gluten will be tolerated. It is also possible that their digestive system has more healing to do.

For my daughter, the Trienza alone was not enough. I called the very helpful staff at Houston Enzymes and they helped me troubleshoot the problem. It turned out that she needed help with phenols. If your child's stomach still hurts and emotions persist, check for phenol and other sensitivities. Ask Houston enzymes for a free sample of their No-Phenol" and add one in with the normal dose of two Trienza.

Before natural allergy desensitization, if my daughter ate a meal with gluten in it, such as at a birthday party, I would give her enzymes specific for gluten, such as Trienza. It made me feel better that I was adding protection. Both AFP Peptizyde and Trienza come in capsule or chewable form. These products can be found at www.houston-enzymes.com, 866-757-8627, www.pureformulas.com, and at www.amazon.com.

COMMON FOOD INTOLERANCES IN AUTISM HELPED BY ENZYMES:

- Wheat (gluten as its protein and can include barley and rye)
- Dairy (casein as it is protein, or lactose as it is sugar or carbohydrate)
- Soy (protein and carbohydrates are a problem)
- Phenols or polyphenolic compounds (oxalates and lectins often in fruits and vegetables)

PROBIOTICS FOR GLUTEN AND CASEIN INTOLERANCE

We cannot avoid the healthier foods in our daily lives because we would likely become malnourished. The gluten and casein-free diet is based on ridding the body of these opiate receptors that can react with peptides in the body. We can live gluten and casein free just fine if we need to, but vegetables are necessary for good health and some of us need to eat meat. HLC Mindlinx contains strains that work to digest the vegetable and meat exorphins, as well as gluten and dairy.

HLC Mindlinx is a probiotic supplement that was developed specifically for those with gluten and casein intolerance. "HLC Mindlinx contains specific strains of lactobacillus crispatus and lactobacillus rhamnosus which have been proven in scientific trials to degrade wheat and dairy exorphins, and to attach to and colonize intestinal epithelial cells." Mindlinx is made by a company called Pharmax that has an impeccable reputation.

Of all the products I used to heal my son's GI tract, this one wins my gold medal. Prior to using HLC Mindlinx, Jacob's stomach would hurt him almost every day. If he ate dairy products or foods with gluten, he would be bent over in pain.

Jacob's physical health changed drastically for the better through the use of this product, more than from anything else I had tried. As his health improved, so did his behavior—drastically. I had no idea what a significant impact his GI tract was having on his brain and behavior. He became calmer, less impulsive and reactive, and more socially engaged.

For a short time, I had him taking the enzyme product, Trienza. I wanted him to have additional support for breaking down gluten and other potential problems like fats, carbohydrates, and sugars.

Even more amazing, once his gut healed, it never gave him the same pain or nausea again. Today he is absolutely fine with gluten. His behavior does not seem to be affected by it, and he no longer needs enzymes to digest gluten or casein. Now, years later, I can still say this. He eats pizza and drinks milk, although I limit these foods in our home, and he is completely fine, physically and emotionally.

My daughter has had digestive issues and had problems with gluten for years. The DPP-IV enzymes did not seem to help her. I decided to give her Mindlinx to see if she and I would notice a difference. It was like magic. She felt better immediately. I continue to give this to her when she has anything with gluten in it, and she is completely fine. No stomach aches or headaches, and no emotional issues. Any child or adult, whether they have autism or not, would benefit from using HLC Mindlinx, especially those with intestinal issues.

HLC Mindlinx contains a specifically selected strain of Lactobacillus rhamnosus (CLT341). This strain of organism is proven to degrade wheat and dairy exorphins and to attach to and colonize intestinal epithelial cells (Figures 1 & 2).

Figure 1: Breakdown of milk B-caseomorphin-7 by selected HLC lactic acid bacteria

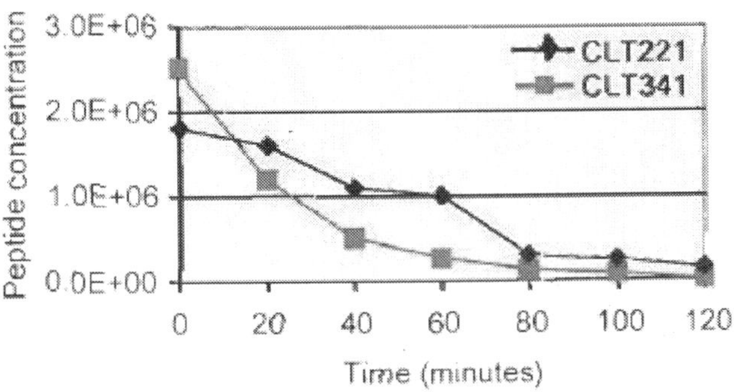

Figure 2: Breakdown of wheat exorphin-A5 by selected HLC lactic acid bacteria

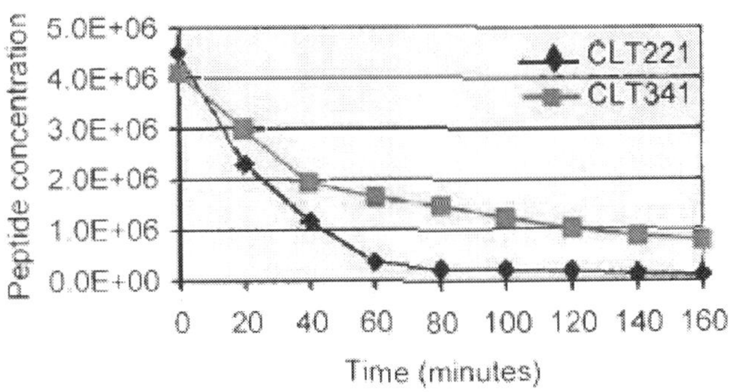

HLC MindLinx has been shown to degrade dietary exorphins in human subjects (Figures 3).

Figure 3: Effect of 21 days supplementations of HLC MindLinx on urinary excretion of opioid peptide exorphin B5 in six normal adult subjects.

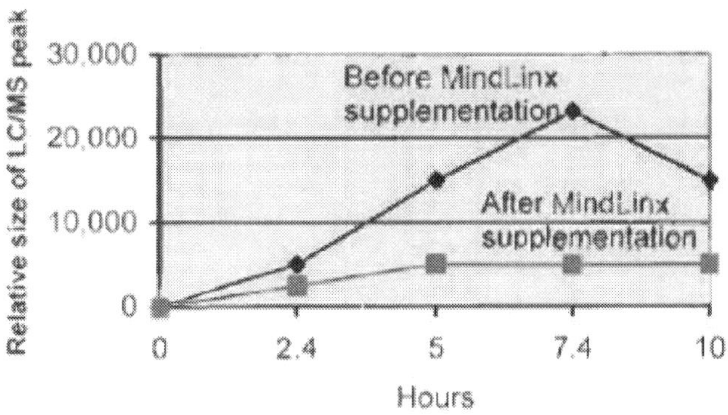

Subjects were provided with a meal of bread and milk and urinary exorphins measured over the next 10 hours. Subjects took Mindlinx for 21 days before being offered the same meal of bread and milk. The differences in the before and after urinary exorphin profiles are clear.

- HLC MindLinx contains the original HLC High Potency specification.
- HLC MindLinx provides a total specification of 12 billion cfu's per day.

Note: For further detailed reading, see Pharmax Technical Monograph titled "Intestinal Effects on Autism and ADHD? Potential for a Novel Probiotic Approach."

Dosage is 1 capsule or 1/4 tsp of powder 2 times a day with meals.

Each dosage also contains L-glutamine to assist in healing the intestinal lining. HLC capsules do not contain FOS. HLC powder does contain FOS (from chicory roots): 8 to 12 billion consortiums of six specifically selected strains. Some individuals have shown sensitivities to FOS, so the company has given you a choice if you would prefer not to give it to your child.

Fructooligosaccharides (FOS) are medium and short-chain sugar molecules that are a form of fiber carbohydrate and prebiotics in the intestines, but many people find discomfort when digesting them.

Note: the amount of L- glutamine in HLC Mindlinx is far below harmful levels. Occasionally, a child will have some excitability even from this low dosage. For those children it may not be the best choice, but this is very rare. Muscle testing can be used to ask the body if the product is compatible with it. I highly recommend trying this product, if possible.

Mindlinx can be purchased for a good price and no shipping charge at www.pureformulas.com. It is also carried in quality healthfood stores. This product must be refrigerated to maintain its potency. When shipped, it should be packaged with an ice pack.

MAINTAINING BALANCE

It is important not to load the system up with gluten. Eating gluten once a day may be tolerable for some. For others, it is a better idea to only give gluten and casein-filled foods once every two, three, or even four days. Beyond test results, you must experiment to see what the tolerance level is for your child. Much of this depends on the health of their intestinal lining.

Once the lining is healed, some children have little or no issues with gluten, while others remain highly sensitive. The highly sensitive are often the ones with true gluten allergies. Remember that wheat is no longer the healthy food it once was. Agricultural tactics have altered this once healthy food and made it into something that even most healthy bodies have trouble digesting. It is best to avoid, or at least minimize, wheat and gluten altogether.

My daughter could not tolerate much gluten at all until we healed her system. Since then she is able to eat some gluten without problems. She does, however, have to watch her intake over the course of a few days. She will know if she has had too much because her stomach hurts. I will know too because she gets dark circles under her eyes, is lethargic, and her behavior becomes very emotional.

GLUTEN TESTING:

- Muscle testing is a simple way to test for any product sensitivity. This can be done by an allergy desensitizing practitioner or by yourself. See "muscle response testing" in the chapter on alternative therapies for more information. Also, see the note below.
- Eliminate gluten from your child's diet. Remember that it can take up to two months for gluten to be completely out of the system.
- www.enterolab.com can provide you with precise results from a stool test done in the home. These results show the degree of sensitivity to gluten from mild to severe.
- For the sensitivity test, place a small amount of gluten mixed with pure water on the inside of the wrist before bed. Check upon waking. If the area is reddish and looks inflamed, then there is sensitivity to it.

Note: To be sure the allergy is to gluten, muscle testing should be done with pure gluten to be sure that any response is not a reaction to additional ingredients. Allergy desensitizing practitioners carry this in their office to test with. Be sure to check your labels.

Common foods that contain gluten:

- Wheat
- Barley
- Rye
- Soy sauce
- Gravy

NON-FOOD BASED PRODUCTS TO BE AWARE OF

Due to the nature of biology, one person can be unaffected by a food or toxin, whereas another is greatly affected by the same product.

Some individuals are so sensitive that merely touching a food with their hands can cause severe reactions because the skin absorbs it.

Seemingly harmless toys can have an effect on a highly sensitive individual. Colored playing dough that children play with contains both gluten and food coloring. Absorbed through the skin, the body's largest organ, it travels into the bloodstream, just as a food particle can that passes through the intestinal lining. Check the labels on shampoos and lotions, too. Many of these products contain wheat, dairy, and soy, another common allergen.

My daughter took gymnastics for a couple of years. I constantly found myself wondering why she became so hyperactive when we were there. Later I found out that she was allergic to talc (talcum powder), another common allergen. This is commonly used on the bars in gymnastics to help keep their hands from slipping off of the equipment. It is also used in climbing gyms.

My daughter had a reaction to paper mache; her hands broke out in a horrible rash from the glue, otherwise known as gluten. Before she was desensitized by our natural allergy desensitization practitioner, she wore gloves if she wanted to use those products. Now she no longer needs to wear them and has no reaction.

There is gluten-free, dye-free playing dough available at www.amazon.com and recipes available online at many sites to easily make it at home.

GLUTEN-FREE AND CASEIN-FREE AND STILL NOT BETTER

Gluten can take up to two months to remove itself from the system, casein about three weeks. I sometimes hear, "My child is already on a gluten-free and casein-free diet, and they're still not better." If the GF/CF diet has been done in 100% compliance for at least three months and there has been no improvement in their symptoms then it is likely that:

- Their gut is not getting what it needs to heal the damage that was done before the diet began
- There is an overgrowth of Candida or pathogenic bacteria that needs to be addressed

- Mercury toxicity still remains and is preventing the gut from healing
- Additional food allergies exist (see natural allergy desensitization in the chapter on alternative therapies)
- Their brain is in need of additional support (see the chapter on supporting the brain)

JUST BECAUSE IT'S GLUTEN-FREE DOES NOT MEAN IT'S GOOD FOR YOU.

People go on the gluten-free diet only to substitute their carbohydrate cravings with different starches such as potato flour and tapioca flour. The digestive system is having trouble with more than gluten and casein. The gut flora (bacteria), is usually so out of balance that it cannot successfully digest starches, but more importantly, the starches and sugars feed the bad bacteria in their gut. This only makes the problem worse.

One thing no one wants to waste is time. If you only remove gluten and casein from the diet, there is a strong likelihood that your child's gut will not get the chance to heal completely. If their gut does not heal, neither will their brain and behavior.

Some higher fiber, healthier gluten-free alternatives are:

- Millet
- Teff
- Coconut flour
- Almond flour and almond crackers
- Lentil products, including chips

REMOVING ALL STARCHES

This should really be the first step, but so many parents are overwhelmed with the thought of removing even gluten and casein that they cannot comprehend removal of all starches. Often this is your answer and it must be done.

When the gut flora ratio of friendly bacteria to unfriendly bacteria gets out of balance, as is the case with children on the autism spectrum (and often ourselves), all starches and sugars need to be removed. This does not, however, mean forever.

For a temporary period from two days to two months (depending on the individual), we cannot allow anything in that feeds the pathogenic bacteria. It is also crucial to give time for the intestinal lining to heal. The pathogenic bacteria have bored holes in the lining of the intestines (leaky gut). These holes must be healed and sealed so that toxins and undigested food can no longer enter the bloodstream, and therefore, the brain.

When undigested particles of gluten enter the bloodstream, they trigger an immune response in the body. The body then begins to see gluten as a foreign substance or danger. This builds gluten intolerance or a developed allergy.

Pathogenic bacteria in the gut thrive on sugar. These carbohydrates turn to sugar in the body and end up being a food for the bad bacteria just as sugar itself is. Sugars, even natural ones, should be avoided at first. We do not want to feed anything to the bad bacteria that will allow it to strengthen and survive.

Many gluten-free substitutes are starches or bad, processed carbohydrates. All forms of starch must be removed such as rice, peas, potatoes, soy, tapioca flour, etc.

In turn, we want to eat foods that help to starve the bad bacteria, reduce inflammation, heal the lining of the intestinal tract, and feed the good bacteria what it needs to grow.

SUMMARY

When on the gluten free, casein free diet there is roughly a sixty percent noticeable improvement within a short period of time. Gluten is the protein in wheat and wheat products, and casein is the protein in dairy. Today's crops in the U.S. have been bioengineered to have ninety percent more gluten in them than they did a century ago. The human body cannot easily process this much gluten.

If a person has a weakened digestive tract and leaky gut, which is common for those on the autism spectrum, the large undigested proteins make their way into the bloodstream and trigger an allergic reaction. These reactions can cause severe physical and behavioral problems. At home testing can be done to find your child's level of sensitivity. Muscle testing can also be done for this.

A gluten free/casein free diet is a good way to begin healing and notice changes in health and behavior. Specific enzymes are needed to break down gluten. They are often too low in numbers to do the job for people with a compromised GI tract. These enzymes can be taken as supplements to assist digestion of these foods. Sometimes removal of all starches must happen during the healing process in order to allow the body full recovery.

The products found in this chapter can be found at http://naturallyhealingautism.com/a-healthy-home/

CHAPTER 19

ADDITIONAL COMMON CHILDHOOD EPIDEMICS

Our kids are vulnerable to many toxins that weaken their immune system. This breakdown can allow for weaknesses creating additional illnesses. We will cover autism, allergies, and behavioral disorders throughout this book. In addition to these epidemics, there are increasing numbers of children with other common ailments.

ASTHMA

Between 1980 and 1993, the CDC resolved that, "An estimated 15 million Americans suffer from asthma, including 4.8 million children and adolescents."

Although anyone at any age can suffer from asthma, those that are affected the most are children. Asthma is often believed to be an inherited sensitivity to environmental factors such as smoke, pollens, dusts, molds, or pet dander. The prevalence of asthma among children ages 5 to 14 rose 74% from 1980 to 1993, and continues to grow today. Let's look at some possible reasons why.

ASTHMA AND VITAMIN D DEFICIENCY

Once again, vitamin D has been shown to help more than bones. It has recently been linked to depression, autoimmune disorders, and now asthma.

In one study done in Washington, D.C., researchers found that 86% of children in the study with asthma were deficient in vitamin

D. In contrast, of non-asthmatics, only 19% showed the same level of deficiency.

Most babies should get their vitamin D levels from breast milk, but today, most mothers are deficient in this vitamin also. For those babies born in the winter months, there can be an even greater deficiency due to less sunlight. Our bodies convert sunlight into vitamin D through our skin. Researchers are now recommending that most babies take a vitamin D supplement. Ask your doctor to check your child's vitamin D levels.

The overuse of the wrong sunscreens is one cause of this deficiency. I know of one sunscreen that blocks out the harmful, cancer-causing UVA rays, but allows the much-needed UVB rays in. The UVB rays are the ones our bodies need to convert sunlight into vitamin D. This product can be found at www.mercola.com, or call 877-985-2695 to order. This sunscreen is also environmentally friendly, so if you swim in oceans and lakes, you can be assured you are not affecting the delicate balance with poisonous toxins.

ASTHMA AND GLUTEN

Food is more important to understand than the typically thought of dusts and pollens. You are more likely to control your foods and your fungus yourself. Asthma is due to chronic inflammation of the airways, but what factors trigger this inflammation in the first place. One cause for these attacks may be gluten sensitivities.

A study done in November 2001, in the *Journal of Allergy and Clinical Immunology* 108 (5), showed that children with celiac disease (24.6%) had a much higher prevalence of asthma than those without celiac (3.4%).

One study done in March 2001, "A Major Allergen in Wheat-Dependent, Exercise Induced Anaphylaxis," in *Clinical and Experimental Allergy* (31) 3, found that those on a gluten-,free diet continued to be free of symptoms. Other clinical studies have been done reporting scientific cases that give strong evidence of gluten sensitivity to asthma.

It is also common to get hives or skin rashes, especially on the hands, when some gluten sensitive people eat gluten. This is the case with my daughter.

Please remember that many commonly used tests, such as blood tests, do not show positive for gluten even if there is a sensitivity or allergy to it. A more precise test for this can be done through www.enterolab.com.

The simplest and cheapest way to find an answer is to go on an completely gluten-free diet. Completely remove any traces of gluten from their diet. It may take a week or more to see results, but remember that gluten can take up to two months to be completely removed from the system.

At first, look for any changes in the frequency of your child's attacks. See if you notice connections to gluten or anything else in particular. People have been known to no longer need inhalers or medication for asthma when on a gluten-free diet, even if they have had asthma their entire life.

When the gluten-free diet works but is too hard to keep your child on continuously, there are two options. First, I recommend seeking out a natural allergy desensitizing specialist (see the chapter on reducing inflammation). Second, you can try using an enzyme product called Trienza.

There is a specific enzyme in this product called DPP-IV that is capable of breaking down the gluten in your child's stomach so that there may not be a reaction to it. We talk about this in greater detail in the chapter "supplements to Heal the Gut". Trienza can be purchased at www.amazon.com, www.pureformulas.com, www.houston-enzymes.com, or by calling Houston Enzymes directly at 866-757-8627.

ASTHMA AND CANDIDA/FUNGAL GROWTH

"It is well known that the sensitization to fungi is higher in the early years and declines rapidly as we age." (Kauffman, H.F., et al.).

The other aspect not often known is the correlation between asthma and fungus growth within the body. The use of antibiotics and the increased use of sugar, processed foods, and food coloring in our diets, all assist fungal growth. When fungal growth invades the intestines, it then invades the bloodstream. Once in the bloodstream, fungus can reach any organ of the body including the lungs, therefore increasing the likelihood of asthmatic attacks from fungal infections.

This is known as bronchopulmonary candidiasis. Each year in the U.S., fungi cause more pulmonary infections than bacteria.

Once in the lungs, it is a living parasite and requires food. Those cravings your child has for sugar and carbohydrates are from this parasite's need to be fed. These foods will weaken the immune system and have molds of their own that only perpetuate the problem. The best thing to do is starve the parasite of what it needs most. This is where limiting or removal of sugar and refined carbohydrates is greatly helpful.

Some have implied that one cause of asthma is due to stomach acid from the esophagus that has made its way into the lungs and caused irritation to the bronchial tubes, commonly known as acid reflux. "The most common cause of Candida albicans bronchopneumonia is from aspirations of oral secretions." (Doug Kauffman, "The Fungus Link, volume 1.")

While we are sleeping, we all aspirate small amounts of stomach fluids or oral secretions. Acid reflux secretions can be caused by yeast, just as the yeast can cause lung irritation. We are inhaling molds from our own gut. If there are molds in your home or at school, your child can also inhale molds from there.

ASTHMA AND CRANIOSACRAL FAULTS

The most common subluxation, or bone imbalance, caused at birth is when the bone at the lower portion of the back of the head (called the occiput) slips off of the first vertebrae in the neck known as cervical one. This area is also called the atlas. When these bones are out of place they can pinch a branch of the vagus nerve, which can cause both breathing and digestion to be affected. It is also another reason for colic in a baby. This can easily be balanced by a good chiropractor, osteopath, or craniosacral therapist.

ASTHMA AND VACCINATIONS

There seems to be a correlation in timing with the increase in asthma and the increase in immunizations. A survey published in The Journal of the American Medical Association reported that children who had received the pertussis vaccine were six times more likely to develop asthma than those who had not received the vaccination.

ASTHMA AND ENVIRONMENTAL TOXINS

We do not realize how many toxic chemicals we and our children are exposed to on a daily basis. Household cleaners, pesticides, lotions and soaps can all play a significant part without us realizing it.

The daughter of a friend of mine had been on an inhaler for nine years. The mother changed her home over to all natural disinfectants, cleansers, and detergents, (and she ran a daycare in her home). Within three weeks her daughter no longer needed her inhaler and has been without one since. They discovered that the child had been having an asthmatic reaction to the phosphates in the dishwashing detergent she had used previously. The vapors inhaled can trigger asthmatic reactions.

For a list of non-toxic, safe household cleaning agents please visit my website at www.naturallyhealingautism.com, and look under "my healthy home."

RESOLVING ASTHMA

- Asthma and migraines have been linked to low magnesium levels
- Asthma has been associated as a possible reaction to MSG, and it is best to avoid this toxin
- Asthma has been linked to many household cleaning agents such as phosphates in dishwasher detergent, fabric softeners, and much more. See the chapter on environmental toxins.
- Decongest the liver
- Candida cleanse: see the chapter on Candida
- See your allergy desensitizing practitioner. They will help you find additional causes through muscle response testing. This tells you if something is a trigger for your child. With food colorings, sometimes it will be one or two colors that there is sensitivity to but not others.

- Go gluten free and avoid refined carbohydrates, such as bread, pasta, beans, and potatoes
- Go dairy free (dairy builds mucus and triggers inflammation)
- Reduce or remove sugar from the diet and follow the diet used for removal of fungal overgrowth from the body (see the chapter on Candida). Also, be aware that cane sugar is known to carry mold. When we eat foods with cane sugar in them, it is likely that we are ingesting molds.
- Remove yeast (both bakers and brewers) from the diet
- Have IgE antibodies checked
- Look into possible mold/ biotoxin illness through www.survivingmold.com
- Grapefruit seed extract nasal spray has been known to be helpful with sinus issues. Make this yourself in a nose spray bottle with two to three drops of grapefruit seed extract in two ounces of distilled water, or purchase an already made tincture. Citricidal grapefruit seed extract is available in liquid drops or a nose spray at www.pureformulas.com.

ASTHMA ACCUPRESSURE POINT

One method I have shown to other parents is very helpful at the onset or during an attack. There is an acupressure point just below the Adams apple on the front of your neck. We all have one. Your Adams apple is the lump that sticks out so well on a man's throat, but is a bit more concealed in women. To find it on your child gently place a few fingers over the front of their throat and ask them to swallow. The Adam's apple will jump up and then come back down. Swallowing will help assist the bump outward. This is helpful if you have trouble finding it.

Once you have located the Adam's Apple itself draw your finger downward just slightly, about ¼ to1/2 an inch, until you feel a slight dip. Allow your finger to settle into the dip and hold it there. There is no need to apply much pressure at all. Only the gentlest touch is needed here. This point is very sensitive and very effective whenever you have any trouble breathing, or any bronchial issues such as bronchitis. I have successfully used this point to stop the beginning of an asthma attack on a child. This point also brings energy into the system.

Continue to hold your finger on this point for as long as you need to. Usually within a few minutes you will see it working. It is helpful to place your other hand on the back of their neck for support and because this area on the head can create a calming effect on the brain as well.

HELPFUL NATURAL AIDS

BIOPURE PROPOLIS VAPORIZERS

Biopure propolis vaporizers are essential for killing indoor airborne microbes. An Italian study showed 70% of asthma was cured in children in 6 weeks with the use of vaporized propolis.

Propolis is a resin-like composite derived from bees. When vaporized, propolis destroys pathogenic microbes and air pollutants. Inhaling the properties of propolis allows it to quickly reach the cellular level via the bloodstream. The flavonoids in propolis are strongly anti-inflammatory and reduce type one allergies. It is all natural, free of chemicals, and eliminates mold, fungi, bacteria, and viruses.

The active flavonoids in propolis vary due to the regions in which the bees travel. The propolis sold by the company Bee Healthy Farms, www.beehealthyfarms.com, is certified to contain the necessary active flavonoids. They also carry vaporizers. The Biopure propolis vaporizer is small and can travel with you. They even make a car model that plugs into the cigarette lighter or power source in your vehicle.

HEPA FILTERS

Purifying the air in the rooms of your home, office, or school is always a good idea. We do not realize how many contaminants we inhale on a daily basis. Air purifiers filter dust, smoke, pollen, pet dander, mold spores, and other airborne particles as small as 0.3 microns in diameter. HEPA stands for high efficiency particulate arrestance. The most efficient HEPA filter removes 99.7% of particles as small as 0.3 microns. ULPA or "ultra" HEPA filters are available too. They are designed to remove 99.999% of air particles at 0.3 microns. Select your HEPA filter by looking at the efficiency in which it removes airborne particles. In order for the efficiency to filter at these high levels they need to be "true" HEPA filters and will say so. Otherwise, you are likely to get an inferior substitute.

True HEPA filters are easy to find. They are carried in many department stores and online sites including, www.amazon.com.

VASAKA

Vasaka is an ayurvedic herb that has been used for centuries to calm bronchial passageways, the lungs, and overall respiration. Banyan Botanicals makes a certified organic powder form. It is sold at www.amazon.com.

N-ACETYL-CYSTEINE (NAC)

This amino acid is derived from L-cysteine and can assist your lungs in many ways. It is a precursor to glutathione, so it increases the levels of this vital antioxidant in your lungs, strengthening their defense mechanisms. NAC also causes the breakdown of mucus, and it inhibits the inflammatory protein TGF-beta-1, which is crucial in assisting your body's responses to asthma. It is also known to be incredibly helpful with chronic obstructed pulmonary disease (COPD).

It is best to clean the diet and clear Candida before using N-acetyl cysteine, as it has a tendency to worsen Candida if there is strong Candida overgrowth.

TURMERIC/CURCUMIN

Derived from the curry spice turmeric, curcumin is extremely powerful in lung support. Studies have shown that curcumin decreases allergy-related cells by inhibiting the inflammatory signaling component NFkappaB. The study resulted in an effect on white blood cells, eosinophils, and IgE antibodies. Curcumin also aids the natural killer cells (NK cells) in the body that are crucial to a healthy immune system. Additional added benefits of curcumin are improved cognitive health, including memory, it acts as an aid to digestion, enhances liver function, and helps purify the blood.

For best absorption, take curcumin with oil (the good oils), such as omega-3 fatty acids, (fish or krill oils) olive oil, coconut oil, or avocado. Look for turmeric that is organic and at least 95% curcuminoids.

MULLEIN

Mullein tea is made from the dried leaves or flowers of the mullein plant. Mullein tea or capsules are helpful for treating respiratory problems like asthma, bronchitis, congestion, pneumonia, and whooping cough. It is also helpful with insomnia to calm the mind, and aids with diarrhea, urinary tract infections, cleansing the blood, and the removal of parasites.

QUERCITIN

Often used by those with allergic reactions. Quercetin can be useful against asthma because it blocks histamine and reduces inflammation.

PYCNOGENOL

A strong, safe antioxidant that is derived from plants, pycnogenol has the capability of crossing the blood-brain barrier, therefore also helping neurons in the brain. Due to its ability to reduce inflammation and fight free radical damage, it can be quite helpful fighting asthma.

Mucostop by Enzymedica is one of my favorites. I have found this product to be extremely helpful if there is a problem with excessive mucus, especially during or after a head cold. Another great product to help loosen mucus is Air Power by Enzymatic. Remember that when enzymes are used therapeutically, they must be taken one hour before eating or two hours after.

CORDYCEPS

Cordyceps is a medicinal mushroom used by both traditional and non-traditional medical practitioners. It dilates the lung airways and is anti-inflammatory to the bronchial tubes. It has been shown in clinical studies to enhance respiratory disorders such as asthma, bronchitis, chronic obstructed pulmonary disease, and helps with cough. (Holliday JC, Cleaver MP. Medicinal value of the caterpillar fungi species of the genus Cordyceps (Fr.) Link (Ascomycetes). A review. Int J Med Mushr. 2008;10(3):219-234.) (Zhu JS, Halpern GM, Jones K. The scientific rediscovery of a precious ancient Chinese herbal regimen: Cordyceps sinensis : part II. J Altern Complement Med. 1998;4(4):429-457.)

Cordyceps is also used by many athletes to increase recovery time. It stimulates the immune system. Laboratory studies show cordyceps to stimulate immune cells. It is so helpful for the liver that it is used by people with hepatitis B, and animal studies show it to improve kidney function. It increases energy and reduces fatigue increasing oxygen in the blood and circulation. It is also known to reduce blood glucose levels and help balance insulin sensitivity.

Although cordyceps is a fungus it is not known to have any contraindications for those with fungal issues. First consult your health care practitioner regarding its use for your child.

There is a liquid form of cordyceps available at www.pureformulas.com.

A FEW HELPFUL FOODS

Foods that can be helpful to the lungs are pine nuts, and white fruits such as apples and pears (as long as you are not on the strict part of the Candida diet). Pears are known to be highly beneficial for the lungs. Radishes are an excellent choice to assist in reducing the over-production of phlegm.

To reduce coughing and open the air passageways high quality eucalyptus oil rubbed into the bottom of the feet and on the chest can be very helpful.

ADDITIONAL INFORMATION

See the chapter on environmental toxins, and pathogenic microbes for more information on mold allergies and air pollution pertaining to asthma and other respiratory issues.

SEIZURES

Diet is a big issue for those with seizures. A ketogenic, or high-fat burning diet, is often used for epilepsy when drug treatment does not work. Essentially, it is a diet high in good fats, medium protein intake, and very low carbohydrates. It is the same diet that is in this book for gut healing and reducing inflammation in the brain.

Eliminate excitatory foods. Do not ingest any MSG, aspartame, caffeine, or anything excitatory. Also see information regarding supplements that protect against excitotoxicity (see excitotoxins) and calms the brain such as GABA.

Hypoglycemia can also trigger a seizure. There is something known as nocturnal hypoglycemia. When we sleep, we go for many hours without food. There are some people whose systems cannot tolerate this, and it triggers seizures. Proteins take longer to digest, and they stay in the system a lot longer than other foods. Eating some form of protein before bed can help, such as almonds or a hard-boiled egg.

There is a book called *Silent Seizures* written by a mother. It explains the common misdiagnosis of autism for those with seizures. These children then lack proper treatment.

MERCURY TOXICITY

DIPTHERIA, PERTUSSIS, TETANUS (DPT) VACCINATIONS

A correlation has been found between the diphtheria, pertussis, tetanus vaccination (DPT) and seizures. Pertussis is one of the most toxic substances found and has been known to cause many problems. Have your child muscle tested by a natural allergy desensitation practitioner to see if their body is reacting to any remaining viruses or bacteria from vaccinations, especially the DPT shot. See the chapter on alternative therapies for more information on natural allergy desensitization.

THE GUT/BRAIN CONNECTION CONTINUES

After a couple of months of detoxifying and the seizures have diminished, you may want to do a Candida cleanse. Cleaning up the diet and the GI tract has shown to greatly improve seizures and even stop them in some cases. Parasites are often found in people with seizures.

GABA

The amino acid GABA is known to be extremely calming to nerves and the brain. It balances the firing of neurons and reduces hyperactivity within the brain itself blocking excitatory messages. There are many pill and capsule forms available in healthfood stores and online. I found a sublingual form from Source Naturals called GABA Calm Sublingual Orange available at both www.swansonvitamins.com and www.pureformulas.com.

See the chapter, a short lesson in the brain, for more information including brain SPECT imaging and clinics.

COMMON VITAMIN AND MINERAL DEFICIENCIES INDICATED IN SEIZURES:

- Vitamin D
- Vitamin B3
- Vitamin B6
- Magnesium protects the brain from glutamate toxicity and calms brain cells. Low levels of magnesium are implicated in the onset of seizures for those susceptible to them.

Hypoglycemia or low blood sugar is also a known trigger for seizures

For specific indicators for brain activity, a SPECT image from the Amen Clinic would be most helpful. www.amenclinics.com. Also, see the chapter on brain support for more information.

CANNABIS OR MARIJUANA AS TREATMENT FOR SEIZURES AND MUCH MORE

One lesser known fact about children with autism is that roughly fifty percent start having seizures around the onset of puberty. The best news lately for this issue is that there is a solution for it that works for many individuals.

Some of the newest and most enlightening studies regarding seizures, Crohns disease, pain, Parkinson's disease, and cancer is in cannabis, that's right, marijuana. Specific strains are used for specific needs. Before you think about it as only a drug that people use to get high, think again.

Decades ago, in the 1970's, Israel became the medical marijuana research capitol. There are two ingredients in cannabis; THC and CBD. Israel was the first to isolate the psychotropic portion of cannabis called THC, from the medicinal, non-intoxicating, CBD portion. Medical marijuana can have less than one percent THC and it has the potential to treat many diseases with NO SIDE EFFECTS! This is opposite of what the medical prescription drugs are doing. Every nineteen minutes there is a fatality due to accidental prescription medical overdoses. There are no reports of fatal marijuana overdoses, and it is less harmful or addictive, (less than nine percent), than alcohol.

The science behind it tells us so far that the CBD or cannibal diol modulates chemical and electrical activity in the brain that quiets excessive activity causing seizures. Specific strains are used for different illnesses. In Israel over 10,000 patients are licensed to use marijuana medicinally. There are more than a dozen studies to treat illnesses such as post-traumatic stress disorder, Crohns disease, pain and cancer. Depending on the age or need of the patient marijuana can be used like an herbal tincture in liquid form with only a few drops put under the tongue or it can be added to food.

Although the FDA has approved studies there are organizations who say there is no evidence that it is effective. These organizations include the American Academy of Pediatrics and the National Institute of Drug Abuse. They block out the studies that are positive because it is not in their scope of beliefs. This can be the case with any organization. Changing beliefs is a difficult thing to do. I strongly encourage you to make your own educated decisions.

There is a great story of a five year old little girl with almost constant seizures whose parents had exhausted every other route. Cannabis worked for her and has given her life back. She went from 300 seizures a week to one every seven days! For the full story on this go to, https://www.youtube.com/watch?v=B4GUkzTnFG0. In Colorado more than forty one children are using cannabis with significantly positive results.

Cannabis is now legal in Colorado and California. If it is not legal in your state get involved in the movement with your legislature to help get it legalized. Cannabis works so well for so many people who have tried everything else with no success that if it were my son and my state did not allow it legally I would move to wherever I needed to.

There is an informative book on the subject edited by Julie Holland called, The Pot Book: A Complete Guide to Cannabis; Its Role in Medicine, Politics, Science and Culture, 2010. There is an organization called The Realm of Caring that can help you to gather information for your child's needs. They can be found at http://theroc.us/.

To learn more about high quality medical grade cannabis refer to www.actnowprogram.com, 877-396-4245, and www.harborsidehealthcenter.com.

To receive an evaluation for your child or yourself contact, www.meadowmd.com. Also, please listen to my informative podcast interview with a medical grade cannabis expert at www.naturallyhealingautism.com.

SUMMARY

Additional childhood epidemics such as asthma and seizures have risen greatly. Asthma alone has increased more than seventy-five percent in the last three decades. Possible varying factors include vitamin deficiencies, food allergies, candida/fungal growth, and vaccinations. There are several natural ways to assist in resolving asthma including diet, detoxification, and supplementation. Become educated in all forms of help for your child including cannabis and other non-traditional remedies that have a strong success rate.

Diabetes is also among the newer childhood epidemics. This was covered in detail in chapter eight, Balancing the Body's Chemistry.

The products found in this chapter can be found at http://naturallyhealingautism.com/a-healthy-home/

CHAPTER 20

A SHORT LESSON IN THE BRAIN

As a craniosacral therapist, I study and have an ongoing fascination for the brain. It is an amazing organ. Whether an individual has autism, ADD, depression, anxiety, anger, or any other emotion, it is a result of brain functioning. How the brain is affected by toxins, chemicals, or cranial bone imbalance determines behavior. I thought that giving you some education about its functioning would be helpful in understanding what may be going on for your own child and yourself.

Individual supplementation that has been helpful for specific conditions will be discussed in its own chapter in step four of the four healing stages. Brain supplementation can begin at any time.

As you read, it may be helpful to know that studies show the brain of a person with autism is most affected in the cerebellum, limbic, and pre-frontal cortex.

HYPOTHALAMUS

The hypothalamus is part of both the endocrine and nervous systems and is responsible for messages between the two. The hypothalamus releases many hormones and neurochemicals including:

- Gonadotropin-releasing hormone (GnRH) telling the pituitary to stimulate the ovaries stimulating egg follicles to begin the female menstrual cycle
- Growth hormone (GHRH)
- Corticotrophin releasing hormone (CRH), comes as a response to stress and can cause anxiety and depression

- Thyrotropin releasing hormone (TRH), stimulating the thyroid, metabolism, and the endocrine system
- Somatostatin, affecting secretion of acid in the digestive system and can inhibit the release of growth hormone
- Dopamine, a neurotransmitter affecting reward-based motivation, decision making, ADHD, Parkinson's disease, Restless Leg Syndrome, lack of focus, motor control, and also affects a part of the brain called the prefrontal cortex
- Oxytocin is released via the pituitary due to hypothalamic functioning and is the hormone involved with the ability to bond with others after birth, especially the mother

Via the parasympathetic nervous system, the hypothalamus tells us if we should feel calm or fearful, also known as the fight-or-flight response. This is subject to how we individually perceive an incident. Messages are interpreted via the hypothalamus and sent to the pituitary which alert the adrenal glands. If the message is regarding fear then the adrenal glands release stress hormones. When we are stressed the frontal portion of the brain called the pre frontal cortex which is responsible for decision making will shut down. All blood is sent to the arms and legs to fight or flee. The stress hormones also shut down the gut and the immune system because digestion and immunity are not the top priority when we are in immediate danger. Thus, we are more susceptible to colds, flu and diseases when out system is under stress.

The hypothalamus holds within it the areas responsible for aggression, territorial defense, and sexual pursuit. It is also controls sleep and appetite cycles along with the limbic system. Estrogen receptors in the hypothalamus affect food intake, energy, and the distribution of body fat.

The hypothalamus has no protective blood-brain barrier. Toxins can easily enter this area causing damage and it is often injured in people on the autism spectrum. Lead exposure under 10 µg/dL has been shown to cause dysregulation of the hypothalamic-pituitary-adrenal (HPA) axis in children. Gump, B., P. Stewart, et al. (2008). "Low-level prenatal and postnatal blood lead exposure and adrenocortical responses to acute stress in children." Environmental Health Perspectives 116(2): 249-55

Gump, B., P. Stewart, et al. (2008). "Low-level prenatal and postnatal blood lead exposure and adrenocortical responses to acute stress in children." Environmental Health Perspectives 116(2): 249-55

What helps the hypothalamus? Zinc, vitamin D, proper iodine levels, and exercise are crucial to the proper functioning of the hypothalamus.

CEREBELLUM

The cerebellum is involved in voluntary (large movement) motor control, and small fine motor control, and balance. It modifies and relays information to the muscles. The cerebellum is also involved in cognitive function including language. The cerebellum is located at the back of the brain just above the brain stem where the brain meets the spinal cord.

PREFRONTAL CORTEX (PFC)

The control center for the brain, often called the brain's CEO, the prefrontal cortex (PFC) is the center for making judgments, and in seeing the consequences of our actions. The PFC stops impulsive reactions, rules the emotions, and calms the fear center of the brain called the amygdala. When the PFC has decreased activity, it increases problems with impulse control and distractibility.

When underactive, the PFC is often the hidden cause behind ADD. These people have little or no filter to the sounds and visual stimuli in their environment. The PFC has the ability to calm other areas of the brain. An underactive PFC means that both the internal, or emotional, and external environment can easily overwhelm the individual.

The PFC is the last part of the brain to develop with completion at about 25 years of age for males and 23 years of age for girls. The PFC is not yet fully developed prior to the early 20s, which is why kids and teenagers take so many risks. Their brain is not yet capable of seeing the consequences of their actions.

There is something known as PFC deactivation. When a person is stressed, as in the case of a test or a social situation, the PFC will temporarily turn off. This can result in a loss of memory for the information studied for in the test and embarrassment when one suddenly cannot remember what they were talking about in conversation. It does not mean the person is stupid. This can be triggered by anxiety which may also lead to loss of impulse control, procrastination, difficulty with self-expression or communication, short attention span, and poor judgment. These are the people others can see as unfeeling because they shut down in stressful situations. The PFC controls how you speak your thoughts.

Note that the PFC is commonly affected by the mold biotoxin illness (see the chapter on pathogenic microbes). The effects often cause symptoms of increased irritability and anger.

The amino acid L-tyrosine can help to build the neurotransmitter dopamine, which helps the prefrontal cortex to stay balanced. More information is available in the chapter on supplementation for the brain.

ANTERIOR CYNGULATE GYRUS (ACG)

The anterior cingulate cortex is part of the prefrontal cortex. It is the decision maker and the center for worry. The ACG motivates us to make a decision and keeps us aware of our own behavior and self-consciousness. It is larger in women.

Problems with the ACG causes trouble shifting attention and hyper-focus. These people tend to get stuck on negative thoughts and behaviors, and are compulsive and very oppositional. This often comes from over-activity in the frontal lobes of the brain.

Damage to the caudate nucleus from inflammation or injury may cause sensory disabilities, trouble with motor skills, cognitive function, problem solving, learning, attention, memory, and mental flexibility.

St. Johns Wort and 5-HTP both help to build serotonin, which can be helpful balancing the anterior cingulate gyrus. L-tyrosine is often helpful along with St. Johns Wort and 5-HTP to help balance low dopamine as well.

BASAL GANGLIA

The basal ganglia integrate feelings, thoughts, and movement. It regulates levels of anxiety and motivation and is often underactive in those with ADD. When overactive, the individual may freeze in a stressful situation.

The basal ganglia is the part of the brain involved in handwriting and motor coordination. Their writing looks sloppy and it is hard for them to get feelings out of their head and onto paper. There is often a need to increase dopamine levels in these individuals to help balance the basal ganglia. Dopamine is increased with the amino acid L-tyrosine. This often improves their handwriting.

LIMBIC SYSTEM

The limbic system lies deep in the center of the brain and is one of the oldest parts of the brain. It helps us to express emotions, create rational thought, plan, organize, and solve problems. It is involved with emotional ups and downs.

The limbic system involved in memories tied to an emotional response. The limbic system stores old memories. Good or bad, the stronger the emotion involved, the stronger the memory. It drives the way we emotionally interpret our daily events. It is our emotional filter. When overactive, the limbic system creates negative feelings and behavior. These people tend to generally be very negative in their thoughts and actions.

Depression is very common in those with overactive limbic systems. These people also have low motivation. The limbic system is involved with the hypothalamus in sleep and appetite cycles. When sleep is lost, it leads to even lowered motivation and depression.

Important for those on the autism spectrum is the connection with the limbic system to social connectedness and the ability to bond with others. The hypothalamus is part of the deep limbic system which is also involved with the release of the hormone oxytocin allowing for emotional bonding.

There is a strong connection between the limbic system and the prefrontal cortex (PFC). The limbic system being the emotional driver and the PFC being the area of rational thought leave much to personality. If there is poor integration between these two areas of the brain, one acts either irrationally, driven only by emotion, or alternately, robot-like with only logic and no emotion.

To help with mood, depression, and focus, the supplements DL-Phenylalanine, L-tyrosine, and S-Adenosyl-Methionine (SAMe) have been known to be helpful.

AMYGDALA

The amygdala is the center for instinctually sensing danger, creating fear, and emotional impulses. It starts the fight or flight response and is larger in men.

PITUITARY GLAND

The pituitary produces hormones relating to nurturing and fertility. These hormones are also involved in the production of milk during pregnancy and after birth. Hypothalamic and pituitary activities are involved in the release of the hormone oxytocin, which is involved in the ability to bond with others.

INSULA

The insula is the center for gut feelings and is larger in women.

TEMPORAL PARIETAL JUNCTION (TPJ)

The TPJ seeks to solve issues relating to others with emotional involvement and empathy. This is the center for the male brain's desire to quickly "fix" the problem.

ROSTRAL CINGULATE ZONE (RCZ)

This is where we recognize social approval and disapproval. It is how we recognize what makes us different from others. The RCZ is how we recognize our social errors.

VENTRAL TEGMENTAL AREA (VTE)

Located in the temporal area, this is the main center for motivation. It makes the neurotransmitter dopamine, which assists with focus, motor control, and reward. It is more active in the male brain.

MIRROR-NEURON SYSTEM (MNS)

This is the main area for emotional empathy. This helps us interpret nonverbal expressions such as facial expressions and tone of voice. It is larger in the female brain.

TEMPORAL LOBES

Located behind the ears, the temporal lobes are indicated in mood instability and anger. They also affect language, speech, ability to understand words when reading, and many learning disorders.

PARIETAL LOBES

Located above the temporal lobes on the posterior lateral portion of the head, the parietal lobes are indicated in extreme sensitivity to light, noise, and touch.

HORMONES

- Testosterone is the aggressor and is present in both males and females
- Estrogen is mostly known as the powerhouse in women but is also a strong controller of the male brain; it stimulates the release of oxytocin when receiving and giving affection
- Progesterone calms the effects of estrogen fluctuating in volume throughout the month
- Vasopressin is instinctively protective and responds when our children are present and our home invaded
- Cortisol is the stress hormone secreted by the adrenal glands

- Oxytocin is the calmer and creates feelings of trust, love, affection, and of safety and security; it is released with feelings of love and affection and allows us to bond with others

NOTED STUDIES ON OXYTOCIN AS RELATED TO AUTISM

A 1998 study showed significantly low levels of oxytocin in the blood plasma of autistic children. Modahl C, Green L, Fein D et al. (1998). "Plasma oxytocin levels in autistic children (http://psychcentral.com/news/2010/02/26/autistic-children-benefit-from-sensitive-moms/11735.html)". *Biol Psychiatry* 43 (4): 270–7. doi:0.1016/S,0006-3223(97)00439-3. PMID 9513736.

In a 2003 study, when oxytocin was given intravenously, there were reduced levels of social anxiety and repetitive behaviors. Hollander E, Novotny S, Hanratty M et al. (2003). "Oxytocin infusion reduces repetitive behaviors in adults with autistic and Asperger's disorders". *Neuropsychopharmacology* 28 (1): 193–8. doi:10.1038/sj.npp.13,00021. PMID 12496956.

WHY MORE BOYS HAVE AUTISM THAN GIRLS

From the time a female baby is in utero, her brain has a large supply of estrogen. Throughout the first 24 months of her life, a female is in a stage known as infantile puberty. During this time, the ovaries produce enormous amounts of estrogen. This also helps to grow and develop neurons in her brain. The greatest numbers of vaccines are given in this crucial time of brain development during the first two years. For the female, estrogen assists in protecting the brain against toxins and heavy metals. This is one reason why so many more boys have autism than do girls. His brain lacks the protective estrogen, and contrarily, is filled with testosterone. The neurotoxicity of mercury is actually enhanced by testosterone.

PUBERTY

Beginning around the age of nine, the body triggers hormones to begin puberty. By the age of fourteen, a noticeable change in behavior happens. Boys become especially territorial as their testosterone levels rise dramatically, which triggers their vasopressin and Cortisol to surge. Girls become extremely emotional. Both sexes become very private and often withdrawn.

If your child, like mine, has been going along peacefully and suddenly becomes incredibly difficult to deal with, more aggressive, angry, moody, and loses all motivation, it is due to hormonal changes affecting his brain.

This surge in hormones makes the teen brain more vulnerable to the effects of chemicals. MSG affects hormones and increases episodes of anger and rage. This is true for all ages, but is heightened during puberty. Take care to feed him healthy foods without dangerous food dyes, chemicals, and bad fats.

A lesser known fact is that about fifty percent of people on the autism spectrum begin having seizures around the onset of puberty. One of the safest and most effective forms of treatment has become cannabis or marijuana. I know this will sound strange to you if you have not read the studies on medicinal marijuana but it works for many people with seizures and has no side effects. The intoxicating portion of the cannabis can be almost completely removed leaving only the healing properties. For detailed information on this and the Youtube link to an amazing story please see "seizures" in the chapter on Additional Childhood Epidemics.

Everything will become boring to him. The teen brain, especially in boys, is difficult to stimulate because his reward center has been almost desensitized. Below I talk about supplements to support the brain (and therefore the hormonal system), and brain scans that saved our home life when puberty hit. Fortunately, both punishment and reward centers are heightened during this time, so they can be used for motivation. More motivation is needed due to testosterone washing out their reward center. Offer strong rewards so that everything is not punishment based.

Testosterone receptors also change the clock schedule in his brain. Teens are not lazy. They actually need at least ten hours of sleep per night. They are becoming programmed to stay up later and sleep until noon. If you are homeschooling, your child has the privilege of getting this extra needed sleep. Traditional school schedules do not allow for our kids to properly adjust to their new internal time clocks. For people on the autism spectrum and those with ADHD, getting up in the morning and going to sleep at night can be very challenging. It is difficult for the brain to slow down.

Remove video and computer games at least one hour prior to settling down for the night as they stimulate the brain. In contrast, the electronic reading device known as Kindle from www.amazon.com has a different light source that does not stimulate the part of the brain that keeps them awake. If they cannot go to sleep, let them read their Kindle or a printed book.

HORMONE TESTING

Most doctors, including naturopaths offer hormone testing (saliva test), if needed. Testosterone analysis is also available at www.mgeier@comcast.net, or ASDcenters.com, 301-989-0548.

NOTE: It is important to note that females who act with above average aggression may have excessive testosterone imbalance, (but never rule out heavy metal toxicity with aggression).

SUMMARY

This chapter offers an educational baseline of knowledge regarding the brain's different areas, chemical influences, and the parts they play in behavior.

The products found in this chapter can be found at http://naturallyhealingautism.com/a-healthy-home/

CHAPTER 21

WHAT MAKES THE BRAIN BEHAVE THE WAY IT DOES?

Therapy or discipline is far more challenging, and sometimes impossible, for any child or adult whose brain is not working properly. The way the brain works is somewhat due to hereditary issues. Most of us can pick out which family member talks excessively, is impulsive, angry, lacks focus, or is hyperactive. Autism is not hereditary. If it were, there would be millions of children born before the 1980s with it. It is not possible to have so many people go undiagnosed.

Brain imbalances can be genetic when triggered, physical due to injury, including cranial faulting as early as birth, damage due to toxic exposure, poor diet, lack of absorption of nutrients, caffeine, alcohol, other physical trauma, or severe emotional injury.

Stress is also a strong factor in creating an imbalance in brain chemistry. Stress reduces brains chemicals such as serotonin. This can cause depression, weaken the adrenal function, and increases cortisol levels, which cause irritability, causes insulin resistance, creating hypoglycemia, which then goes back to creating more imbalances in brain chemistry.

Exercise, eating a balanced nutritious diet, and learning ways to cope with stress are all crucial factors in healthy brain chemistry, but sometimes we need more help. What we do not need are negative or even dangerous side effects.

OUR JOURNEY TO BRAIN SUPPLEMENTATION

We began taking my son to therapists when he was 5 years old. Jacob was not diagnosed with Asperger's Syndrome, agitated depression, and oppositional defiance disorder until two months before his 11th birthday. It was extremely frustrating during all of those years for my husband and I to parent a child whom therapists told us simply needed more disciplining.

Not one therapist we had taken our son to throughout all of the years had ever picked up that it might be Asperger's, let alone guide us to ways we could help our child. I knew drugs were not the answer for Jacob. Most would have said that his "window" period was closing, however I believe it is never too late—and it wasn't!

When a therapist told me that I would be helping my son if I were to give him medication, I almost panicked. They also said that I would be hurting him by not doing it. I was in one of those places where what I wanted most was to help my son, yet I knew in my heart there was another way. My problem at that moment was in not knowing what the other way was.

When this happened to me, I left the office of the therapist who made the suggestion and went straight to the office of my holistic medical doctor. I explained that I had been told to drug Jacob, but that I refused to do so. I asked if he had another solution.

I was offered a product called Serene Plus by Neuroscience, Inc. www.neurorelief.com, 800-342-7272. Serene Plus was a compound of a few B and C vitamins along with magnesium and zinc, but included 5-HTP (5 hydroxytryptophan) and Suntheanine (L-theanine). I began researching neurotransmitters at depth and the supplements that can be helpful in building each of them.

My son began taking Serene Plus, and within a few weeks I noticed how much calmer he was. Tantrums and impulsivity seemed to be dissipating more each day. He took the product for about a year, but he complained often of nausea. I hadn't even connected it to the Serene Plus because I was giving him other supplements, too. In this particular product, the one component, 5-HTP, was too strong for him per dosage. This did not harm him, but it did make him nauseous. (We will discuss enteric-coated 5-HTP and dosages later.)

If your child is already taking medications or supplements, it is recommended to seek the advice of a practitioner who is educated in both. Natural supplementation is known to be just as effective as prescription medication for many psychological disorders such as depression, anxiety, and more, but much safer.

NEUROTRANSMITTERS

Neurotransmitters can be thought of as the brain's messengers. Neurotransmitters are chemicals made by the body or in the brain. They are the transmitters of messages vital to our brain's ability to function properly, our body's muscle movements, and more. They regulate our moods, appetite, and sleep. They even control our body's response to pain. If the volume of these chemicals is too low or too high, the message is not sent properly and we experience symptoms.

When neurotransmitter levels are too high or too low, they are felt by imbalances of different parts of the brain and cause disturbances in our ability to function properly. The level of deficit corresponds to the level of the disorder. For example, if your serotonin is a little bit low, you may have mild depression. If it is extremely low, you might be suicidal.

There are ten neurotransmitters, and each has a different job. The three main groups are single amino acids, neuropeptides, and monoamines. Neurotransmitters that are in the brain are mostly made from amino acids. Amino acids are made from proteins, so protein foods will raise levels of neurotransmitters in the brain as long as we are assimilating our food properly.

We need proper nutrition, especially proteins, to build neurotransmitters. Twenty different amino acids build the proteins our body needs to function at optimum. There are eight essential amino acids that the body cannot make them on its own. This is why diet is so important.

The eight essential amino acids are:

1. Isoleucine
2. Leucine
3. Lysine
4. Methionine

5. Phenylalanine
6. Threonine
7. Tryptophan
8. Valine

Protein foods in our diet should vary so that we get a complete protein to include all eight. Some good sources of protein are eggs, poultry (especially turkey), fish and seafood, meat, dairy, beans, grains, nuts, and seeds. Eggs and turkey contain higher levels of tryptophan, which builds serotonin. We will talk more about this in a moment.

Vegetarians need to be especially careful to eat the proper combinations of vegetable, fruits, and grains to get all eight of the essential amino acids.

Sometimes the body is deficient in the vitamins and minerals necessary to make neurotransmitters. When this happens, any problem can arise from anxiety and depression to autism or schizophrenia. Though it may have started with a deficiency of only one nutrient, through an event of chain reactions in the body, it becomes a deficiency of many. It is never just one thing alone. Malabsorption can then occur and metabolism breaks down. Your child's body is deprived of even more than it started with and his brain does not get what it needs to work the way it is supposed to.

Eating these foods will help if proteins are properly assimilated, but this is often a problem for children on the autism spectrum. Neurotransmitters are made from protein. If the GI tract is not functioning properly, the body lacks the resources to build them in the brain. Heavy metals such as mercury interfere with protein synthesis. Whichever neurotransmitter or neurotransmitters are deficient results in the behavioral aspects of the brain.

THE THREE GROUPS OF NEUROTRANSMITTERS ARE:

1. **Single amino acids**: directly affect neurons
2. **Neuropeptides**: known commonly as endorphins, they are very powerful protein chains made up of two or more amino acids; these regulate the body's pain response

3. **Monoamines**: single amine groups that contain additional molecules that enables them to do their jobs. These are extremely important to the proper functioning of our brain

The monoamines we need to discuss most are serotonin and dopamine.

EXAMPLE OF NEUROTRANSMITTER IMBALANCE

Low dopamine levels affect our ability to write by hand due to its effect on a part of the brain called the basal ganglia that helps fine motor coordination and gets our thoughts out of our head and onto paper. The prefrontal cortex may not have enough dopamine, so it cannot organize thoughts or plan future events. Large numbers of serotonin-producing neurons are found in the limbic system, the part of the brain that controls emotions. Low levels of both serotonin and dopamine can create problems in the prefrontal cortex causing behavioral problems. We will go into further detail on this in a moment.

TESTING FOR NEUROTRANSMITTER LEVELS

Your practitioner should have these tests available, but if you do not have insurance or prefer to do it yourself without the added expense, there are online sources available. The company NeuroScience Incorporated has many products for different needs. They also have tests that they provide to learn more about what your child's neurological needs are, such as neurotransmitters. Contact information: www.neurorelief.com or (888)342-7272.

These brain abnormalities will not show up on EEGs or MRIs. If you would like truly educated experience, please see the information on the Amen Clinic and all they offer in the chapter on Natural Supplementation for the Brain. Additional brain scans will be discussed soon.

SEROTONIN: THE KING OF NEUROTRANSMITTERS

Serotonin is the neurotransmitter most involved in the cause of multiple medical and psychiatric problems. Inflammation reduces tryptophan, which is needed to build serotonin. Serotonin is prone to disruption from mercury toxicity. It is also disrupted by imbalance in the mucosal lining of the intestines.

Serotonin receptors in the GI system play a critical role in irritable bowel syndrome (IBS). There are cells in the stomach, small intestine, and large intestine called enterochromaffin (EC) cells. They hold 95% of the body's serotonin. IBS and its symptoms of abdominal pain may be due to hypersensitivity of the GI tract to normal stimuli. Disturbances in the serotonin pathway and a direct impact on the central nervous system would create behavioral disturbances such as anxiety and depression. Symptoms would vary due to molecular make-up. You can imagine what an impact gut dysbiosis has on the release and regulation of serotonin. It is no wonder our kids usually have issues associated with serotonin imbalance.

A part of the brain called the dorsal raphe nucleus (DR) contains serotonin neurons. These effect the cortex and limbic system, therefore effecting cognitive function and behavior. Peptides present in the neurons are thought to effect circuitry in the (DR) to effect the 5HTP system. The "T" in 5HTP is a peptide that influences the serotonergic neurons.

Symptoms associated with low serotonin levels in the brain are headaches of all kinds, including migraines, extreme fatigue, anxiety, aggression, ADD, carbohydrate cravings (including alcohol), lack of satiety with food, chronic pain, chronic fatigue, epilepsy, hyperactivity, insomnia (an inability to fall asleep or stay asleep), muscle twitching, Restless Leg Syndrome, low pain tolerance, obesity and other eating disorders, obsessive compulsive disorder, hyperfocus, panic disorders, premenstrual symptoms, schizophrenia, seasonal affective disorder, depression, suicidal thoughts and behavior, and night terrors.

NIGHT TERRORS

A common issue with children on the autism spectrum is night terrors. They awake in the middle of the night screaming from nightmares. They can also be prone to grinding their teeth while sleeping. This is often an emotional response, unless provoked by parasites in the gut. Low serotonin levels can be the cause of these problems. Candida/yeast may also be a factor in trouble sleeping.

DIGESTIVE ISSUES

Serotonin receptors are present in the cells of the digestive tract, which helps regulate secretion of stomach acid and digestive fluids. It also helps food move through the digestive tract by stimulating the muscles that do so. A poorly functioning digestive tract can be due, at least in part, to low serotonin levels.

OBESITY

There are certain times of day that serotonin levels drop. Commonly this is between 3:00 and 4:00 p.m. This is when we tend to get tired and have the afternoon munchies, especially for something sweet. Snacking on sweets and carbohydrates can increase the levels of serotonin in your brain, but only if you have eaten a protein food with tryptophan in it first, such as turkey or eggs. However, sugar is a bad habit and one that can lead to weight gain and diabetes. Sweets can create swings in blood sugar (insulin) levels that can lead to insulin resistance.

When serotonin levels are low, the brain senses that it is starving and signals us to start eating, especially carbohydrates that increase blood sugar. Obese people often have low serotonin. They may continue to eat, never feeling full, because there is not enough serotonin in their brain to signal satiation. They are always hungry.

Dieting causes serotonin levels to drop, which signals the brain to tell us to eat as though we are starving. Our appetite becomes uncontrollable, and we gain the weight back and often add on even more.

MIGRAINE HEADACHES

I see a lot of children in my own craniosacral practice with migraine headaches who are on the autism spectrum, and also in children who are not on the spectrum.

Migraines can be due to an inflamed trigeminal nerve (see “Craniosacral Therapy” in the chapter on Alternative Therapies for more information). The key areas are the back of the neck and the upper palate. Besides cranial faulting, low serotonin is also implicated in migraine headaches. Serotonin constricts blood vessels which can help relieve the pain.

DOPAMINE

Dopamine is a neurotransmitter. A child who has ADHD and cannot focus or complete a task easily is showing signs of low dopamine. They also tend to have low motivation. Parkinson's disease symptoms show the behavior of a brain that has stopped making dopamine. We mentioned above how dopamine can be helpful with handwriting as it affects the part of the brain called the basal ganglia which involves fine motor coordination.

In contrast, too much dopamine can create hyperfocus. People with too much dopamine will lock onto a task or get stuck in negative thoughts and behaviors, seemingly unable to pull themselves out of it. They tend to be grudge holders. Elevated dopamine levels can also create confusion, behavioral changes, and trouble with social connections.

Although dopamine is the pleasure chemical and is increased when we do pleasurable activities, current research has shown that when children spend time in front of a computer screen, their levels of dopamine are reduced. This is likely due to the heightened anxiety level that most games create and is not a pleasure response at all. Dopamine is prone to disruption from mercury toxicity.

SIGNALS THAT DOPAMINE IS LOW:

- Trouble focusing
- No sense of pleasure or reward
- Inattentive
- Low motivation
- Trouble with fine motor skills such as handwriting
- Trouble with follow through

Too much dopamine can be a problem, just as too little can be a problem. Too much dopamine with phenylalanine can cause behavioral disorders such as schizophrenia and seizures.

SIGNALS THAT DOPAMINE IS TOO HIGH:

- Hyperfocus
- Stuck in negative behavior patterns

SUMMARY

The behavior of the brain is greatly affected by chemistry. I learned through personal experience with my own son the severity at which neurotransmitters, the brains' messengers, affect the brain. Along with toxic impact, the brain's chemistry must be balanced in order for it to be capable of functioning properly.

The products found in this chapter can be found at http://naturallyhealingautism.com/a-healthy-home/

CHAPTER 22

BRAIN SCANS; WHAT'S REALLY GOING ON IN MY CHILD'S BRAIN?

We were told for years that we just needed to be firmer with discipline with our son. Our society has trained us to believe it is only about behavior without considering biology.

WHY CAN'T I BEHAVE THE WAY I WANT TO?

This is where parents, teachers, therapists and caregivers seem to trip-up the most. Increasing discipline does not work, so he gets punished, sometimes beaten, because he is not doing what he is told to do. How can we expect any one, let alone a child, to listen, and follow directions if they have imbalances in their brain that do not allow them to comprehend what they are being asked to do? How can they sit still if they have impulse issues or stay calm if there are neurological issues causing them anger or anxiety?

These people struggle internally. They feel that they are stupid, lazy, or just plain weird. It doesn't help to have their teachers, friends, therapists, and family members saying the same things that they are saying to themselves inside. "Why can't I do it right? Why can't I behave the way I want to? What's wrong with me?" When my son was young he would say to me, "I want to, but I can't."

Often they end up with very low self-esteem by the time they are teenagers because this is what they have heard and felt their entire lives. They have anxiety because they are always afraid of not being able to do things right. Parents, teachers, and caregivers have always tried to control these children, so they often marry someone who is controlling. They feel that this is what they need to stay on track. With oppositional behavior, do they argue just to argue, or is it a way simply to not look vulnerable?

The reason they cannot do what they would like to do is because their brain is overactive in some areas and underactive in others. When you find the answers to those pieces, you will find your solutions. Symptoms are your best guide when looking for supplementation with anything, but especially the brain.

I explained earlier how I thought Jacob was ignoring me when I would speak to him until I realized that he could not hear me. This was not an auditory issue, but one of hyperfocus. We don't know what he hears. His surroundings did not exist when he was locked in and focused on something. Alternately, if he was doing something that needed to stop, he would not react and listen to us or anyone else. You can imagine how frustrating this can be to ask someone to stop doing something, especially if it is dangerous, and not have them listen. Sadly, some children are beaten for this type of behavior. Physical punishment will not help a child who is literally unable to comprehend the information properly and follow through.

It is uncertain what the true needs of your child are until his gut is healed, inflammation reduced, and the heavy metals and other toxins have been cleared from his body. Damage may remain that warrants support for the brain. Neurotransmitter levels can be too high or too low. Sometimes the brain is overactive in a state of concentration but underactive in a state of rest. Psychotherapy will not work for those who need brain support; my own son is a testimonial for this.

I was told to medicate my son, but I refused. I was told that I was hurting him by not giving him drugs. This was my choice because I wanted to find answers to heal or assist his brain without negative side effects. Our family knows someone who was depressed and was given an antidepressant by his general practitioner doctor. The drugs made him worse and he committed suicide.

It may come to it that your child needs medication, but wouldn't it be worth it to try safer avenues first? What I offer you here are alternative choices. Please remember the importance of a good diet along with these choices.

One thing I know is that it is never too late. Scientists used to believe that the brain could not be healed, but current research has proven otherwise. The brain is a constantly regenerating organ. I have seen enough changes in my own child to know that this is true. All it needs to function better is some natural support without harmful side effects.

Knowledge of symptoms is critical. Read Daniel Amen's book *Healing ADD* to help assist you. Getting a brain SPECT image from the Amen Clinic and testing for neurotransmitter levels can all be critical in helping you know exactly what is going on in your child's brain and how it is or is not functioning.

OUR STORY

Jacob had his issues with violent and oppositional behavior, but he kept it at home. Ever since pre-school, he would keep it together at school, and then have a meltdown at home. He has an extremely kind and gentle heart. Perhaps this sensitivity is what made it so hard then.

He got through the tumultuous middle school years mostly frustrated and sad over the behavior of his long-time friends toward him. He just could not understand why they would suddenly start being mean toward him. I explained the difficulties of the age, hormonal changes, and the need for maturity in everyone. I let him know that I knew it was hard, but that they would eventually grow out of it.

He maintained good grades as he always had. Luckily, he is exceptionally bright and school academically was fairly easy for him. The classroom could become overwhelming with the sensory overload, but he knew to excuse himself to get a break from the class. Exercise also seemed to help. Organization was a challenge, but he seemed to figure it out. He would never take help from anyone including his dad or myself. We tried therapy with a specialist in autism spectrum disorders for about a year, but Jacob was just too oppositional. He would not cooperate, so we finally stopped. There was no need to continue if he would not comply, and it was costing us a lot of money.

Finally, it became time to begin high school. I felt my concern regarding the change of schools, but for the first month he seemed to do all right. His friends were maturing a little, and he was calming down. Suddenly, one month later, in October of his freshman year at high school, he just stopped caring. Whether it was social pressures or a new surge of testosterone in his system, we have never quite figured out for certain what happened. He would not do his homework or tests at school. We tried everything to no avail. We had regular meetings with his counselor and teachers trying to adjust his 504 plan so that he would not fail. This is a child who had always been a good student with mostly As and a few Bs.

He was getting older and bigger and violent episodes at home concerned me. I was alone most of the week since my husband worked out of town. I had two kids to care for, one who was oppositional, and his sister who was five years younger than him. I had concern for my daughter around him since impulsivity was a severe problem. There were no friends or family who really seemed to understand the severity of what we were dealing with. Some thought they did, but as you know, they cannot unless they have a child of their own who is like this. I felt alone, helpless, and a concern for my own health due to the stress. I had to find an answer to Jacob's behavior for the good of the entire family. With all of my knowledge, I still had a piece missing from the puzzle due to this sudden onset of new and increasing behaviors.

My husband wanted to medicate him, but I just could not do it. I had read too much about the negative side effects. I didn't want a zombie for a son or one who became more depressed or more violent due to the drugs. I wanted to find out what was wrong and fix it, naturally. Deep in my heart, I knew there was an answer. I knew it.

In the winter of Jacob's freshman year, I had a craniosacral class on the brain. During the class, I heard another student talking with our teacher about a man named Daniel Amen and his work. Dr. Amen had written several books on healing the brain. One they spoke highly of at the time was *Change Your Brain, Change Your Life*.

I purchased this book that evening and began to read it. It was everything I had known existed. Dr. Amen does brain SPECT imaging to find the exact cause of the issues instead of a guessing game. He works naturally first. If after a period of time the natural supplementation does not meet your expectations, he will offer medications, but they are based on precise knowledge from the brain scan. It made so much sense.

Treatment involved some of the natural supplements I had used in the past with Jacob that had helped, but due to increased nausea with one supplement I had discontinued use. I later learned why. Dr. Amen told multiple stories of people of all ages that had been helped tremendously. I looked into it on their website www.amenclinics.com, and decided we had to go.

The clinic offers consultation with scans or without them, but I suggest getting the scans if at all possible to know exactly what is going on. Dr. Amen's book, *Healing ADD*, gives detailed information regarding the six different types of ADD and the supplements that have been helpful for those symptoms. I highly recommend reading it. We scheduled the three-day trip letting Jacob's counselor know what we were doing. He was excused from school on a doctor's note, and we drove five hours to the nearest clinic.

We did 2 scans, each done 24 hours apart. The results were important enough for me to move forward. They took one scan the first day after having him play a computer game to put his brain in working mode. On the second day, they had him rest for about 10 minutes prior to the scan. The brain acts very differently when it is working and when it is at rest. This gives a much more thorough explanation to how his brain functions at different tasks.

On the third day, we were given the results, and Jacob was handed the pictures of his brain. I think the visual aspect of the scans had the greatest impact. He was able to see for himself a difference in the photo that the doctor could tell him about. The doctor explained to us in detail what was going on in Jacob's brain. An overactive cingulate system in his brain was the cause of most of his issues.

We were give a specific treatment plan of SAMe, 5-HTP, L-tyrosine, St. Johns Wort, 1,500 to 2,000 mg per day of omega-3 fatty acids, and multi-vitamins and minerals. Prior to going to the Amen Clinic, Jacob had been taking some of these supplements, but the dosages were not high enough. I also learned that the 5-HTP dosage in the original product I had given him was really high for a single dose. This did not hurt him, but it made him nauseous. I now buy 5-HTP that is enteric coated so there is no nausea. I purchase it at www.swansovitamins.com.

They schedule a follow-up appointment three weeks later. If the results are not what you desire, they ask you to continue for a longer period of time, perhaps on a higher dosage, or offer you prescription medication. They like to go natural first. Remember, natural supplementation can take up to three weeks to see results, and those results will continue to improve over a period of more time.

Jacob's results from this treatment regimen have been nothing short of amazing. He became social, calm, pleasant, happy, engaged, and his grades returned to As and Bs. The following year at school, he was given an award for the most improved student. His previous freshman year had been his worst ever. By his sophomore year, he was back on track and has stayed there. He will be moving away this fall for college where he will study computer engineering. Today, he is a happy, healthy, and has a lot of great friends. He continues to take his supplements daily.

Note: If supplements are discontinued symptoms will return. They must be continued ongoing.

THE AMEN CLINIC AND BRAIN SPECT IMAGING

Daniel Amen is a psychiatrist who has clinics in the United States. The Amen Clinics specialize in brain-health diagnosis and offer various treatments for people of any age. First, they like to offer a natural supplementation program, unless the client chooses otherwise. If within a specific amount of time you are not satisfied with the results of the natural supplements, a prescription program may offered. This is very specific to the needs of the individual from the results of the SPECT imaging brain scan.

Dr. Amen's clinics use an imaging technique called SPECT. SPECT stands for single photon emission-computed tomography. There is a very thorough explanation of this on their website at www.amenclinics.com. Generally speaking, it is neuro-imaging where they take a picture of the patient's brain, revealing any excessively high or low activity. The image is given in different color shades which give the information. You and your child will be able to see this picture for yourselves.

For Jacob, this let him see what was going on in his brain. It allowed him to realize the truth, which in itself made a huge difference in his belief and behavior toward what was going on. Instead of mom and dad just telling him there were things he needed to know about the way he behaved. it made it real to him.

MRIs, EEGs, and blood tests will often show normal results. This can be very misleading and can cause dangerous mistakes. The SPECT image shows precise brain activity.

At the time of this writing, the Amen clinic has done over 70,000 brain SPECT images. We needed real, educated, and precise answers for my son immediately, and this gave them to us.

Instead of the usual scenario of a ten-minute talk with a doctor before treatment is prescribed, the Amen Clinic has a four part process:

- Phone consult and questionnaire
- SPECT imaging scans done in both a resting state and a concentrating state
- Evaluation of SPECT images with treatment recommendations
- Follow-up appointment

There are six Amen Clinics in the U.S. They are located in:

- San Francisco, CA
- Newport Beach, CA
- Bellevue, WA
- Washington, D.C.
- New York, NY
- Atlanta, GA

Important: At the Amen Clinic please use the referral code "Karen Thomas" when you call to get a 10% discount on any evaluations and SPECT imaging scans, (866)260-8227. Amen brain supplements and a free four minute brain questionnaire can be found at http://naturallyhealingautism.com/a-healthy-home/.

NEUROQUANT BRAIN SCAN

A new MRI type of software called Neuroquant precisely measures brain volume. It is capable of detecting shrinkage in specific areas of the brain. Neuroquant is most helpful in gauging changes over time. The good news is that the brain can and does heal once toxic exposure is eliminated and proper treatment is given. The price of this scan at the time of writing this book was $96. For more information on Neuroquant, go to www.radnet.com, or call 800-975-4674.

TO DRUG OR NOT TO DRUG

After seeing Jacob's brain scan from the Amen Clinic, we saw that a drug such as Ritalin would have made his symptoms and behavior a lot worse. Everyone thinks Ritalin is the answer, but pharmaceutical drugs are not for everyone. SPECT imaging rules out the cookie-cutter approach, which is used all too often. Due to the nature of biology, there are no two people exactly alike, and multiple symptoms cannot be fixed with one drug or supplement.

Prescription antidepressants can inhibit the brain's ability to rebuild weakened areas. The brain is an adaptive organ. We do not want it to adapt to a drug that may leave it vulnerable. What about naturally assisting it to rebuild itself?

First of all, if your child is already on drugs and you are feeling any guilt, please leave that right here and move on. We do what we think at the time is the best for our child. Often we are not always completely educated as far as what all of our options are. What we need is knowledge of other possibilities. I have found that not many conventional healthcare providers possess the necessary knowledge of natural alternatives, nor do they wish to learn about them. Self-education is the best way to learn about what you really need to know, which is why I wrote this book for you.

Is it possible to keep my child off of drugs? This is the big question, isn't it? Sometimes the answer may be "no." Many times the answer is "yes." My story is the perfect example. What if it were possible to help your child naturally, without any drugs? What if he could feel even a little bit more calm, happy, and communicative without the use of any drugs or their negative side effects? Would it be worth it to try? Natural supplementation has an overall, long-term, higher level of success. Alternatives are often more effective.

THE PROBLEM WITH DRUGS

The greatest concern with prescription drugs are their side effects. When we drug, we do not repair the problem, but mask it. Often the drugs make people worse. Why mask symptoms when we can repair and safely balance the cause of the problem? I know the doctors have told you that drugs are the best way to go, but this is not always true. My own son is a perfect example. I was told how I would be helping him if I gave him drugs and that by not giving him medication I was doing him a disservice. If I had not refused and started digging for more answers, I would have a son who never would have received the real help from natural supplementation that I was able to find for him, and that changed our lives. (Not to mention that he would now be addicted to a drug that would have done him more harm than good.)

The brain doesn't want too many messages at one time or it gets confused. For example, if too much of any one neurotransmitter (the brain's messengers) is released, the receptors for that particular neurotransmitter will shut down. This is called down-regulation. If the brain is in need of more neurotransmitters, it will also open up more receptors, which is called up-regulation. This is where drugs get dangerous. The brain will open or close receptors for messages from neurotransmitters.

Have you ever known someone that has taken drugs and after a while they need more of that drug to feel the same way. An example is someone taking Prozac for depression. At first, 20 mg may lift the depression and make them feel better. In time, the depression comes back and they need a stronger dosage to alleviate the depression. In the long run, they may never feel good for any length of time, and again, they do not receive the help they need to relieve the cause.

ONE MORE REASON NOT TO DRUG

The brain is not completely finished developing until the age of 25. The last part to develop is the prefrontal cortex (PFC). It is undergoing a process of myelination that protects neurons in the brain to make them more efficient. The PFC is the area of the brain that is responsible for organization, planning, impulse control, and judgment among other things. Drugs can injure the PFC while it is still developing. If this happens during this stage, it can potentially cause permanent brain damage. If the PFC is damaged, it can also negatively affect the cerebellum, another part of the brain in the back of the head that affects our ability to think. Many drugs are known to stunt the growth of children by inhibiting normal hormonal functioning.

SIDE EFFECTS

Of course, the biggest and very real concerns of prescription drugs are their side effects. Actually, they are not really side effects at all—they are additional effects of the drug. If you have seen the drug commercials, you have heard the long list of dangers behind most prescription medications. Sometimes I feel like I'm watching a *Saturday Night Live* skit. Would someone really prefer to get cancer, heart disease, or die, rather than have a skin rash? The big question is, "Is it worth the risk?" Absolutely not!

Common antidepressant medications known as serotonin re-uptake inhibitors, also called SSRIs, create suicidal and homicidal side effects. The school shootings that have occurred have been done so by individuals taking psychotropic drugs. Another common drug, Ritalin, when combined with excitotoxins, can cause distorted thinking, apathy, and rage.

A DOCTOR'S INCENTIVE

We don't want to assume that all doctors only give medication for the financial kickback; however, they are an incentive. The American Medical Association considers it ethically acceptable for medical practitioners to receive payments from drug companies. Most people I have talked to over the years have a hard time getting their doctor to help them get off of the drugs they are on, even when they are experiencing negative side effects.

GETTING HIM SAFELY OFF OF DRUGS

Safety in this matter is of utmost importance. It is important that if you do not feel that you are receiving the proper advice from anyone that you seek additional help. Drug withdrawal is no simple matter. Reduction and elimination of prescription medication should be done very slowly and done under guidance from a knowledgeable professional.

There is a company called True Hope, whose focus is to assist people in natural, non- invasive nutritional sources to help with mental illness. Symptoms from ADD and bipolar to depression and nervous system disorders are addressed. They have a complete product line to help build up the natural resources your body needs to make neurotransmitters and keep them in balance.

True Hope sells products from their own line but also sells products from Natural Factors. Natural Factors products are among the very best. Dr. Michael Murray, N.D. is part of this Canadian-based company. They use only the finest ingredients and are of the highest quality.

Please remember that as brain functioning improves with the help of nutrients and natural supplements, the need for prescription medications will lessen. In order to not over-medicate, it is important to be under proper care. It is also important to know that there are specific nutrients such as certain amino acids that can help with withdrawal symptoms. If you are needing additional assistance than that which you are receiving from your caregiver, then the people at www.truehope.com can help.

If additional assistance is needed, there is another helpful source with this matter, www.drugawareness.org. No one needs to feel alone when going through withdrawal symptoms with a loved one, especially your child.

SUMMARY

Children often cannot behave the way they want to due to an imbalanced brain. Until their brain is free of toxins and supported by necessary supplementation they may not be able to do what is asked of them.

Safer avenues exist to balance the body's chemistry, including the brain. Brain scans can offer an insight into the specifics of an individual's brain. They take out the guessing game of behavioral issues and what can be done for them.

The products found in this chapter can be found at http://naturallyhealingautism.com/a-healthy-home/

CHAPTER 23

NATURAL SUPPLEMENTATION FOR THE BRAIN

Natural supplements can work just as well as medications do, without any of the harmful side effects often obtained from drugs. Most people become frustrated if they do not see immediate results. We are a society of "quick fix" people, but this is not always the best way. It is important to realize that natural supplementation takes about three to six weeks to really begin noticing the greater differences as the brain's chemistry rebuilds and balances. After three to six months, even greater results are achieved.

If within three to four weeks there are no noticeable changes, then it is time to increase the dosages or do something else. If you are with the Amen Clinic program, there will be a follow-up appointment with the doctor and you will be given specific information.

When you have found the right program for your child, they will be on it forever. Going off of the program will slowly reduce improvements made. Specific guidelines are given in step three of the healing stages.

With my son, we noticed differences in the first week. Jacob was calmer, happier, more social, and his moods were more balanced. The improvements in the first few weeks were subtle, but they existed and gave us hope. Over the next three to six months, the differences became much greater, and they have continued to strengthen over time. Our experience with natural supplementation has been exceptional. Our family has gone from living in crisis to living a happy, well-adjusted life. These products can be purchased at www.naturallyhealingautism.com under "healthy home products."

Always check with your doctor if you are currently on medication because some supplements will interact with them.

OMEGA-3 FATTY ACIDS

We have already talked in detail about the benefits of omega-3 fatty acids. Omega-3 fatty acids protect the brain and help to rebuild damaged areas. They contain the omega-3 fatty acids that are essential for the health and functioning of the brain. Deficiency in omega-3 fatty acids can cause issues with moods such as depression, hyperactivity, lethargy, memory loss, cell energy production, and cognitive learning ability.

The neurotransmitters most affected by omega-3 fatty acids are dopamine, affecting motivation and drive, and serotonin, important in sleep, mood, and appetite. This is also why omega-3s are significant when used in treating depression, anxiety, violent and aggressive behavior, and even schizophrenia.

SEROTONIN AND 5-HTP

The best way to build serotonin is by supplementing with 5-hydroxytryptophan (5-HTP). This is the amino acid tryptophan in its already-converted form. Tryptophan must be converted in the body to make 5-HTP. The 5-HTP then makes serotonin, so taking 5-HTP cuts out a middle step. 5-HTP is as powerful as prescription medications for depression, behavioral and mood issues, and sleep disorders, but it is much safer. 5-HTP also helps to build pain relieving endorphins.

Heavy metals such as cadmium reduce levels of 5-HTP and acetylcholine, but increase levels of dopamine. Too much dopamine can be a problem, too.

In order for tryptophan to be converted into 5-HTP, it must be broken down in the digestive tract, and more so, in the liver and the brain. Factors that inhibit the development of serotonin from tryptophan to 5-HTP include:

- Stress causes cortisol levels to rise, which depletes the liver of the enzymes needed to make 5-HTP
- A weak liver

- Poor digestion
- Vitamin B deficiency, especially B6 and niacin
- Low magnesium
- Genetics
- Improper insulin regulation

About 70% of 5-HTP is taken up into the brain versus only 3% of tryptophan. 5-HTP bypasses the liver, so the liver is not needed to convert it into serotonin and serotonin is easily built and quickly reaches the brain. Also, 5-HTP is known to be more effective when taken with St. Johns Wort.

In the case of depression, if the benefits of 5-HTP begin to reduce, it may be due to a drop in dopamine and norepinephrine. In this case, adding the supplement L-tyrosine or DL- phenylalanine may restore the effects. Phenylalanine builds tyrosine, so taking tyrosine is best for this job. I have found the results of L-tyrosine to be extremely beneficial and safe for many mood and behavior issues, especially problems with focus.

DOSAGES OF 5-HTP

5-HTP is generally taken about 20 minutes prior to eating. It is best absorbed on an empty stomach, or with a small snack. When 5-HTP is first taken, it can cause slight nausea for some people, especially in higher doses. This usually dissipates after a short time. Serene Plus has 300 mg of 5 HTP in one dosage, which was the cause of the nausea for Jacob. We now take an enteric-coated 5-HTP. Enteric coatings prevent release in the stomach so there is no nausea, but they are only in pill form. To prevent nausea in other forms, start with very low levels and work your way up. Although absorption is best on an empty stomach, a small amount of carbohydrate food such as fruit can help reduce any possible nausea.

For children, the dosage of 5-HTP depends on their weight. Commonly, 4.5 mgs per kilogram or 2.2 pounds per day is helpful. Consult a practitioner educated in natural supplementation for more guidance.

Helpful dosages for insomnia are 100 to 300 mg at bedtime.

For symptoms of insomnia and depression 100 to 200 mg three times per day with the last dose about 45 minutes before bedtime has been known to be helpful. These are common adult dosages, so a larger teenager may need this amount. For a child of smaller weight, follow the guidelines above for children.

Note: If you are taking antidepressant drugs or other medications, consult your practitioner before taking anything new or adjusting any dosage levels.

Generally, the dosage of 5-HTP for adults is 50 to 300 milligrams per day. Children start at half dose. I purchase the enteric coated 5-HTP through www.swansonvitamins.com. These are in the form of a small pill. Capsule form is available, but they are not enteric coated. For non-pill takers, there is a 5-HTP powder available by Lifemode sold at www.amazon.com. If a form of

5-HTP is taken that is not enteric coated, it can be taken with a small snack.

DOPAMINE AND L-TYROSINE

The best supplement for building dopamine is the amino acid L-tyrosine. Commonly deficient, L-tyrosine is an inexpensive amino acid and it is known to be safe. It is sold in all healthfood stores often in capsule form. One site for this is www.swansonvitamins.com. I did find a liquid form of L-tyrosine at www.tjclarkinc.com, 800-228-0872, and a powder form made by NOW Foods at www.soap.com. 500 to 1500 mg per day is often helpful.

Note: If someone has hyper-focus (see Type 3 ADD), do not give them L-tyrosine alone without 5-HTP because this would make their symptoms worse. For some conditions, such as hyper-focus with oppositional behavior, it is often most helpful to give both L-tyrosine to build dopamine along with 5-HTP and St. Johns Wort to also build serotonin. The balance of both is needed and are best taken away from food.

ST. JOHNS WORT

St. John's Wort, as mentioned above, is more effective when taken with 5-HTP. It is very helpful with depressed moods, anxiety, when one needs a more flexible attitude, and is commonly used in Germany for depression instead of Prozac. When used with 5-HTP, it can be essential for those with insomnia. St. Johns Wort has a long history of being safe and effective.

Be sure the St. Johns Wort product you purchase contains 0.3% of the active ingredient, hypericin. There are many capsule forms available that can be opened up into food or a beverage. Alcohol is often added to liquid tinctures. If your child has a problem with alcohol affecting his gut or brain, there is a standardized, alcohol-free liquid tincture with 0.3% hypericin by Nature's Answer available at www.swansonvitamins.com, 800-824-4491.

Note: For those taking medications that can be metabolized by the enzyme cytochrome P450 3A4 (CYP3A4), do not take St Johns Wort with hypericin, as hypericin induces this enzyme. This enzyme reduces the blood levels of medications that it metabolizes. Contact your doctor if your child is taking medications. St. Johns Wort can also create skin sensitivity to the sun.

The starting dosage for St. Johns Wort is 300 mg per day for children, 300 mg twice per day for teens, and 600 mg in the morning and 300 mg in the evening for adults.

Note: Temporal lobe imbalances (see Type 4 ADD) must be stabilized before using St. Johns Wort as it increases serotonin but decreases dopamine and can make symptoms worse. See the brain symptom categories for more on temporal lobe imbalance.

DL-PHENYLALANINE (DLPA)

DLPA helps form proteins and is a precursor for tyrosine. It is used to assist in symptoms of depression, and helps with mood, focus, and energy. Individuals with PKU (phenylketoneuria) should not take DLPA. These people lack the enzyme necessary to metabolize it.

Phenylalanine causes the release of norepinephrine and dopamine which control the release of the pituitary hormones:

- Growth hormone
- Thyroid stimulating hormone

- Luteinizing hormone: triggers ovulation in women and produces testosterone in men
- Vasopressin: regulates fluids in the body such as water, glucose, salts, and blood
- Prolactin: helps regulate the immune system, fluid balance, the hormonal reproductive system, growth and development, the release of dopamine, and behavior
- Oxytocin: involved in sexual reproduction, bonding after birth, social recognition, social traits, anxiety, the behavior of trust and empathy, and aggressive behavior

L-tyrosine will help to build dopamine.

SAMe (S-Adenosyl-Methionine)

S-Adenosyl-Methionine, or SAMe is derived from the amino acid methionine. It helps the brain to function properly helping to synthesize critical neurotransmitters such as dopamine and norepinephrine. It helps the body to regulate hormones, assists protein synthesis, increases glutathione levels by fifty percent, boosts the methylation (detoxification) process, including brain cell methylation, and helps with joint and liver support. Studies have shown SAMe to protect liver tissue from toxic injury. It also increases the neurotransmitters involved with depression such as serotonin. SAMe is extremely helpful for depression and grief, and does not cause addiction. It is one of the best natural antidepressants available, but is not suggested for those diagnosed with bipolar disorder or manic depression. It is also helpful with low motivation or drive. SAMe is often used by those with chronic muscle pain and disorders associated with it.

SAMe has been shown to have a high level of safety in clinical trials and is well tolerated. It can be purchased at health food stores and at many online sites. For those who take pills, SAMe should be purchased in a sealed blister pack to protect it from inactivation, not in a bottle. Be careful about the ingredients in the products you choose. Many SAMe products I looked into contained FD&C Yellow # 5 dye.

Source Naturals is a great company with quality products. Their SAMe comes in a blister pack and is free of all dyes and allergens. It is available in stores and at www.pureformulas.com. SAMe also comes in liquid form. I also found one from Lumina Health called Cellfood SAMe liquid formula. It is available at www.swansonvitamins.com. Helpful dosages can be 200 to 400 mg, 2 to 4 times per day for adults (depending on individual needs), children get half that.

GABA (gamma amino Butyric acid)

The GABA system is one of the first to develop after conception within the first two months. Specific neurons produce GABA because it is needed by the central nervous system. GABA mediates the activity between nerves. When this system is not working properly and GABA is diminished, the nerves become overexcited and cannot calm down. GABA is greatly affected by chemicals, especially pesticides.

GABA is an amino acid known to be extremely calming to nerves and the brain. It balances the firing of neurons and reduces hyperactivity within the brain itself, blocking excitatory messages. It is helpful for anger, anxiety, irritability, and memory. It also helps regulate muscle tone. There are many pill and capsule forms available in healthfood stores and online. I found a sublingual form from Source Naturals called GABA Calm Sublingual Orange available at both www.swansonvitamins.com and www.pureformulas.com.

Source Naturals is a great company and sublingual forms act very quickly. They are absorbed under the tongue directly into the bloodstream. This could be a parent's best friend during a child's tantrum or time of anxiety and stress. There are also chewable and powder forms available at both online sites. A good dosage is 100 to 500 mg per day. For extreme cases in adults, 1,500 mg per day may be needed.

L-THEANINE

L-theanine is an amino acid derived from green tea. It is known for its relaxing properties without causing drowsiness. Research shows that L-theanine crosses the blood-brain barrier within 30 minutes after being ingested. The effects quickly calm the brain and allow for concentration and greater cognitive ability. L-theanine is also known to reverse neurotoxicity. Dosages up to 200 mg have been known to be helpful for adults, while children get half that.

MELATONIN

Melatonin, the brain's sleep hormone that controls the sleep wake cycle. It is made from serotonin, so you have the choice to eitehr take melatonin alone or with 5-HTP if you would like its added benefits. Remember, 5-HTP builds serotonin and is extremely effective in assisting falling asleep and staying asleep (see 5-HTP).

Melatonin is released by the pineal gland. Light can put the brakes on the pineal's release of melatonin. It is best to remove any light from a room for sleeping. If your child fears the dark and will not go to bed without a night light on, I suggest allowing the security of the light, but try to use the lowest level of light possible. If he tends to sleep through the night, you may be able to turn it off once he is asleep.

There are sublingual melatonin supplements available in liquid or melt-away tabs available at www.pureformulas.com. A dosage of 0.5 to 1mg for children and 1to 3 mg for adults has been known to be helpful.

PHOSPHOTIDYL SERINE

Phosphotidyl serine gives the added benefits of helping with focus, cognition, judgment, and reasoning. It may also help to build new cell membranes and improve memory, behavior, and mood. Dosages of 150 mg have been helpful for adults, while children receive half that.

CHOLINE VS PHOSPHOTIDYL CHOLINE

Contained in krill oil, choline is needed by the brain for building its chemistry. Choline is a precursor to the neurotransmitter acetylcholine which helps cognitive learning, and memory. Phosphotidyl choline repairs neurons in the brain. Phosphotidyl choline is a derivative of soy lecithin, so it is best to avoid it if there is possibility of a soy allergy. If you are taking krill oil, then adequate amounts will be ingested.

ACETYLCHOLINE

Acetylcholine is a neurotransmitter involved in memory. Supplementation can be very helpful for people with learning disabilities associated with memory problems and lack of mental clarity. Heavy metals such as cadmium reduce acetylcholine receptors. Phosphotidyl choline is a precursor (building block) of acetylcholine. Recommendation: Captain's Krill Oil.

NOREPINEPHRINE

Norepinephrine acts as both a hormone and a neurotransmitter. It can reduce inflammation in the brain and increase its oxygen supply. Via its effect on the part of the brain called the amygdala, norepinephrine can trigger the fight or flight response. It also increases the heartrate when under stress and is involved in shifting attention. It is prone to disruption from mercury toxicity.

Note: Both acetylcholine and norepinephrine are greatly reduced by MSG (see dangerous food chemicals).

Norepinephrine is made from dopamine. When staying focused becomes difficult, there is usually a deficiency in dopamine. The amino acid L-tyrosine is the best way to naturally build this neurotransmitter.

EPINEPHRINE OR ADRENALINE

Let me clarify the difference between epinephrine and norepinephrine. Epinephrine is also known as adrenaline. Adrenaline is the hormone that causes the fight or flight response. It tells the body that it is in danger and reacts by increasing the heart rate, activating the lungs, and sending blood away from our brain and digestive tract to our extremities so that we can fight or flee. This is commonly used to stimulate a fight reaction from the body when one is having a life-threatening allergic reaction, such as from a bee sting.

BETA-ENDORPHINES

Beta-endorphins or endorphins are neurotransmitters that help with pain reduction. They are also known to affect feelings and behavior. Too much pain, too much stress, and long-term sickness or inflammation can cause us to run out of these endorphins. Luckily, 5-HTP can restore your endorphins by building serotonin, which regulates both the production and release of endorphins.

SUPPLEMENTS THAT INCREASE BRAIN ENERGY

Supplements that increase brain energy also protect it from excitotoxicity. Some of these include alpha lipoic acid, CoQ10, acetyl L-carnitine, creatine, vitamin E, all of the B vitamins, magnesium, vitamin D, and DHEA.

STRESS RELIEF REMEDIES

Aside from supplements such as GABA and L-theanine that we just discussed, there is some additional help for stress.

DRENAMIN

The product Drenamin from Standard Process is exceptionally helpful to the health and functioning of the adrenal glands. This helps the body and brain handle stress better.

PHOSPHORYLATED SERINE

Along with 5-HTP, there is another supplement that can be helpful for those who fall asleep but wake up between 1:00 and 3:00 a.m., unable to get back to sleep. Phosphorylated serine is the active form of phosphotidyl serine and acts as adrenal support. The stress hormone cortisol is released by the adrenal glands when we are under stress. Cortisol is also necessary to reduce inflammation. When too much cortisol is released on an ongoing basis, the body becomes less sensitive to it and begins to stay in stress mode all the time.

Phosphorylated serine reduces this resistance to cortisol. It is also known to be very helpful with memory because stress affects memory. To retrain cortisol responses, take phosphorylated serine for a minimum of three months but no more than nine. Three months will usually do the job. Take one capsule about an hour before bed or within an hour prior to known stressors. Capsules can be opened up and added to a beverage. It is best taken 30 minutes before a meal or an hour or more after for best absorption. The product Interplexus Seriphos is an excellent choice for this. It can be found at www.pureformulas.com.

PURE TRANQUILITY LIQUID

There is a product called Pure Tranquility Liquid by Pure Encapsulations. It contains GABA, L-theanine, and glycine to assist with stress. It is available at www.pureformulas.com, and is alcohol free.

ASHWAGANDA

Ashwaganda helps with focus, memory, cognition, energy, and supports the immune system. It is known to be helpful with stress by reducing cortisol levels up to 26% while also helping maintain blood sugar levels. It is also neuroprotective. Many products are available including liquid forms. An alcohol-free liquid tincture is available at www.swansonvitamins.com. They can also be found at healthfood stores. Dosages up to 250 mg have been known to be helpful for adults, and children get half that.

RHODIOLA

Rhodiola helps the body, specifically the adrenals, adapt to stressful situations.

RESCUE REMEDY

A well-known and simple solution to momentary stress is the product Rescue Remedy. It is sold in all healthfood stores and at most online sites such as www.pureformulas.com. This product does contain alcohol.

Note: Some of the liquid tinctures contain alcohol. Alcohol is used as a way to help preserve the herb, but is can be a problem for children on the autism spectrum or those with gut dysbiosis. The yeast in their gut is releasing a type of alcohol into their body that is already a problem. Also, the alcohol feeds the pathogenic bacteria in the gut. Use supplements that do not contain alcohol.

Use caution when choosing supplements because many contain soy derivatives, such as soy lecithin. They also may contain yeast, wheat, and casein/dairy, which are all common allergens. Purchase only dye-free with no fillers.

MAGNESIUM

Supplementing with magnesium can be very relaxing to the system. Natural Calm/Natural Vitality is the best product for adequate absorption.

EPSOM SALTS BATHS AND CREAMS

Epsom salts baths are like bathing in magnesium. They are very relaxing to the system as the salts are absorbed into the entire system via the pores. The water should be warm enough to dissolve the salts and allow the pores in the skin to open up for best absorption. One to three cups Epsom salts added to the water has been known to be helpful. A mixture of Epsom salts dissolved in any natural cream is also helpful when rubbed into the skin.

EXERCISE

Aerobic exercise where you increase your heart rate for 30 to 45 minutes, 5 times per week, is crucial for increasing blood and oxygen in the brain and for releasing and building neurotransmitters, especially serotonin. When we exercise, it increases the brain's ability to build serotonin. This is one of the reasons we feel calmer after exercise. This is also why exercise is so helpful with depression.

Martial arts are a good way to train the brain. It uses concentration that forces coordination of the attention centers of the brain which are the cortex, cerebellum, and the limbic system. It is often a recommended sport for children on the autism spectrum. It helps that it is an individualized activity verses a team sport, which can be difficult for our kids.

Cross crawl is another great way to connect the hemispheres of the brain. This lifts energy levels and also brings back the ability to focus. Touch your right elbow to your left knee and then your left elbow to your right knee. Repeat several times back and forth right then left. For a helpful cross crawl video with Donna Eden, see www.happiness.com/brain-gym-exercises.html#cross-crawl.

Lack of exercise increases symptoms of ADD. The less exercise an individual gets, the greater the symptoms. Limiting computer and television to an hour at a time can be very helpful. No one should sit in front of a television or a computer for more than an hour without a break, and this is even more important for our kids. Have them get up and get some form of exercise.

One of the prescriptions for my son was aerobic exercise. This means biking, running, swimming, or something similar that gets the heart rate up and keeps it up. For every hour on the computer, he had to exercise for an hour. Exercise helps rebuild dopamine levels, serotonin levels, oxygenate the brain, increase the blood supply to the brain for better focus, reduce stress hormones, and increase beta-endorphins. Increased endorphins and serotonin help to elevate mood. Studies have shown that exercise is as effective as antidepressant drugs in the treatment of depression.

FOODS THAT FEED THE BRAIN

In the 1970s, when the book *Orthomolecular Psychiatry* by the Nobel Prize-winner Linus Pualing was released, it showed that mental illness on any level could be affected by nutrition as well as medication. At that time, the medical profession, especially psychiatry, disclaimed this knowledge that nutrition was helpful to health, especially emotional health or the functioning of the brain. Today, the information in that book has become elemental in treating chemical and physical disorders that lead to brain dysfunction as well as mental illness.

Medication and supplements are not enough. In order to build the proper levels of neurotransmitters in the brain, certain nutritional needs must be met. Chemical balance relies on enough of the good coming in and the bad being greatly limited.

Hypoglycemia should be avoided at all cost. Hypoglycemia is low blood sugar caused by a drop in blood glucose levels. This can also cause diabetes. It is caused by eating too many refined carbohydrates, such as foods and beverages with white sugar like soda, refined cereals, pastries, etc.

The body responds by releasing hormones that help regulate glucose, such as cortisol from the adrenal glands that help combat stress in the body and growth hormone. It causes depression, irritability, anxiety, fatigue, headaches, blurred vision, slurred speech, mental confusion (brain fog), excessive sweating, emotional and behavioral problems, and sleep disorders. As discussed in the chapter on "Balancing the Body's Chemistry," hypoglycemia causes an excessive release of glutamate in the brain which can lead to the death of neurons in the brain.

The December 2011 issue of *Neurology* stated that diets high in vitamins C, D, E, Bs, and omega-3 fatty acids are less likely to have brain shrinkage. The essential fatty acid component DHA builds serotonin and dopamine in the prefrontal cortex.

Eating plenty of high-protein snacks every couple of hours helps keep blood sugar levels balanced. Whole grains and complex carbohydrates also help to balance blood sugar and promote sleep if a bedtime snack is necessary.

HIGH PROTEIN

For most people, eating a high protein and low carbohydrate diet is the most beneficial way to eat for their brain and helps promote concentration. It also keeps blood sugar levels in balance. Protein helps build dopamine, serotonin, and norepinephrine, which help improve focus, motivation, and mood.

Keep high protein snacks around such as string cheese, hard-boiled eggs, protein bars, and celery with almond butter on it. Reducing simple sugars and carbohydrates is also essential to brain health and behavior. Sugar causes anxiety, irritability, and anger.

DIET TIPS TO REMEMBER:

- Good protein choices are chicken, fish, eggs, cheese, cottage cheese, beans, and lentils.

- Complex carbohydrates are best because it takes the body longer to break them down. Good choices are vegetables and whole grains.
- Sugars and simple carbohydrates, as a rule, should be kept to a minimum. This means fruit juices and even most fruits. Fruit with lower sugar content are pears and apples. Apples also help to build dopamine. Higher sugar content fruits are grapes, dates, and bananas. Carrots tend to have high-sugar content also, so their intake should be kept to a minimum. Reduce or remove processed carbohydrates from the diet.
- Healthy fats are essential for brain health and function (omega-3 fatty acids, avocado, nuts, olive oil, coconut oil)
- Vitamins A, C, and E help concentration by increasing blood flow to the brain. Antioxidants are also helpful (antioxidants were covered in the chapter on basic nutrition).
- B complex vitamins can be helpful too, especially vitamin B6 which has been as effective as Ritalin in improving focus.

Additional resources can be found at www.amenclinics.com and in Dr. Daniel Amen's book, *Healing ADD*. See www.addresources.com, (253)759-5085.

Note: A diet high in protein is necessary to help with focus. Refined or processed carbohydrates will worsen symptoms. Protein increases concentration, so those with hyperfocus issues (see chapter 24) need more carbohydrates than other people.

SUMMARY

Natural supplementation can work as good as or better than many prescription medications, but are far safer. The right diet is crucial for overall body and brain health. There are specific foods that feed the brain for its various needs.

The products found in this chapter can be found at http://naturallyhealingautism.com/a-healthy-home/

SECTION III:

THE HOW—3 STEPS TO WELLNESS

CHAPTER 24

WHERE TO BEGIN

PRE-HEALING

Premature diagnosis is rampant, and behavioral issues are often not psychiatric at all. The body must be healed to reduce inflammation, opiates, and parasitic infection in the central nervous system. First, treat the problem, and then see which behaviors are left.

DECIDING TO START BRAIN SUPPORT SUPPLEMENTS NOW OR LATER

If learning or behavioral issues are extreme, you may wish to muscle test now and see if your child's body is accepting brain support supplements. This is covered in detail in this book. You can jump ahead and read that information to see if you would like to choose some support supplements even prior to the diet stage. Remember that after his gut has healed, some of his symptoms will diminish or even disappear. You can adjust dosages as necessary if you have used brain support supplements first. It is a personal decision.

TEST YOUR NEWBORN OR CHILD'S MICROFLORA

In the first few days after birth, have your child's fecal sample tested for any microflora by a reputable laboratory such Genova Diagnostics. Genova tests can be purchased at www.crohns.net, 877-240-7528. Once ordered, it comes to your home, you collect the sample, and it is sent to the company from your doorstep via FedEx.

A qualified practitioner from www.crohns.net will get back to you with the results and information on what you can do.

Genova Labs are thorough. They grow the cultures to get all of the information on the strains of bacteria found. This can take up to three weeks, so be patient; it's worth it.

A urine test is also a good idea to check for metabolites (byproducts of metabolism). Genova Labs urine profile also shows any heavy metal excretions that may have also passed on from the mother. This is also sold at www.crohns.net. If you have questions about which tests to buy, just call them; they have excellent customer service. Ask if the test also covers the bacteria H. pylori. This is common in Candida overgrowth, so it is wise to test for it.

If your child's microflora (gut bacteria) are imbalanced, or you presume it may be, then their immune system is suppressed. In this case, *do not vaccinate*. He will not be able to fight off viruses and heavy metal toxins with lowered immunity, and they can invade his still rapidly growing brain. This is a big problem.

If you are choosing to vaccinate; all vaccines should be postponed until his GI tract is healthy and clear. Even then, be very picky about which vaccines you allow and when. Once his gut is clear, only give single viruses, one at a time, and spread them out over a period of several months. Remember that his brain is still developing rapidly until the age of four, and the protective blood-brain barrier is not yet developed to protect it against toxins. Any toxic exposure during these early years puts him at a higher risk for injury to his neurological system.

Meanwhile, breastfeed, eat a healthy diet, and include krill supplements and probiotics into your own diet that your child will benefit from through your breast milk.

While eradicating Candida, we want to do our best to make our body the least hospitable environment possible. Certain foods should be avoided at first, about two to four weeks, although individuals vary. Some may need to be on the diet longer than others. Symptoms are your best guide; however, it is important to continue the diet for additional weeks beyond just feeling good.

I know that people can get very emotional about their food. When it comes to our kids, we think changing their diet must be impossible, but it's not. For the first one to two weeks of an initial Candida diet, do your best to follow the food lists below. After physical and emotional symptoms subside, if your child is noticeably better, you can slowly add other foods. Never overload his diet with refined sugars and carbohydrates; they are not healthy choices and can cause inflammation and Candida to come back.

The amount of time each child needs to strictly adhere to the diet varies greatly, but know that children bounce back faster than adults do. Your job is to watch for symptoms. Know that the die-off of bad bacteria from the diet alone can cause symptoms to flare up. He may get worse for a few days before he gets better.

Remember that there are often sensory issues around the tastes and textures of food that can contribute to discomfort at mealtimes. When your child refuses to eat, it is helpful if you can get even a few teaspoons of broth into him. Bribery, or negotiating, can help here. If he refuses to eat, then you can offer him a bite of something he wants in exchange for a bite of something you are asking him to eat. As his gut and brain heal, his likes for food and eating will get much easier. For a reassuring story on this, see the article fussy eaters at www.gaps.me. This is Dr. Natasha Campbell-McBride's website that goes with her book, *Gut and Psychology Syndrome*.

I know how difficult it can be to get enough good bacteria into a person with gut dysbiosis. The numbers need to be high enough to really crowd out the bad bacteria and allow the good to flourish. For this reason, I rely on the intake of quality probiotic supplements instead of only fermented foods to do the job. Most children will not eat many fermented foods due to their taste, and most yogurt is high in sugars along with strong allergens such as casein.

I prefer to add prebiotics (food for the good bacteria) and probiotics that include the strain E. faecalis or TH10 to break down the biofilm. Biofilm is the protective coating on yeast cells, and it must be destroyed in order for the cell to die. TH10 is proprietary to Dr. Ohhira's probiotic formula by Essential Formulas. Their probiotics also naturally contain prebiotics in them.

THE ONLY SUPPLEMENTS TO TAKE NOW

During the initial three weeks on the diet, there is a rebuilding process. We do not want to overwhelm the system, so wait on most supplements. Prior to the diet, many nutrients are often not properly absorbed anyway.

Along with probiotics, I believe enzymes, liver support, adrenal support, and a product with glutamine, (such as Glutagenics), should be started before the strict portion of the diet to assist healing the digestive tract. My experience is that this works profoundly better. I have done it both ways, and I will offer a sequence for these supplements to assist you. These products can be purchased at www.naturallyhealingautism.com under "healthy home products."

The only other supplements (other than those listed above) that should be taken during the rebuilding process are omega-3 fatty acids, vitamin B12 sublingual drops, and liquid vitamin D. These are supplements that are crucial to your child's health and should continue to be taken for the rest of his life.

Any "away from food" supplements can be taken with other "away from food" supplements, just not within 30 minutes prior to eating food or 90 minutes after.

Do not take any Candida cleansing products yet. The diet must be cleaned up and probiotics slowly increased for several weeks before beginning actual cleansing products.

Note: There should be at least three weeks of gut restoration and bowel support with probiotics before starting any other multi-vitamin, multi-mineral, or antioxidant supplements as they can feed any parasites.

DIE-OFF REACTION

When yeast dies off, it releases toxins that can enter your bloodstream. This is also known as Herxheimer's reaction. It means that the liver cannot keep up with filtering out the toxic waste being released by the dying pathologic organisms.

This can cause headaches, fatigue and flu-like symptoms. Some people also experience either diarrhea or constipation. This waste also produces inflammation and injures the intestinal lining. These toxins injure the immune system, kidneys, bladder, and liver, and they do especially significant harm to the brain and nervous system.

There may be heightened emotional outbursts or hyperactivity. If this reaction becomes too intense, then stick to the diet, but reduce the dosage of any supplements that may create a faster die-off. At this stage, the only supplement that may increase the die-off would be probiotics. They need them, but may need a lower dosage or a few days off to let their body catch up. The yeast is dying faster than the liver can keep up, and too many toxins are in the bloodstream. Watch his symptoms. Muscle test and lessen the amount to one that is tolerable for the individual and slowly build back up over time.

The diet alone can cause the die-off because the yeast is starved and dying. In this case, when it is not due to supplements, just support your child in any way that you can. Chicken broth can be very soothing. He may not want food for a day or so, which is common in this stage, but it will pass.

Remember that this is a sign that the yeast is dying, and that is a good thing. It is wise to anticipate the possibility of behavioral issues accelerating for a few days, to possibly a week, on and off. Know that this means that the process is working.

HAVING SUPPORT

Always refer back to the chapters on muscle testing and natural practitioners for help. By now, you likely have found a few practitioners to assist you with the process when needed. A natural allergy desensitization practitioner is essential during this process.

THE ONLY SUPPORT SUPPLEMENTS TO TAKE NOW:

PRIOR TO AND WITH THE DIET

Always muscle test to see if the supplement you are trying is right for your child. Remember, you can ask the question of which product is best or if it is needed (and if it will be assimilated by the body), before purchasing. See the chapter on "alternative therapies" for more on muscle testing.

Muscle test for dosages from beginning to end always as they can continuously change. Less may be needed as your child's health improves. These products are safe. Remember, no cleansing products yet, those will be added later.

SUMMARY

There are specific supplements for the brain and the GI tract to take now to prepare your child's body for the healing stages. These supplements offer support for the entire system.

The products found in this chapter can be found at http://naturallyhealingautism.com/a-healthy-home/

THE THREE HEALING STAGES

CHAPTER 25

STAGE ONE: HEALING THE GUT

1. LIVER SUPPORT AND ADRENAL SUPPORT- DAY ONE (AND CONTINUE ONGOING)

The liver is the organ of detoxification, and I would venture to say that all children on the autism spectrum need better liver health. It must be healthy and not congested in order to do all of its jobs effectively. It will need support prior to and during the diet to assist in the dying off of Candida and other parasitic microbes. Liver Life by Bioray is an excellent choice. Muscle test for beginning dosage and weekly thereafter for increases.

The adrenal glands are often over taxed. The detoxification process will add burden to them so it is a good idea to offer support. An easy saliva test from Diagnos-Techs is a great way to identify the health of the adrenals.

Drenamin by Standard Process is great but it is in pill form. This can be crushed for non-pill takes. A liquid form homeopathic supplement to assist the adrenals is Ribes Nigrum Gemmo by Seroyal.

RESTORING BALANCE IN THE GUT

At this time begin very slowly easing into dietary changes.

WEEK ONE: BEGIN VERY SLOWLY EASING INTO DIETARY CHANGES

It is easier for you and your child to slowly begin making dietary changes, rather than to immediately restrict everything he is used to. Begin slowly easing into the diet below, but allow time for probiotics to begin balancing his digestive tract and liver support to kick in before engaging in a more strict diet. The bad foods will continue to damage his gut and prevent healing and inflammation reduction if prolonged for too long. You are the judge of this timeline.

1. PROBIOTICS –WEEK TWO (AND ONGOING)

A must during any cleansing or Candida program is the use of probiotics. The product must contain a variety of multiple strains of Lactobacillus, Bifidobacterium, and the strain E. faecalis. These are the key bacteria needed to crowd out, kill, and eat up the pathogenic bacteria in your system and help build up the good.

Yogurt is not enough. Heat during pasteurization kills the live bacteria. You need a supplement that can increase the positive numbers of bacteria, feed themselves through a prebiotic involved, create lactic acid, and survive the stomach acid to make it to the colon alive.

DOSAGES DURING THE DIET STAGE

Probiotics are best taken away from food, but if your child does not take pills, it is fine to puncture the capsule of Dr. Ohirra's probiotics and squeeze the contents into food or beverage. You may want to ask your child if he would chew on the capsule and swallow it; the flavor is fairly benign. I recommend Dr. Ohhira's because I feel it is superior to anything else on the market. The best price is at www.crohns.net, and they also carry the professional formula that is hard to find in stores. Healthfood stores carry the original formula. See the chapter on reducing inflammation for more on these products and dosage guidelines.

Probiotics should be started today. It is best to take probiotics for about two weeks before becoming very strict on the diet. This will give your child's body a chance to strengthen, build up his good bacteria, and help you begin making subtle changes to his diet. Less processed food, less dairy, and less sugars now can ease the transition to a more strict diet.

Depending on the weight of your child, you will begin with one capsule in the morning and one at night. Muscle test along the way, but slowly build up the dosage. An average 5 year old can take as many as 5 in the morning and 5 at night. When I started, I was told to take 20 per day in split dosages.

Dr. Ohhira's probiotics are very safe. What you will want to watch for is a die-off reaction. If the dosage causes strong die-off symptoms, back off by one or two capsules per day for a few days. When he is balanced again, try adding one back in strategically until you know it is all right to increase another. You will be the judge of how much is right for your child.

The higher dosage will be continued for at least a couple of months. As your child heals, you may slowly reduce the dosage, but he will always take a minimum of one in the morning and one in the evening. If the need arises, such as a cold or flu, or he has ingested foods you know will weaken his system, add one or two capsules per day for a few days or until symptoms subside.

Dr. Ohhira's Professional Grade Probiotics

Your child will be better off if he has already been on the probiotics for about two weeks prior to beginning the diet. Dosage guidelines have been discussed previously in Chapter Eleven. It is a gradual increase working your way up from one in the morning and one at night to whatever the maximum daily dosage is for your child per his weight. This is usually between one and three twice per day for children and up to five twice per day for adults. Muscle testing is an excellent way to gauge dosage needs as they change. Monitor dosages because with die-off you may need to reduce dosages along the way. They are best taken away from food, if possible. Your best price is at www.crohns.net.

2. BROAD SPECTRUM DIGESTIVE ENZYMES:

WEEK TWO AND A HALF TO THREE.

Enzymes are good always, at any time. We just want to be sure we know what reactions come from the probiotics. If all is well after a few days to a week on the probiotics, then begin enzymes. They are immensely helpful.

Broad spectrum enzymes are the ones that are taken just prior to eating a meal for the assistance in digesting food. Broad spectrum means that they cover all of the basic foods such as proteins, carbohydrates, fats, and fiber. There are several great products available such as Omega-Zyme by Garden of Life, Digest Gold by Enzymedica, and Trienza by Houston enzymes. You will only need to choose one brand at a time. I do suggest using up one bottle and then purchasing another brand to use next. Switching up enzymes is beneficial because when the same blend of one enzyme brand is used ongoing the body adapts to it and it becomes less effective. Alternating back and forth between two brands is fine if you find ones you really like.

All are sold at www.amazon.com and www.pureformulas.com. Omega-Zyme and Trienza come in powder form. Digest Gold is in a capsule but can easily be opened and added to food or a beverage. The capsules are also handy when traveling. The size of the meal often determines the dosage, so follow directions on the bottle. If digestion is still a problem, seek an enzyme product that contains hydrochloric acid (HCl) as an added ingredient (see below).

If the enzyme is taken in capsule form, it is best if ingested 10 to 30 minutes before eating if that can be incorporated into your schedule. If not, don't stress over it. This simply allows for the capsule to be digested in the stomach and the enzymes to be released before the food gets there. Opening up the capsules or taking powder forms are best for this reason.

3. GLUTAGENICS: THIS MAY BEGIN WITH ENZYMES

Glutagenics by Metagenics is a sweet tasting powder that contains L-glutamine, which is critical in helping heal the intestinal lining.

Glutagenics also contains deglycyrrhizinized licorice root to help soothe the digestive tract and aloe leaf extract (laxative properties removed), which helps to relieve inflammation. One teaspoon, three times per day, is helpful for adults. Children may need half that. Muscle test for dosage. Glutamine should only be used short term while healing the gut lining. It increases levels of glutamate which increase excitotoxicity. Two to four weeks should be sufficient. This is sold at most healthfood stores or can be purchased at most online sites such as www.pureformulas.com.

4. CHLORELLA:

Chlorella may begin with enzymes and Glutagenics

Chlorella assists in cleansing toxins from the blood. This can be very helpful in the prevention of die-off. It also makes the gut environmentally friendly for probiotics to grow, and supplies a high concentration of beta-carotene, mixed carotenoids, vitamin C, iron, and protein. It is anti-inflammatory and contains vitamin B12. Chlorella vulgaris, such as Yaeyama Chlorella from Jarrow Formulas, is a strain that is easier to digest and has higher chlorophyll. It comes in both capsule and powder form. It is available in healthfood stores and online at www.naturallyhealingautism.com.

One dosage can be put together into a beverage. My family takes probiotics with a small glass of water containing liver support, glutagenics, and chlorella all in one glass. It can be added to a small amount of juice if necessary.

ADDITIONAL SUPPLEMENTS THAT MAY BE HELPFUL:

In an effort not to be too overwhelming with supplements I have left the following as additional options. They are all extremely helpful when needed. Muscle testing is always helpful when determining necessity.

HYDROCHLORIC ACID (HCl)

In addition to digestive enzymes, HCl may be helpful in the digestion of protein. If there is acid reflux, people tend to think that they have too much acid. It is often to the contrary. The gut does not make adequate amounts of HCl when there is dysbiosis, so there is often not enough acid to break down proteins. If digestive enzymes are not doing the job alone, try adding some HCl.

The production of HCl is usually impaired in those with gut imbalance. We think acid reflux or GERD is due to too much acid in the stomach, but it is often a need for more. Take one or more pills, depending on the size of the meal, just prior to eating. HCl can be very helpful while the gut is healing to assist in the digestion of proteins. I like the product GastroDigest II by Vervita because one pill has broad spectrum enzymes, HCl, pepsin and more. It is a small pill that can be crushed with a pill crusher and added to any food or beverage. See www.vervitaproducts.com.

I have also had great success with the product Metagest by Metagenics, but it is only HCl, and it is a large pill, sold at www.amazon.com and www.pureformulas.com. The product Zypan by Standard Process is also used for this purpose. They are small pills that can be crushed. (Pill crushers are found in drug stores and online.) Zypan is commonly sold by natural practitioners but can be found at www.amazon.com. Lastly, several companies make a capsule form of Betain HCl with pepsin that can be opened up and added to any food or beverage. See www.pureformulas.com. As with enzymes, the size of the meal often determines the need. One or two per meal is common.

MORE INFLAMMATION FIGHTERS

All of the ingredients in Glutagenics will help with inflammation, healing, and soothing the gut lining. If you feel that you need more assistance, see the chapter on reducing inflammation for more information.

ALLERGY ELIMINATION NOW

We discussed allergy elimination in the chapter "alternative therapies". If you have not done this already, now would be a good time. By doing this before the diet, you may not have to cut out all of the foods. Dairy and grains, especially gluten, have likely become foreign agents to your child's body. His immune system is using a lot of its strength to unnecessarily fight certain chemicals. We do not want to get false reactions at this point. You need to know what is real and what is not. Candida will still need to be normalized so do not add in a lot of processed carbohydrates or sugars, regardless.

Let your N.A.E.T or other practitioner know that you are in the process of doing a Candida cleansing and gut-rebuilding diet (not yet on cleansing supplements). Bring in all supplements your child is taking, and those you are planning on giving him if you would like the practitioner to muscle test your child for them. The practitioner will also be able to strengthen his organs through treatment.

Wait to test on the post-diet cleansing supplements (found in the next chapter), as your child's body is likely not ready for them and will test weak. When the diet is well underway, after about a month, and results show enough to move forward with cleansing products, then it is time to muscle test. You can do it yourself or bring them in to a healthcare practitioner that is proficient in doing so such as a chiropractor or a N.A.E.T practitioner.

When introducing anything new, first rub it on the skin or do the overnight sensitivity test. Then try only a small morsel of that food on the end of his tongue to look for any reactions. Remember allergic reactions are not just in the digestive system but behavioral, mucus-producing, or skin-irritating anywhere on the body, etc.

Wheat is a food in the U.S. that has become so bioengineered that I do not deem it safe for consumption by anyone. It has 90% more gluten in it that when I was a child. Depending on the practices in your country or its distributor, this will vary. As far as Candida goes, do not overpower the diet with a lot of refined carbohydrates. Processed carbohydrates are particularly bad and feed the pathogenic bacteria. Fiber and good carbohydrates can come from fruits, vegetables, and nuts.

THE DIET-WEEK THREE

Before you begin, take into account the process of changing a diet. Hopefully, you have already begun slowly reducing items from your child's diet. As the diet becomes a bit stricter, he will crave sugars and starchy carbohydrates because Candida uses them as food. There will be a couple of days that can be difficult here. The strictest part of the diet may only need to be about two weeks, more or less, depending on the individual. The closer you adhere to the diet, the faster the results will be. If needed, use bribery to get him to eat as noted above (a bite of bad for a bite of good).

I have strictly followed this diet myself. Do your best to cut out sugars and refined carbohydrates. The better the diet is adhered to, the faster the results. We need to starve the bad bacteria while we heal the gut and reduce the inflammation. There is a lot of nutrition offered from the foods listed below.

We discussed metabolic typing in the chapter on balancing the body's chemistry. Every individual is different; however, the following anti-brain inflammation diet has been shown helpful for those on the autism spectrum, those with seizures, ADHD, bipolar, and other behavioral disorders. It is even beneficial for those with dementia and Alzheimer's.

This diet mainly consists of a higher intake of good fats, medium protein, increased green vegetables and very low carbohydrates with no processed food, dairy, gluten or soy. We want to heal the gut and balance blood sugar levels. This is for gut and brain healing, and is always a good way to eat. Once your child has cleared some of the Candida and his gut has healed, he will likely be happy to eat this way on his own. We have discussed the best diets for different behavioral types in the section on brain support. Refer to it for later use.

If it needs a name we could call it the anti-inflammation, gut healing, brain healing, blood sugar balancing diet.

FOODS TO AVOID (that feed Candida and create inflammation):

- **Drinks:** Alcohol and any products containing it (especially beer and wine because they contain yeast), carbonated drinks, and caffeinated beverages

- **Sugars:** Sucrose, maltose, dextrose, fructose, (anything ending in "ose"), all syrups, molasses, agave, and honey (honey is only removed initially)
- **Artificial sweeteners:** None are allowed
- **Fruits:** Fresh, dried, frozen, or canned
- **Refined carbohydrates:** Anything containing yeast or white flour, including bread, crackers, brewers yeast, malt, pasta, cookies, crackers, etc.; white rice
- **Grains:** Wheat, rye, barley, buckwheat, spelt, millet, quinoa, rice, corn, oatmeal, and cereals
- **Lactose/Casein:** The sugars and protein in milk, and everything that contains it, ghee may be tolerated (see below)
- **Starchy vegetables:** Yams, potatoes, artichokes, peas, soybeans, garbanzo beans, and chickpeas
- **Mold foods**: Cheeses, flavored or commercially cultured dairy products, mushrooms (because they are fungi, avoid them initially); also scrub the skins on fruits and vegetables before peeling and cutting to minimize the possibility of mold ingestion
- **Soy**: a highly allergic food that interrupts natural hormonal activity, reduces thyroid function, and is high in glutamate which increases excitotoxicity.
- **Vinegar**: (avoid initially for candida issues), anything made with vinegar such as mayonnaise, mustard, salad dressing, sauces, soy sauce, pickles, tamari, and rice vinegar
- **Peanuts and pistachios**: These nuts carry fungus so they are not allowed initially, including any products containing peanuts such as peanut butter
- **Bad oils and margarines**: imitation spreads or shortenings; trans or hydrogenated oils such as corn, canola, sunflower, safflower, peanut, and soybean
- **Processed meats**: cured or dried, most pre-packaged lunch meats, bacon, sausages and hot dogs

- **Supergreen food supplements**: initially, before allergy desensitization, be aware of the possibility that these may contain gluten "tags" that trigger the system for an allergic reaction

FOODS YOU CAN HAVE:

Remember that proteins and fats (good fats) are not easily utilized by yeast, so they are very beneficial to have in the diet.

- **Drinks**: Decaffeinated herb tea (one cup per day), pure water, coconut water, almond milk, lime, or lemon juice
- **Carbohydrates**: Vegetables (see below), all nuts (except peanuts and pistachios), almonds, sunflower seeds, pumpkin seeds, and Brazil nuts are best. Navy beans, string beans, lima beans, and lentils. Limit your quantity of beans at first due to starch content, and do not eat processed beans as they contain a lot of sugar. Gluten-free oatmeal, oat bran, and brown rice may be eaten in small amounts after the first week if tolerated. Almond or other nut flours such as coconut are great substitutes for recipes.
- **Protein**: organic eggs, poultry, fish, grass-fed beef or lamb, and soup broth made from animal meats; if diarrhea persists, temporarily omit eggs
- **Vegetables**: All non-starchy vegetables are allowed, preferably organic. (See "foods to avoid" for a list of starchy vegetables). Beets and carrots should be eaten in moderation. I would suggest waiting until after the first week because they have a naturally high sugar content. Be aware that vegetables, especially raw, can be painful to digest if the gut is inflamed. It is best to steam them to allow for easier digestion and to kill off any remaining bacteria. Note: If digestion of vegetables is painful, the gut is too inflamed to handle the fiber. Stay on the diet, but eliminate vegetables until you notice a marked improvement, and then try one to two tablespoons of one that is cooked. Check labels of frozen foods and beware of hidden sugars, vinegar, and additives.

- **Good oils and fats:** avocados, coconut oil, cold pressed olive oil, macadamia nut oil, sesame oil, almond oil, and organic butter or ghee, if tolerated (see dairy below), and animal fats
- **Condiments:** Herbs, sea salt (Himalayan salt is best), wait on spices as they can tend to irritate the gut lining at the early stages
- **Natural sweetener**: Stevia ONLY; it is a natural sweetener that is a "0" on the glycemic index and will not affect yeast growth. NO other sweeteners are allowed—NONE! Try NuNaturals stevia for the best flavor and limit use initially.
- **Fermented foods**: Only small amounts are needed, a tablespoon or two can assist the gut.

A simple snack can be celery with almond butter or a hard boiled egg. Cooked beans or lentils are also good.

If after about ten days you notice symptoms have disappeared, you can offer cooked fruit such as cooked apples with cinnamon. If that goes well, try slowly adding raw green apples with the skin on. Then try berries; they have fiber so they are lower on the glycemic index, but it is important to note if the fiber still disturbs his digestion. Fruit should be eaten very ripe as the ripening causes the starches to become a more absorbable form of monosaccharide sugars.

Phenols can trigger symptoms. They are in dark vegetables and fruits such as blueberries which also contain a lot of fiber. They are health benefitting foods so, if phenols are a problem, you can desensitize your child to them through your natural allergy desensitization practitioner. Phenols were discussed in detail in chapter 10. There are also non-Phenol enzymes by Houston-ensymes.com.

For some, the duration for the reduction of anything containing sugars, including fruit, may need to be much longer. If you notice symptom flare-ups, such as diarrhea, constipation, digestive pain, or emotional outbursts, then it is too soon to add fruit. Wait at least three weeks before re-introducing a new food back into the diet if you are doing an elimination diet. Very slowly add new foods to his diet. Do this one at a time so you are able to tell which food is causing any issues if they arise.

Note: I do not advocate soy for any purpose. Almost all soy is genetically modified, it is a common allergen, and it can interfere with hormone levels and cause excitotoxicity. See the chapter "allergies and the gut/brain connection for more information on soy.

EATING UP THE BIOFILM AND TOXIC WASTE

Muscle test your child before and during the initial diet phase to see if he is ready for the following supplements. They are very helpful with destroying the biofilm, but he may not be ready for them until after the diet is well underway and possibly until he begins the Candida cleansing products. If his body tells you it is ready now, continue to test dosages.

Interphase by Klaire Labs (not Interphase Plus, which contains mineral-binding EDTA). Interphase is a blend of specific enzymes used systemically that are capable of getting into the biofilm (mucosal lining) and breaking down the cell wall of the yeast. It was developed by some of the world's leading authorities on biofilm. Commonly, one capsule taken three times per day in divided doses on an empty stomach is helpful. The capsules can be opened up and added to food or beverage, but are best taken away from food. Limit the food intake with them because these are used systemically. We don't want them to concentrate on the food in the digestive tract, but on the yeast cells. It is sold at www.pureformulas.com and www.amazon.com. This product is essential if H. pylori is detected in the stool sample and for a duration of about six months.

AN ADDITIONALLY HELPFUL STRAIN OF BACTERIA

Saccharomyces boulardii is healthy yeast that acts as an antagonist to pathogenic bacteria. It binds to toxic microbes, helps the inflammation response, strengthens the intestinal lining, assists the immune and respiratory responses (beneficial with asthma), helps prevent candida from invading other parts of the body such as the lymph nodes, and is helpful with removal of parasites. This product can be extremely helpful in regulating bowel movements within an hour or so, whether from diarrhea or constipation, but is commonly known to be very helpful especially in cases of diarrhea. Commonly one taken first thing in the morning and one at night is helpful. Many brands are available, and I have had personal success with the product from Klaire Labs sold at www.amazon.com and www.pureformulas.com. Be sure this product is shipped in a cold pack and is refrigerated continuously. Read labels as some other products contain fructose and lactose.

INTRODUCING DAIRY

The sensitivity test can be used to check for toleration prior to ingesting any food. Using only organic foods will help assure that in the case of a reaction there are no complications arising from hidden pesticides, hormones, antibiotics, or other additives.

Dairy has been avoided up to this point because it contains natural sugars and casein, the problematic protein in milk. Dairy is an issue with most sensitive children. When testing for dairy tolerance (lactose or casein), most children on the autism spectrum may need to wait one to two months before introducing it back into the diet (gluten can take as long as three months) unless it has been cleared by a natural allergy elimination specialist such as a N.A.E.T. practitioner. If the allergy was known to exist prior to starting the diet, then always be sure to minimize its use.

With each introduction you can first try the sensitivity test, but also only use one new food every few days so you know which food is doing what. This causes less need for backtracking. If a food tends to cause sensitivity now, wait a few weeks and try again. Always begin slowly using only a teaspoon to begin.

Clarified butter, also known as ghee, is the gentlest form of dairy to start with. It is possible for some to tolerate this from the beginning because all of the whey, lactose, and milk proteins have been removed. The milk sugars can also encourage yeast growth.

Commercial ghee may contain additives, so read your labels and purchase only from a quality healthfood store. Remember to buy organic. If you are unable to find untainted ghee, you can easily make your own (see recipe at the end of this chapter). If ghee is not tolerated now, wait a few weeks and try again. If ghee cannot be tolerated after a few weeks on the, then dairy may need to be completely omitted from the diet. If all goes well with ghee, then try using butter next.

Organic butter is the next choice to test. It contains only a small amount of whey, but it does have traces of lactose and milk proteins. Butter, contrary to popular belief, is a vital and necessary food containing important fatty acids and vitamins. Avoid margarines as they are mostly chemical in nature and can be harmful to your health.

If butter is tolerated, then try cultured dairy such as homemade yogurt or organic plain yogurt from a quality healthfood store (no fruity or flavored ones). You may add some stevia to the yogurt if you need to sweeten it a bit. Stevia has a "0" on the glycemic index and will not feed yeast. Yogurt is the first product to add to test proteins from dairy. Homemade yogurt is best, but you should be on a sufficient amount of probiotic supplements at this time to eat a quality organic product. This choice is only to add variety to the diet. Heat processing during pasteurization of commercial yogurt often destroys its live bacteria. See the chapter on "recipes" if you would like to make your own.

If yogurt goes well you may try a small amount of kefir if you like. This is the reason for the loading of probiotics from the beginning. Without sufficient probiotics in your system, cultured food such as kefir will likely cause a die-off reaction. Start with only about a teaspoon.

I personally had a lot of dizziness and fatigue when I started kefir the first time I did the diet because my probiotic intake had not been sufficient enough. The next time, I went through the sequence with a lot more education. My probiotic intake had been sufficient and I had almost no die-off at all the entire time. This had been unheard of for me before. I also believe that the Liver Life product was helping my body with detoxification (see "die-off" below). This is the information I need before I put my child on any program.

Lastly, I added cheese. Due to the sugars in dairy and the difficulty in digestion, especially with cheese, it is wise to limit its intake. There are a few cheeses that are best and some that are best to avoid. Common cheeses that are better are Brie, cheddar, colby, Monterey jack, Gouda, Muenster, Parmesan, Romano and Swiss.

Avoid anything that is processed, such as cream cheese. Mozzarella came up for me as one of the avoided cheeses. I still, occasionally, eat small amounts of it because I enjoy it, and I feel no ill effects. Additional cheeses to avoid are cottage cheese, feta and ricotta. Test your child's tolerance to each. Sometimes goat or sheep cheese can be tolerated.

I always try to keep my family away from drinking cow's milk, and I greatly limit dairy in general. Cow's milk is not easily digested by the human body, and it causes inflammation. Most of the enzymes are destroyed during pasteurization, and it can contain harmful pesticides, hormones, and antibiotics. We take calcium supplements and probiotics daily for those health requirements. Almond milk and coconut milk are a far better choice if the need for a milk-type liquid is desired. Goat milk is much easier to digest than cow's milk and *may* be more easily tolerated if casein has been an issue in the past.

CLARIFIED BUTTER OR GHEE RECIPE

Heat the butter in a small skillet. Once melted, the milk sugar (white residue) will separate from the clarified butter (the yellow liquid). Skim off and throw away the white portion. When cool, pour the yellow liquid into a glass storage container with a tight-fitting lid and refrigerate.

SUMMARY

Follow the diet and eat a lot of gut-healing healthy fats such as homemade chicken, beef, or fish broth made from organic ingredients and organic cold-pressed olive oil. You will also be taking probiotics, Liver Life liver support, Glutagenics, and chlorella away from food, and adding broad spectrum digestive enzymes with your meals. Muscle test along the way for help with dosage amounts.

If you need additional assistance with digestion, especially protein, add hydrochloric acid just before mealtime. S. boulardii and Interphase can be helpful for eradication of pathogenic bacteria when taken away from food. First muscle test to see if these are compatible with your child's body at this time.

Have your child tested by an allergy elimination specialist such as an N.A.E.T. practitioner to see what sensitivities exist. See the chapter on alternative therapies for more information.

If after following the diet for roughly 10 to 14 days and symptoms have improved greatly, try offering one new food every 2 to 3 days to see if it is tolerated. Food allergy reactions can take up to 3 days to show up. After about a month on the diet and support supplements, it is time to muscle test to see if your child is ready for the cleansing supplements to be added. Cleansing supplements are covered in the next chapter.

The products found in this chapter can be found at http://naturallyhealingautism.com/a-healthy-home/

CHAPTER 26

CANDIDA/BACTERIAL CLEANSING PRODUCTS (AROUND WEEK SEVEN OR SO)

I have left the timeline here a bit vague because some children will be ready for this stage before others. It can be much longer for some, and that's okay. This is not an exact science and no two people are the same. Always muscle test with products or questions for the body to see if it is ready to receive what you wish to offer it. Keeping a journal is helpful too.

After many years of trial and error and money spent researching, I finally found a great Candida product that works. There are a variety of Candida cleansing products on the market, but the problem with most is that they do not complete the job. Results can be minimal at best and the yeast comes back more quickly than it should. You can go through life bouncing in and out of yeast overgrowth.

Stress, poor diet, and the use of antibiotics are among the many reasons why yeast periodically comes back. Once you have done a thorough job eradicating the yeast from your system, be on the lookout for symptoms of its return. The difference now is that you are far better prepared. If you catch it right away, it will be a much simpler job with a far shorter duration required to bring back balance. There are also some products that when used at an ongoing maintenance level can help prevent any flare-ups.

THE SEQUENCE

After one month on the initial diet and gut-healing supplements, it is likely time to add the following two Candida cleansing products.

I say "likely" because you always want to muscle test to see if the individual is ready for this. Symptoms are your friends. Does he have headaches or extreme fatigue? If so, see what results come from the muscle testing against the products you wish to add.

I was surprised at how strong the die-off was for me when I started the cleansing product Candelim before being on a strict Candida diet. My body was not prepared for yeast die-off before my gut was balanced. I needed weeks of probiotics, Liver Life, and Glutagenics before I could even start these additional products.

Detoxification pathways should be clearing up and liver support and Candida down to a minimum prior to the use of any cleansing products or heavy metal removal. Below you will learn about the need to remove mercury from the system to assist in Candida eradication as one of the products assists with it.

There are countless Candida cleansing products on the market. I have personally used the majority of them on myself, my son, or my daughter with no better than short-term results at best. The Candida always came back.

In my research, I came across a company that uses energetic frequencies in their products. This would be the same principle as is used by Dr. Shari Tenpenny's vials used in allergy elimination (discussed in the chapter "Alternative Therapies").

This company has a Candida cleanse that is the first one I can say worked thoroughly for us and many others. I had implemented the diet and probiotics along with whatever past products we were trying, but it never completely did the job for the long term.

The company that makes and carries the products I recommend is called Get Healthy Again. There is a lot of information behind these products. They act differently than most because they are infused with frequencies that kill the yeast cells. They assist in energetically removing the spores out of their protective hiding places. Remember, spores hibernate in tissues.

Let me explain frequencies a little further. Quantum physics explains that we are all interconnected through universal energy. Each of us constantly emits frequencies or vibrations in every part of our body down to our cells. There is communication between these cells.

Robert Harrison is the founder and owner of the company Get Healthy Again. He has deeply studied, developed, and learned the skill of energy testing. He compares energies of products to energies of the human body. He asks for the energetic "rating" of each. The results that come from the products are the best way to assess their value.

The energetic testing scale goes from 0 to 100, with 0 the weakest and 100 the strongest. An example would be a food that is genetically modified (GMO) and rates at about 10. The majority of health products have a rating of 30 or less.

Always muscle test before using a product to be sure it is compatible with your child's body. Muscle testing is also helpful to find what dosage to begin with. Often it is much less than what is recommended on the package, especially for those on the autism spectrum.

Continue on the same supplements as you were on with the diet at the same dosages, especially probiotics, but now add the following two supplements:

1. **CandElim or CandiCalm:** With autistic children use CandiCalm first to 6 years old, starting with CandElim at 7 years old at just a drop a day. With a younger child older than 3, after 6 months on CandiCalm they can switch to CandElim if there still is some candida around.
2. **CandiClear5:** A chalky tasting powder that mixes with juice or can be put into a smoothie. The carbohydrates in the fruit actually draw out the yeast and set them up for attack from the product. It also absorbs and eliminates waste from Candida and assists in removal of mercury.

These products can be purchased at www.naturallyhealingautism.com under "healthy home products." Additional information on the products and an explanation of frequency ratings per each product, and an explanation of dosages can be found at www.Candida-yeast-infection-relief.com.

For more detailed information on frequencies go to: www.gethealthyagain.com.

From their website:

CandElim fights Candida in three different ways. It uses a set of vibrational instructions encoded into the water that fight Candida and Candida spores. Plus, they supercharge anti-Candida essential oils and herbal extracts to better kill Candida. These also boost the immune system response so that it will more effectively fight Candida.

The energetic frequency instructions make the oils and herbs in CandElim work much more effectively than they do on their own, without the instructions.

CandElim kills Candida, bad bacteria, viruses, and other pathogens, with the focus on Candida. The frequencies it carries to your body deactivate Candida spores, and gradually eliminate Candida hiding in parts of the body where the immune system, herbs, oils, extracts, and other Candida remedies cannot access.

Use one bottle per month for at least three months, or until the Candida overgrowth has been eliminated throughout your body.

I was personally so sensitive to CandElim that I had to back off to one drop every couple of days in the beginning. Muscle test for appropriate dosages.

It is a proprietary blend of the following:

> Frequency Enhanced Purified Water, Herbal Extracts of: Olive Leaf, Magnolia-Officialis, Yucca, Astragalus Root, Pau D'Arco, and Dandelion Root.
>
> Flower Essences of: Larch, Pine, Oak, Redwood.
>
> Pure Organic Essential Oils of: Cedarwood (Thuja), Clove Stem, Fir Needle, Juniper Berry, Lemon Grass, Oregano, Pine, Spruce, Peppermint, Cinnamon Bark, Orange, Lemon.
>
> Minerals: Volcanic origin ORMUS, Humic and Fulvic Minerals.

Although they offer guidelines remember to muscle test for dosages. If one drop per day is too much, then ask about one drop every two days, and then every three days until you get a strong answer.

Candiclear5 offers 5-way support for effective Candida control:

1. Ruptures and destroys yeast blooms.
2. Absorbs and removes toxic debris.
3. Balances pH levels.
4. Provides nutrients that fight Candida.
5. Nutritionally supports intestinal repair.

The main ingredient in CandiClear5 is a fossilized freshwater phytoplankton that shreds any parasites and Candida that come in contact with it. Its porous structure absorbs toxins and waste debris to help reduce unpleasant symptoms due to Candida die-off.

You get a large amount (8.4 grams) of plankton per 20 gram serving, as well as 4.6 grams of air-filtered pyrophyllite powder. The primary function of pyrophyllite in CandiClear5 is to remove toxins and heavy metals from the body. It does this because of its high mineral content that bonds to the heavy metals in the body and pulls them out of the body.

The mineral and electrolyte content also help to rebalance the body's nutrients and provide protection against future toxicity, as a sufficient nutrient balance in the body will continue to bond with freestanding heavy metals and convert them into benign or beneficial compounds.

CandiClear5 also contains 400 mg of vitamin C, 60 mg of vitamin B6 (with P5P), 280 mg of zinc (picolinate), supplying 56 mg of elemental zinc, all of which serve to boost the immune system's response against Candida or directly kill the yeast. Note: Zinc picolinate is 20% zinc, providing 56 mg or 350% of the RDA, an effective but still a relatively low therapeutic level.

Yet another part of this product's Candida-fighting ability comes from a proprietary blend (5,220 mg) of 12 other ingredients, with immune boosting, Candida-killing, anti-inflammatory properties, including organic burdock root, organic cinnamon, arabinogalactans (10% DHQ) from Siberian larch, xylitol (a sweetener that does not feed Candida and actually helps to kill it), extracts of barley grass 4:1, broccoli sprouts 4:1, parsley 10:1, astragalus 5:1, polycil humic/ fulvic acid (to help eliminate toxins, kill pathogens, and increase mineral absorption), apple cider vinegar powder (to fight Candida by increasing pH), Alterra seabed mineral powder (to increase the absorption of these ingredients), and astragalus 5:1.

CandiClear5 comes in a 1.5-pound container that will last one month when taking 3 scoops a day. Start out at just 1 scoop a day and gradually increase to full dosage. CandiClear5 is quite potent.

A low-carbohydrate diet (versus no carbohydrates) helps fight Candida faster. If you are thin, consider mixing or baking CandiClear5 in with carbohydrates, which could include juice, oatmeal, pancakes, muffins, or even cookies. CandiClear5 will shred more Candida as they are attracted to the carbohydrates. It is best in a smoothie or other hiding place as the taste and consistency is very chalky.

These products should be used at a full dose level (whatever your personal full dose level is) for four to six months to completely eradicate the pathogenic bacteria. After this initial period, an ongoing maintenance dosage should be used. This can be as little as one drop per day or one drop per week. As always, individual dosages vary.

As you already know, I recommend Dr. Ohhira's probiotics. The company Get Healthy Again also makes a quality probiotic, but theirs also offers the infused frequencies for Candida removal. Together they can be very helpful.

FLORA 15

This is the probiotic supplement from www.gethealthyagain.com. It contains 15 different strains of probiotic bacteria, but it also has frequencies infused to assist in killing the Candida.

When doing a Candida cleanse, I like using Flora 15 for about two months along with Dr. Ohhirra's probiotics. This offers all of the benefits of Dr. Ohhira's and the infused frequencies that come with Flora 15.

SATISFACTION IS GUARANTEED WITH THEIR PRODUCTS.

REMEMBERING DIE-OFF

If the die-off reaction is extreme, you may want to stop all cleansing products and wait two or three days before beginning again at a much lower dosage. Give the body a chance to recover and keep up with the toxins being released. Just watch your child for signs. You will be able to tell what is right and when. It is not necessary to put your child or yourself through this process too fast. I have found muscle testing very helpful during this time.

I thought I was working my way up slowly enough, but I was wrong. As my fatigue became overwhelming, I called the owner of the company with questions. I needed to stop taking the products all together for a few days to a week so my body could catch up.

If you are taking CandElim and the die-off is extreme, you may want to switch to CandiCalm for a while.

DIE-OFF SUPPORT

Continue with probiotics as they will support the immune system, build the good bacteria, and assist with die-off. Below are a few helpful detoxification suggestions.

CoQ10/ UBIQUINOL (converted CoQ10)

The supplement ubiquinol is the converted form of CoQ10. It can be additionally helpful to assist energy levels with any die-off fatigue.

CHLORELLA

Chlorella binds to toxins and assists their removal from the body. Chlorella is exceptional in helping the body excrete toxins and in cleansing the blood. During die-off, it can be very helpful. It is also anti-inflammatory. Chlorella vulgaris, such as Yeayama chlorella from Jarrow Formulas, is the strain that is easier to digest and has higher chlorophyll. It comes in both capsule and powder form. It is available in healthfood stores and online at www.pureformulas.com.

BETA-SITOSTEROL

Beta sitosterol by the company Pharmax is helpful in capturing and eliminating neuro toxins. See the chapter on detoxification support for additional suggestions on assistance with detoxification, such as clay baths, baking soda baths, and far infrared saunas.

IF SYMPTOMS OF CANDIDA RETURN

Not to worry because now you will be prepared and know how to treat it immediately. By doing this, you will save a lot of agony. If you jump on it right away, the yeast will not have a chance to grow in numbers and likely a few days or a week of treatment will get it back under control. The best thing to do is do an ongoing Candida prevention program.

CANDIDA MAINTENANCE

If I stay on the CandElim daily (one drop per day), it keeps things balanced. Only the holidays or too much of the wrong things will throw me or my children out of balance.

When my Candida is "up" (the numbers of yeast have grown and are large enough to be causing problems in my system), I become much more irritable, tired, and I tend to crave sweets. I also wake in the middle of the night feeling very hungry and anxious. I know then that it's time, once again, to treat it.

Pay attention to any physical or emotional changes in your child during the holidays or during festive times when foods include more sugars, refined carbohydrates, and processed ingredients. Sometimes I hear people talk about the physical issues that came up suddenly for their child. It may be a knee that swelled up for no apparent reason or an earache or sinus issue that has quickly come up. My son's teachers noticed a sudden inability to concentrate in class and abrupt defiance after one Halloween holiday when he had eaten a lot of candy.

MY INTERMITTANT CANDIDA CLEANSE

This is a strict diet with no sugar, fruit, or starches of any kind, but includes a lot of organic olive oil, chicken, fish, broth, and green vegetables. The addition of increased probiotics and a small daily dosage of products from the company Get Healthy Again such as a drop or two per day of CandElim and the use of CandiClear5.

My son is a teenager now. He generally eats pretty well, but he doesn't eat only what I would like him to eat, so things can become imbalanced. It's a real world we are living in, and we can only do our best while simultaneously keeping our sanity.

My entire family takes probiotics daily, one in the morning and one at night. If I notice behavioral changes in my children, I increase the dosage of probiotics to two twice per day for a week or two, and I can always give them some CandElim while keeping them away from bad foods. It usually only takes a week or so to be completely back on track if you catch it right away. You can then go back to the maintenance dosage of probiotics but watch the diet.

The maintenance dosage for Dr. Ohhira's probiotics is usually one or two in the morning and one or two at night. This strengthens the overall positive bacteria on an ongoing basis. Some people need more than two twice a day on the maintenance level. It is important to find what your child needs. If they have strayed from their regular diet or have extra stress, increase the dosage for a few days. You will be able to find what you know is the best balance over time. Individual needs vary, so remember to muscle test or ask for the help of a practitioner.

Watch for symptoms and muscle test or do the morning saliva test along the way. If my kids go to a birthday party or eat higher amounts of sugary or carbohydrate-filled foods, show any sign of a cold or flu, or have increased stress, I give them additional probiotics for a few days.

ADDITIONAL REMEDY CHOICES

COLLOIDAL SILVER OR BIO-ACTIVE SILVER HYDROSOL

An additional remedy commonly used for gut dysbiosis such as candida, irritable bowel syndrome, leaky gut, Crohn's Disease, colitis, and Diverticulitis is Bio-Active Silver Hydrosol, or most commonly known as colloidal silver. Adult dosages are two tablespoons colloidal silver mixed with two tablespoons pure Aloe Vera juice swallowed straight into an empty stomach 30-60 minutes before breakfast, one hour before lunch, and one hour before dinner. Children often take two teaspoons with an equal amount of aloe prior to meals three times per day. Talk to your health care practitioner. This along with probiotics can be very helpful for intermittent cleansing. Generally, this is done for ten days to two weeks for candida issues.

The product Argentyn 23 is of the highest quality colloidal silver. It is available at www.pureformulas.com.

HOMEOPATHIC REMEDIES

I am a true believer in homeopathic remedies, and my children and I have had success with these products. There are homeopathic remedies available on the market to assist with Candida. I have tried several, but only to find that the Candida comes back. We have had no long-term success with these products for Candida. If choosing this method, I would recommend seeing a qualified homeopathic doctor.

SUMMARY

Slowly begin taking CandElim and CandiClear5. Continue probiotics and add chlorella. If you notice symptoms of die-off such as extreme fatigue, increased irritability, or headaches, you may need to reduce dosages of CandElim. Muscle test along the way for guidance to increase or reduce any dosages.

The products found in this chapter can be found at http://naturallyhealingautism.com/a-healthy-home/

CHAPTER 27

STAGE TWO:
HEAVY METAL DETOXIFICATION

Detoxification of heavy metals is a key component in any chronic state of disease or illness. Heavy metals can hide in various tissue, bone, and bodily fluids including the cerebral spinal fluid. They aggravate every medical condition from neurological to arthritis in the smallest joints of the hand. They must not be overlooked. Proper removal of heavy metals from the system is crucial!

TESTING FOR HEAVY METALS

Testing may be a personal choice only to fulfill the question of which heavy metals are in your child's body and at what level. For various reasons I have stated below, no test is completely reliable when it comes to these metals.

For the sake of education I offer you information on the mainstream ways to test for heavy metals. However, not all of the results come up positive, even when there are metals present in the body, because the results depend on how much your body is excreting at that moment. If the body is exhausted and the liver and kidneys are overworked, they may not be able to do their job properly, and the metals will not pass through. The toxins get stuck in the body and are reabsorbed through tissue and blood only to re-circulate in the system. Mercury may react with the plastics in the container used to hold the urine sample, and it evaporates at room temperature so some may be lost. Mercury is difficult to diagnose because it resides in various tissues and in different ionic forms. Furthermore, mercury gets stirred up in the body during testing challenges and concentrates in the brain and liver which can make health matters worse. I personally spent a lot of money on tests that I later learned were unreliable.

Noted reliable testing doctors and their labs are:

1. Dr. Andrew Cutler has extensive knowledge on the proper way to detoxify heavy metals with prescription DMSA and EDTA if you were to choose this route. He has a very specific schedule for the treatment protocol which also involves the use of alpha lipoic acid to naturally assist with chelation. To find multiple websites with the description of his chelation protocol go to www.curezone.org. Here you will also find additional websites to connect you to people already using Andrew Cutler's treatment.
2. Mark Schauss, MBA, DB is an internationally acclaimed lecturer on the effects of environmental toxicity on human health and the use of laboratory testing. He can be contacted at www.labinterpretation.com, and the most reliable tests are available for doctors to purchase at an 80 percent discount. The results can be back in as little as 24 hours. Assistance will be given for interpretation of the tests which is the most important piece. Many doctors and data personnel are not properly educated in test interpretation.
3. Dr. Deitricht Klinghardt's website is very informative regarding heavy metal detoxification, www.klinghardtacademy.com.

HAIR ANALYSIS TESTING

Hair analysis testing has been refined and has become more reliable, but it is still common to get false negatives. Some tests can be purchased online without an expensive doctor's appointment. The ability of the practitioner to properly interpret the results is key. There are practitioners available to go over the results with you when they come in. For more information on this read the book, *Hair Test Interpretation; Finding Hidden Toxicities,* by Dr. Andrew Cutler.

Notable companies who carry hair analysis tests are:

1. www.labinterpretation.com
2. www.arltma.com/HairAnalysis.htm (screens for the level of 20 minerals and toxic metals in one sample of hair)
3. www.annloise.com or www.unikeyhealth.com, 800-888-4353

The mother's hair can be tested for levels of heavy metals before, during, or after pregnancy, but the U.S. Biotek's Environmental Pollutants Biomarker urine test finds metabolites for multiple and various toxins.

NON-INVASIVE NEWBORN HEAVY METAL TESTING

A heavy metal test can be done on a child as young as a newborn through hair analysis.

TESTING PH LEVELS

Litmus paper is helpful to see exactly where your pH levels are. This helps you to know what state your child's body is in when it comes to acidity and alkalinity and therefore, the amount of burden on the liver. The liver is the detoxifier, and a body that is too acidic is already causing stress on the immune system, liver, kidneys, and other organs and glands. It is imperative that your liver is able to handle the job of detoxifying, especially of heavy metals.

First morning urine is an excellent indicator of pH. If this is impossible to get from your child, you can use a saliva test the same way, but urine is a bit more precise. A tiny strip of litmus paper is put into either the running stream during urination or you can collect a sample in a clean cup and dip the paper into the cup to test. If you are doing a saliva test, have your child put a small strip of the paper on his tongue for a moment.

After the strip has your sample on it, put it next to the color codes on the litmus paper dispenser. Match the color on the dispenser to the color that is closest to the one on your test paper, and this will tell you what the pH is.

Litmus paper can be purchased at most healthfood stores. It is important to purchase the kind that shows at least every two tenths of a point change. This is much more specific than one that will only show every five tenths of a point change. For example, you want the one that reads 6.4, 6.6, 6.8, OR 6.25, 6.5, 6.75, etc. You do not want the paper that only reads 6.0, 6.5, 7.0, etc.

The product Cell Power normalizes pH levels, and it also supports the liver and the kidneys by helping clean up toxins. It also strengthens the immune system. It can be found in most healthfood stores and at www.brainchildnutritionals.com.

SUPPORTING THE LIVER

Children on the autism spectrum often already have a congested liver, and with any detoxification process it is crucial to have the liver as strong and healthy as possible.

Metallothioneins are proteins and polypeptides found throughout the body. They are synthesized in the liver and kidneys but must have enough copper, zinc and selenium present to do so. Metallothioneins are in charge of holding in or regulating the transfer of zinc and copper in and out of cells. They also neutralize toxic exposure of heavy metals such as cadmium and mercury. When mercury enters the liver, its cells begin producing large quantities of metallothioneins.

Zinc increases the metabolism of metallothioneins and its overall production. It can be extremely helpful with toxicity, but it must be regulated. Too much zinc in the body has the potential to increase damage from mercury and cadmium. Usually 10 to 15 mgs is helpful.

Liver support is important during any detoxification. We discussed this in detail in the chapter two, on detoxification and organ support. We also discussed some good choices for natural liver support products, such as Liver Life by Bioray. It is sold at most healthfood stores and online at www.pureformulas.com and www.brainchildnutritionals.com. The homeopathic trio by Apex Energetics is also great. See the chapter on organ support and detoxification for more information.

The liver can be checked by your meridian stress assessment (M.S.A.) practitioner, a N.A.E.T. practitioner or by a chiropractor skilled in muscle testing. (See the chapter "alternative therapies" for information on practitioners). A blood test can check for liver health, but it can be a bit more difficult to obtain blood from some children. Using litmus paper can be a much easier way to gather information by checking your first morning urine.

PHARMACEUTICAL CHELATION

Chelation therapy is the use of chelating agents or drugs to remove heavy metals from the body. These agents bind themselves to many different compounds.

A chelation challenge is when you are given chelating drugs to look for quantities of heavy metals in the system. The word "challenge" comes from the fact that your body is put through exactly that—a challenge. These drugs are very hard on the body and results are not always accurate. Both are very hard on the kidneys and the liver.

Depending on the weight of the individual, a certain number of chelating drugs are given. The two main types of chelating drugs are:

1. **EDTA** (edetate disodium) is more lead specific.
2. **DMSA** (diamuric acid with sulfur). DMSA is more mercury specific. Fewer problems are seen with this when chlorella and alpha lipoic acid are used in conjunction. (See Dr. Andrew Cutler's method discussed in the previously.)

THE PROBLEM WITH CHELATION THERAPY

The drugs used in conventional chelation therapy attach to agents in the body, such as heavy metals and other toxic materials. These compounds then enter the bloodstream where they are removed via the kidneys and the liver. The chelation process is known to be very hard on these already burdened detoxifying organs.

Once a bond is made to these toxic agents, it can also be lost, therefore allowing the heavy metals to be freely released back into the bloodstream and allowing them to go anywhere in the body including the brain.

Due to lead harboring itself in the bones, traditional chelation therapy with DMSA may cause an increase in blood levels of lead as it leaves the bones. As this happens, it puts the brain at greater risk from its toxic effects. One study showed that DMSA was as equally ineffective at removing lead from the brain as was a placebo (Toxicology Applied Pharmacology 161(1999): 283-293, Efficacy of Succimer for Reducing Brain Lead in a Primate Model of Human Lead Exposure; Cremin, Luck, Laughlin and Smith).

Chelating drugs are also non-specific, meaning that they may pull out the metals but will also pull out the much-needed minerals in your body at the same time. DMSA binds to zinc leaving the body deficient of it. EDTA can chelate the much-needed metals in the body along with the harmful ones. Children with autism already have mineral deficiencies. They do not need another toxic agent further weakening their systems.

Whatever makes it through the kidneys and liver will then be excreted in the urine. Urine is collected over a course of hours, usually six. The sample is sent to a lab to obtain the results. The negative with this test is that it is very dependent on how much your body is excreting in only those six hours. If your liver is really congested or your body is unable to excrete properly on the day you take the test, then your results can be misleading.

Another concern regarding DMSA and other chelating agents is that they contain sulfur. This can cause additional trouble in the GI tract. Chelation therapy with drugs should not be done until the liver is balanced, Candida is under control, the gut is healthy, and nutrition and supplements are being absorbed well.

The most accurate way to do a challenge, which is far less expensive or time consuming, is through a stool sample. Since metals like to cling to tissue, especially acidic tissue, the stool carries it from the wall of the large intestine or bowel. Again, the results are based on what the body has not already reabsorbed.

Doctors Data, Inc. is a company with over 30 years of experience and provides specialty testing to healthcare practitioners worldwide. Many of their tests specifically look into aspects that address the autism spectrum. They do comprehensive testing on all types of nutritional, gastrointestinal, and environmental issues. www.doctorsdata.com.

Note: Magnesium has been shown to be far more effective than EDTA to chelate lead.

NATURAL HEAVY METAL DETOXIFICATION WITH MODIFIED CITRUS PECTIN

Modified Citrus Pectin with alginates: Modified citrus pectin is known for its safe, and gentle detoxification of heavy metals. The product Pectaclear by Econugenics has been clinically proven to reduce up to 74 percent of dangerous heavy metals, including lead, mercury, cadmium and others within six months, without lowering levels of essential minerals such as calcium, magnesium or zinc, as conventional chelation therapies do. It also includes anti-microbial activity against bacteria and fungi. This soluble fiber binds to toxins in the blood. Peer reviewed research also shows that modified alginates bind to heavy metals and environmental toxins within the digestive tract, therefore preventing reabsorption into the bloodstream, which is a common problem with conventional chemical chelation methods Please listen to my very informative podcast interview with Dr. Isaac Eliaz on heavy metal detoxification and modified citrus pectin at www.naturallyhealingautism.com:

PectaClear is best taken away from food, but the capsules can be opened up and added to a little applesauce or other food for nonpill takers. The alginate portion should be very helpful in supporting digestion and clearing toxins from the gut/bile, etc. Ecodetox is best taken with food. Both can be found on my website, www.naturallyhealingautism.com, on the products page. NOTE: citrus may interfere with absorption of medication or supplementation, so take 30 minutes apart.

Suggested Protocol

Just as it takes years to accumulate high levels of heavy metals and environmental toxins within the body, the process of removing these harmful substances from deep within the tissues and organs will take time as well. For the safe removal of heavy metals it should be a minimum of a 3-6 month course of Pectaclear, accompanied by the use of the phase II liver detoxification supplement Ecodetox by Econugenics during this time.

PectaClear is best taken away from food, but the capsules can be opened up and added to a little applesauce or other food for non-pill takers. The alginate portion should be very helpful in supporting digestion and clearing toxins from the gut/bile, etc. Ecodetox is best taken with food. Both can be found on my website, www.naturallyhealingautism.com, on the products page. NOTE: citrus may interfere with absorption of medication or supplementation, so take 30 minutes apart.

PREGNANCY, BREASTFEEDING AND HEAVY METALS

During pregnancy, most heavy metals cross the blood-brain barrier and get into the fetus. After birth, the mother's heavy metal toxins are released into her newborn baby via breast milk. The greatest release often goes to her firstborn child. This is not to say that formula is better than breastfeeding; I would never say that.

The supplements listed below to help with detoxification can be helpful. The best choice is always to detoxify before pregnancy, if able.

PROTECTION FROM HEAVY METAL TOXICITY

The best ongoing protection comes from eating organic, local, and whole foods because proper nutrition can help your body detoxify. Taking antioxidants such as vitamins E and C, selenium, magnesium, zinc, carotenoids, and alpha lipoic acid can all assist the body in the removal of mercury toxicity. Be sure to support your liver. Liver support was discussed in detail in the chapter on detoxification and organ support.

SUPPLEMENTS THAT ASSIST WITH DETOXIFICATION:

- Vitamin D reduces heavy metal injury to the brain. Low vitamin D levels mean low glutathione levels. Vitamin D enables glutathione to do its job. Glutathione helps detoxify heavy metals such as mercury and lead from the body. Therefore, if vitamin D levels are low you cannot detoxify well. Have your vitamin D levels checked. Often extra D is necessary to bring levels up to balance.

- Alpha lipoic acid
- Selenium
- B vitamins
- Vitamins E and C
- Carotenoids
- Garlic
- N-acetyl cysteine
- Glycine
- Glutathione
- Zinc
- Magnesium
- Chlorella
- Flavonoids
- Taurine
- Molybdenum

NOTE: a quality multi-vitamin/mineral supplement will contain all or most of these. A good one is found at www.brainchildnutritionals.com, and they specialize in autism spectrum disorders. All of these including glutathione are talked about in detail in the chapter on Common Nutritional Deficiencies.

SUMMARY

Heavy metals are present in all of us in different amounts. The commonly used drugs used for chelation are very hard on the body. They pull minerals at the same time as they excrete the metals. The drugs are also very hard on the liver, which is your detoxifying organ, so it must first be decongested (see Chapter Five for liver support).

The natural clathration product PCA is currently unavailable, so the next best thing for heavy metal detoxification is using DMSA with Dr. Andrew Cutler's protocol. His protocol uses alpha lipoic acid at very specifically timed intervals to assist the release of heavy metal toxins, so that they do not bind and stay in the body. There are many natural supplements that can help to detoxify the system.

The products found in this chapter can be found at http://naturallyhealingautism.com/a-healthy-home/

CHAPTER 28

STAGE THREE BRAIN SUPPORT AND REPAIR

SUPPLEMENTATION EXAMPLES FOR INDIVIDUAL BEHAVIORAL NEEDS (timing to begin is based on individual choice)

Every individual is unique, and there is not one program for everyone. For this reason, I have given many examples of symptoms and supplements that relate to them. It is often obvious what your child needs, but not always. The chapter on brain scans offers steps to lead you to a more specific approach with the help of a qualified practitioner.

In one study done by a team of scientists at Stanford University School of Medicine and Lucile Packard Children's Hospital, researchers suggest that the diagnosis of autism may show different cognitive abilities, but does not necessarily signal a disability. These children tend to have more trouble with social interaction, but have exceptionally high math skills. Perhaps this shows us that autism is simply different ways for the brain to function. This could be anyone, diagnosed or not.

It should now be obvious that there is commonly more than one part of the brain or more than one neurotransmitter that is not functioning at optimum. Some areas of the brain are overactive and others underactive. Some neurotransmitters are in excess, and more commonly, others are deficient. Many aspects do overlap and each needs to be addressed. MRIs, EEG's, and blood tests will likely all come up normal.

Deficiencies in neurotransmitters can cause abnormalities in brain function. People with untreated ADD often suffer from low self-esteem. The child is continually in trouble, and people are often angry with him.

Contact your doctor if your child is taking medications to be sure there are no contraindications with any supplements you wish to add. Be sure that your practitioner is educated about the supplements you ask about. Natural supplementation works as well as prescription drugs without the harmful side effects. St. Johns Wort, L-tryptophan, and 5-HTP work so well that they should not be taken with prescription antidepressants without the knowledge and close supervision of your physician. All supplements suggestions are what have been known to be helpful. Each individual may vary. These products can be purchased at www.naturallyhealingautism.com under "healthy home products."

Muscle test for dosage levels or ask your qualified professional.

The staples everyone needs:

- Multi-vitamin/mineral supplement with adequate B vitamins, that is free of yeast, wheat, and dairy with no added colors or fillers. The website www.brainchildnutritionals.com offers quality supplements. Supremely Green from www.herbprod is a whole food vitamin/mineral supplement.
- Omega-3 fatty acids (500 to 2,000 mg per day). Captain's Krill Oil is best. Purchase from www.stillsmilin.com. The company Pharmax makes a quality fish oil supplement in liquid or chewable form with a sweet orange flavor. It is sold at most healthfood stores and at www.amazon.com.
- Vitamin D: 2,000 to 5,000 IU per day, depending on size and age.
- 30 to 60 minutes of intense aerobic exercise every day. This improves blood supply and oxygen to thc brain and minimizes symptoms of ADD.

Important: For results from natural supplementation, it may take up to three weeks to notice results, so stay with it and be patient. If after three weeks you do not see desired effects, their dosage may need to be increased. A knowledgeable practitioner, such as one at the Amen Clinic, can help guide you with this if necessary. After an individual has been on supplements for three to six months, he should continue to improve even more. Improvements will continue over the year and beyond. He will need to take these forever. If he stops taking the supplements he will regress.

BRAIN SUPPORT DIET

Essentially, the diet in this book follows all principles needed to support a healthy fed brain while also minimizing foods that cause inflammation in it. Everyone, except for those with issues of hyper-focus (see below), benefit the most from higher protein, lower carbohydrate diets. Stay away from simple sugars and processed carbohydrates. Eat more meat, poultry, fish, and eggs, and only eat complex carbohydrates such as brown rice, beans, and vegetables. Limit simple sugars and processed carbohydrates that will turn to sugar in your body like breads, pastas, pastries, etc. These foods will make his symptoms worse. Good oils will also help his brain such as olive, avocado, coconut, grapeseed, and most nuts. In general, remember that a diet higher in protein is necessary to help with focus. Refined or processed carbohydrates will worsen symptoms of difficulty with focus and attention.

BRAIN SYMPTOM CATEGORIES:

HYPERACTIVE AND IMPULSIVE OR ADHD

These people are commonly known as hyperactive or ADHD, which stands for attention hyperactivity deficit disorder. They are impulsive, easily distracted, have trouble concentrating, are forgetful, need constant excitement and attention, talkative, have trouble sitting still, are interruptive, have trouble waiting their turn, and have trouble with organization, following instructions, or completing a task.

THE CAUSE

These people have a deficiency in the neurotransmitter dopamine.

SUPPLEMENTS KNOWN TO HELP

L-tyrosine is the amino acid that helps typical hyperactive ADD symptoms. L-tyrosine builds dopamine. It is known to be safe, effective, and is inexpensive to purchase.

Dopamine will also help balance the needs of your child's prefrontal cortex, which is in charge of organization, planning, impulse control, and more. Their prefrontal cortex has normal activity at rest, but decreased activity (more trouble working) when the person tries to concentrate. Remember, when they have low PFC activity, they have trouble filtering, so they are easily distracted. The basal ganglia can also be functioning improperly in the brains of these people. Poor fine motor skills such as handwriting are common.

HOW MUCH?

L-tyrosine: Adults start with 500 to 1,500 mg, two to three times per day. Children start with 100 to 500 mg, two to three times per day. Most teens and adults begin with 1,000 to 1,500 mg per day and go up from there. If after three weeks you do not see enough improvement, then increase the dose with an added 500 mg in the afternoon. Do not give it to him in the evening because it can keep him awake. Take L-tyrosine on an empty stomach for best absorption, one half hour before meals or one hour after. There are no side effects, except for occasional lowered appetite. L-tyrosine can be purchased at any healthfood store and at many online sites such as www.swansonvitamins.com.

Optional: Grape seed extract and pycnogenol are also effective for hyperactivity, and they are great antioxidants to boost his immune system.

LACK OF FOCUS AND MOTIVATION OR ADD

People with a lack of focus and motivation are often thought of as "couch potatoes." This is commonly called ADD, or attention deficit disorder. They are quiet and inattentive. They daydream often, complain of being bored, are unmotivated, easily distracted, have a short attention span, and are thought of as spacey.

THE CAUSE

Although these people have the same original cause as the hyperactive/ADHD person, a deficiency in dopamine, the imbalance is in a different part of the brain. The prefrontal cortex seems to be affected more. There is a similar type of deactivation of the PFC during concentration.

SUPPLEMENTS KNOWN TO HELP

L-tyrosine will help to build their levels of dopamine. SAMe is also helpful with motivation.

HOW MUCH?

L-tyrosine: See hyperactive and impulsive ADHD for dosage levels of L-tyrosine that have been helpful. Dosages of 400 mg, two to four times per day, of SAMe have been shown to be helpful. Children are often half that as it varies with size and age.

HYPER-FOCUSED

People with hyper-focus have the same ADHD and ADD core symptoms but also tend to get hyper-focused. They lock into subjects and have trouble shifting out of them. This is the stubborn child who often throws seemingly endless tantrums. They get stuck on negative thoughts, worry excessively, are perfectionists, have oppositional behavior, are argumentative and defiant, have trouble seeing solutions, are opinionated, and are obsessive compulsive. They hold grudges and can become substance abusers.

THE CAUSE

People with hyper-focus have a deficiency in both dopamine and serotonin. Their anterior cingulate gyrus is overactive, which is the part of the brain that helps us shift our attention. The ACG needs a lot of serotonin, also noted to help those with obsessive compulsive disorder. These people get stuck on one thing because their brain's gear shift is not working. This has been noted as a common trait among children and grandchildren of alcoholics. There may also be issues with the prefrontal cortex.

SUPPLEMENTS KNOWN TO HELP

5-HTP and St. Johns Wort both build serotonin and work better together than alone. They lower activity in the anterior cingulate gyrus and the prefrontal cortex. They also help with depression, moodiness, and trouble shifting attention. Be sure to buy the St Johns Wort with 0.3% hypericin which is its active ingredient.

St. Johns Wort and 5-HTP alone can make some people too complacent, so it is important to add L-tyrosine for stimulation. L-tyrosine is also needed to build dopamine. Note: do not give L-tyrosine alone to people with hyper-focus as it will cause an increase in focus and worsen symptoms. A drug such as Ritalin would aggravate the symptoms of these people. This is why it is important never to use a cookie-cutter approach to psychology. Biology must be considered.

HOW MUCH?

L-tyrosine: Follow the same guidelines for the use of L-tyrosine noted in hyperactive/ADHD.

St. Johns Wort: The starting dosage for St. Johns Wort is 300 mg per day for children, 300 mg twice per day for teens, and 600 mg in the morning and 300 mg in the evening for adults. Note: temporal lobe imbalance (see below), must be stabilized before using St. Johns Wort.

5-HTP: For 5-HTP, the adult dosage is 50 to 300 mg per day. For children, it is half that amount. 5-HTP can cause slight nausea when it is first taken. We use an enteric-coated source that prevents this. I purchase mine from www.swansonvitamins.com.

EXCESSIVE TEMPER AND MEMORY IMBALANCE

This brain imbalance has the same ADHD core symptoms but causes more severe behavioral problems. These people are known to have extreme problems with temper, unstable moods, periods of rage, confusion, anxiety, poor memory, may be suicidal or homicidal, and may have headaches and abdominal pain for no apparent reason.

THE CAUSE

The temporal lobes of the brain lie under your ears. They hold the organs of hearing, balance, reading abilities, affect language and speech, and help to keep moods stable. There is often a combination of temporal lobe dysfunction and an underactive prefrontal cortex, especially during concentration. In my craniosacral work, I often find the temporal bones jammed up in children with ADD, autism and learning disabilities. There seems to be a connection with head injuries or toxic damage.

SUPPLEMENTS KNOWN TO HELP

The best supplement to help calm the neurons in the brain and reduce anxiety is GABA. GABA will not cause addiction as its pharmaceutical prescription counterparts do. Phosphotidyl serine may help with cognitive function, behavior and mood. Gingko biloba helps with circulation, energy, concentration, focus, and memory. It also increases blood flow to the brain. Vitamin E can additionally be helpful with memory.

Note: Do not use St. Johns Wort or 5-HTP if there is temporal lobe imbalance because they increase serotonin levels, which can make symptoms worse.

HOW MUCH?

GABA: start with 100 to 500 mg per day for adults and half that for children.

Phosphotidyl serine: 100 mg, two times per day.

Ginkgo biloba: 60 to 120 mg, twice per day.

Vitamin E: 400 to 600 IU, two times per day.

LONG-TERM OR LIMBIC DEPRESSION

These people have the same core ADD/ADHD symptoms with the addition of depression, negativity, sadness, moodiness, low energy, feelings of hopelessness, chronic low self-esteem, and tend to be socially isolated. The difference between symptomatic depression and long-term or limbic depression is that symptomatic depression will be cyclic where limbic depression will last for a prolonged period of time. Parents will often remember this as the child's personality since childhood. Substance abuse is common as a form of self medication.

THE CAUSE

The deep limbic system is the brain's center for emotion. It creates the emotions behind our experiences and our desires. It is how we interpret events determining whether we feel calm or anxious as the result of a given situation. In limbic depression, if we are already sad during a negative event, we will become depressed. If we are feeling positive, we become happier.

In limbic depression, there is also low activity in the prefrontal cortex during periods of both rest and concentration, and a deficiency in the neurotransmitters dopamine and norepinephrine. An overactive limbic system decreases our motivation and drive. This is commonly depicted as depression. Sleep and appetite are also controlled by the limbic system as is our ability to bond and feel socially connected.

SUPPLEMENTS KNOWN TO HELP

SAMe helps the brain to function properly, and also increase neurotransmitters involved with depression. The body makes SAMe, but it is often deficient in depressed people. It is one of the best natural antidepressants available and shown to be as effective as antidepressant medications. It is also helpful for fibromyalgia and chronic muscle pain disorder. Fibromyalgia is common among people with brain imbalances. DL-phenylalanine (DLPA) helps with mood, focus, depression, and energy and pain control. L-tyrosine assists with building dopamine and norepinephrine.

HOW MUCH?

SAMe: 200 to 400 mg, two to four times per day, half that amount for children.

DL-phenylalanine (DLPA): 400 mg, three times per day, half that for children.

L-tyrosine: See ADHD/ADD guidelines for L-tyrosine.

THE EXTREMELY SENSITIVE

These people have the same core ADHD/ADD symptoms with the addition of anger, aggression, and extreme sensitivity to their environment such as noise, light, clothing, and touch. They have extreme highs and lows, and are inflexible, mean, and set in their ways. There are periods of excessive talkativeness and impulsivity. They may appear anxious or fearful with unpredictable behavior, hyper-focus, and extreme oppositional behavior. This may be related to bipolar disorder.

THE CAUSE

Problems for those with extremely sensitivity stem from an imbalanced brain that has too much activity, especially in the cingulate gyrus, parietal lobes, temporal lobes, and prefrontal cortex.

SUPPLEMENTS KNOWN TO HELP

GABA is calming to the nerves and calms the brain reducing hyperactivity within it. Omegas-3s are especially helpful. It was shown in a study done by Harvard University that omega-3s showed significant improvement in bipolar depression.

Important: Those with extreme sensitivity should not take SSRI antidepressant medications such as Prozac or Zoloft. Stimulant medications such as Ritalin also worsen symptoms for these people. Also, they should not take SAMe, as it may induce manic or excessively impulsive behavior. Use caution with any supplements that increase serotonin such as 5-HTP, and St. Johns wort.

HOW MUCH?

GABA: 100 to 500 mg per day, half that for children.

Omega-3 fatty acids: 500 to 2,000 mg per day. Captain's Krill Oil is best (one to two capsules per day depending on the size and age of the individual).

Magnesium: start with one teaspoon (Natural Vitality, Natural Calm), and work up to bowel tolerance.

DIET: HYPER-FOCUS, THE DIET EXCEPTION

For most people with low levels of serotonin and dopamine, a diet of high protein and low carbohydrates is best. This helps their energy and their focus. For those with issues of hyper-focus, they cannot stop focusing and often become fixated on negative issues. They are specifically low in tryptophan which builds their needed serotonin.

Tryptophan comes from high-protein foods, especially turkey and eggs. It is a small molecule, so it has a hard time making its way into the brain before the larger molecule amino acids. This can cause lowered tryptophan levels, which means an increased deficiency in serotonin and an abundance of dopamine (the focus-building neurotransmitter). This makes their issues of hyper-focus worse.

Foods that contain carbohydrates such as vegetables, whole grains, and yes, pizza, pasta, potatoes, and pastries, also increase L-tryptophan levels but they increase at a faster rate. Hyper-focus individuals need more carbohydrates than other people, but it must be balanced with protein. This can help to raise levels of both serotonin and dopamine.

This does not mean loading up on the bad carbohydrates. It means balancing the two with meals that contain both. Have them eat bites of the protein food first, if possible, as it is easier on their blood sugar levels. Examples are meals with eggs and toast or meat with vegetables or brown rice.

Note: a little pasta or potatoes to their diet should come second to vegetables or whole grain and should be done so only after the gut has been cleared of Candida, and there is no allergic reaction to gluten.

I highly recommend reading Dr. Daniel Amen's book, *Healing ADD*, for a more indepth explanation and case study examples of these categories that he calls types of ADD. Also see his website www.amenclinics.com.

An additional trick to assist with behavior control is offering some type of carbohydrate if you are in need of cooperation. This makes the brain less able to focus but the person more agreeable. Do not do this before a test because they will not be able to think as clearly. If you are in need of greater focus, then protein is your answer.

The exception with this rule is for those with hyper-focus. They need protein to focus for the test but some additional carbohydrate to balance the brain. If these people have too much protein without enough carbohydrate, they can become fixated on one problem or question in a test and not be able to move on. When I want my son to participate with the family in something he does not want to do, I sometimes give him a piece of toast or other carbohydrate so he will be more agreeable. (Oops! If he reads this, he will know my trick.)

INDIVIDUAL BRAIN SYMPTOM QUICK GUIDE

I give my family specific supplements for their specific needs. You can do the same or Dr. Amen has formulated products in categories of brain basics, calmers, enhancers, focus, mood and weight. They are sold through his website at www.amenclinics.com. If you mention the referral code "Karen Thomas," you will receive 10% discount off of all evaluations and SPECT imaging brain scans.

Additional examples and possible solutions:

Compulsivity, worrier = increased anterior cingulate and low serotonin
Solution: 5-HTP and St. Johns Wort

Impulsive, easily distracted = low PFC and low dopamine
Solution: L-tyrosine

Impulsive/compulsive = high anterior cingulate and low PFC, low serotonin and low dopamine
Solution: St. Johns wort, 5-HTP and L-tyrosine

Lacks ability to focus, easily distracted = low dopamine
Solution: L-tyrosine

Depressed, low energy, crave carbohydrates = high limbic activity, low PFC, check vitamin D levels and DHEA levels
Solution: SAMe, vitamin D, with possible need for DHEA

Anxious = high basal ganglia, low GABA levels
Solution: GABA, vitamin B6, and magnesium

Temper, anger, and mood with memory problems, and learning disabilities = problem with temporal lobes
Solution: GABA, vitamin B6, magnesium, ginkgo, and acetyl-L-carnitine

Stuck on negative thoughts/grudge holder = anterior cingulate gyrus issue
Solution: 5-HTP and St. Johns Wort to build serotonin, if hyper focused may also need L-tyrosine.

For more motivation and drive: L-tyrosine and SAMe

WHY SOME TREATMENT PROGRAMS DO NOT WORK

- The wrong diagnosis
- The wrong treatment protocol, i.e. supplements, medications, or therapies. This also means the incorrect dosages
- Citric acid is taken too close to supplement time. Citric acid as is in orange juice, lemonade, preservatives and more deactivates some medications and supplements. Do not ingest it within an hour before or after taking them.
- Stress hormones, namely corticosteroids, damage brain cells, especially the temporal lobes. They may also counteract the effectiveness of some treatments. Reduce stress level.
- Lack of support from family, school, caregivers or therapists; creates stress
- The wrong diet
- Caffeine and nicotine use
- Lack of exercise

- Taking over-the-counter medications or supplements that may interfere with treatment
- Mixing together incompatible medications and supplements
- Not staying on natural supplements for a long enough period of time to allow them to work (minimum of three to six weeks)
- Purchasing cheaper, lower quality products in order to save money
- Not having the right doctor. Using the doctor on your insurance plan may seem cheaper at first, but may cost you far more in the long run.
- Being in denial about what your child really needs and not getting the proper help

SUMMARY

Every individual is unique in their behavioral symptoms. Evaluation of specific needs allows for the right supplement program to assist the brain to be able to function better. Enough time must be allowed for natural supplementation to take proper effects. Diet is important for specific chemical needs of the brain as well as the body. If results are not what were expected there are guidelines to look into for possible reasons why.

The products found in this chapter can be found at http://naturallyhealingautism.com/a-healthy-home/

CHAPTER 29

REBUILDING THE BRAIN; RESTRUCTURE AND REPAIR

IT IS NOW KNOWN THAT THE BRAIN CAN AND DOES HEAL AND REBUILD ITSELF.

Neurons are the ultimate brain cells. They are information messengers that transmit their electrical impulses and chemical signals, known as synapses, within the brain and from the brain to the spinal cord. Sensory neurons carry messages from the five senses: sight, hearing, touch, smell and taste. Motor neurons carry messages from the brain to muscles and control voluntary muscle movement.

A dendrite is a little spiny projection that comes off of a neuron. They are conductors that receive information from other neural cells in the body. Axons look like tails that come off of the neurons. They transmit messages from the cells. We need to protect neurons from damage. A misguided neuron can cause epilepsy, mental retardation, and even schizophrenia. Alzheimer's and other diseases of the brain are also associated with these neural problems. If damage occurs, we must work to rebuild them for normal brain function. Within the brain, new connections can develop and dendrites can travel to different damaged areas.

WHAT DAMAGES NEURONS?

Neurons can be damaged by:

- Free radicals

- Toxins such as pesticides, chemicals and heavy metals are stored in fat cells; the brain is 60% fat, so it acts as a magnet for toxins
- Mercury has been shown, even in small amounts, to kill neurons in the brain. Once the mercury is removed, the dendrites on the neurons may be able to regrow with adequate nutrition.
- Omega-6 fats such as corn, safflower, sunflower, peanut, canola, and soybean oils weaken the brain and its ability to function. They also reduce the protective omega-3 fats.
- Prolonged stress destroys dendrites and memory due to the release of the stress hormones cortisol and adrenaline
- Oxidation
- Excitotoxicity from excess glutamate and aspartate
- Head injury

When starting any new supplement, consult with your healthcare professional. Listed below are supplements that have been known to protect, rebuild, and repair the brain.

We have already gone into detail about neurotransmitters and supplements that can support brain functioning. There are additional supplements that are capable of improving brain function and repairing damage.

SUPPLEMENTS TO SUPPORT REBUILDING DENDRITES AND NEURONS

THE ESSENTIAL FATTY ACID DHA

The component DHA in essential fatty acids (fish oil) builds new brain pathways and is essential for brain health. It also protects the brain and blocks excitotoxicity. These polyunsaturated fats cover neurons, make up dendrites and their connections, and repair damage. Mitochondria, the cell's energy builder, need DHA for health. DHA also increases the neurotransmitter serotonin in the brain.

CoQ10/ UBIQUINOL

CoQ10, or its more bio-available counterpart ubiquinol, is helpful for cell energy which the body needs to function, rebuild, and grow. It protects the cell from damage and builds glutathione within the cells improving antioxidant strength and improving memory. CoQ10 protects mitochondria and neurons from viruses and their damage, including mumps. When taken with niacinamide (vitamin B3/niacin), it protects the brain from excitotoxicity. This is enhanced when taken in conjunction with pyrroloquinoline quinine (PQQ).

PQQ (PYRROLOQUINOLINE QUINONE)

PQQ is naturally found in vegetables and breast milk but it is essential, which means that the body cannot make it on its own. PQQ is a breakthrough in the building and protection of the mitochondria. The brain and the heart are especially abundant in mitochondria because they both use a significant amount of energy. This energy must be replenished. Mitochondria acts to produce the energy for cells.

Some of the benefits of PQQ include:

- Activation of genes that signal mitochondrial protection, production and repair
- Blocks neurotoxicity, including that of mercury
- Improves memory and focus
- Protects neurotransmitters
- Repairs DNA within the mitochondria itself
- It is a powerful antioxidant
- Lowers lipid peroxidation reducing oxidative stress

PQQ works best when taken with CoQ10. There are companies that make a supplement with both. They can be found at www.pureformulas.com. Generally, for adults, 20 mg has been known to be helpful. Children are usually half the adult dosage. This is commonly used for aging adults, but our kids have experienced neurotoxicity and are prone to sensitivities of the brain. This supplement may be very helpful; however, always consult your healthcare practitioner to be in accordance with your child's weight, age, and personal needs.

DHEA (DEHYDROEPIANDROSTERONE)

DHEA is the adrenal hormone precursor that protects brain cells. Levels of DHEA can be tested in the same saliva test used to check adrenal function. When the body is under prolonged stress and the adrenal glands become taxed, it will often lower the levels of this important hormone.

VITAMIN D

Lack of sunlight and poor digestive absorption can easily cause vitamin D deficiency. More has been learned about this essential nutrient that is essential for the health of the immune system and the brain. Vitamin D is involved in brain development and functioning and is neuroprotective. Vitamin D also helps neurons to grow and to survive.

Vitamin D deficiency commonly causes depression, lack of motivation, poor neurotransmission, and even epilepsy and schizophrenia. Deficiency can slow memory and the functioning of the prefrontal cortex (PFC). The PFC helps with planning, impulse control, and making decisions. There are vitamin D receptors in parts of the brain including the hypothalamus, cerebellum, and basal ganglia.

ALPHA LIPOIC ACID

Alpha lipoic acid is one of the best antioxidants available. In the brain, it can block excitotoxicity, helps remove heavy metals, reduces oxidative damage, and protects the mitochondria improving memory.

ACETYL-L-CARNITINE

Acetyl-L carnitine is a protective antioxidant. It helps increase the strength of energy from mitochondria, protects brain receptors, and helps build the neurotransmitter acetylcholine, involved in memory.

THE B VITAMINS

The B vitamins—riboflavin, thiamin, folic acid, B12, B6, and niacinamide—repair, protect, and strengthen the brain.

ANTIOXIDANT VITAMINS

Vitamins C and E protect the brain.

MAGNESIUM

Magnesium is the key mineral that protects the brain. see details in chapter-------.

THE ANTIOXIDANT ENZYMES

Manganese, selenium, zinc, and copper protect the brain in their correct amounts. Each of these must be monitored to avoid excess, which can injure the brain. Consult with your healthcare practitioner for your child's particular needs.

GINGKO BILOBA

Gingko biloba is one of the most extensively studied and safest herbs. It protects and strengthens blood vessels and improves oxygen and glucose levels in the brain. It also protects synapses in the brain. It is known to be very calming and improves memory. Ginkgo is an anticoagulant and thins the blood. For those looking for these benefits without the negative aspects related to drugs such as aspirin, it is a healthy substitute. If you are taking anticoagulation drugs, first consult your healthcare practitioner.

See the chapter on Alternative Therapies for information regarding the benefits to brain function from craniosacral therapy and neurofeedback.

PHOSPHOTIDYL SERINE

Phosphotidyl serine maintains cell membranes, memory, and cognitive function.

GRAPE SEED EXTRACT

Grape seed extract supports brain structure and brain cell networks.

ADDITIONAL BRAIN HEALERS

Homeopathy, neurofeedback, and craniosacral therapy are all essential components to healing the brain. For further information on each please refer to chapter two. Below I have given an example from one homeopathic treatment we used successfully with my son.

SEROYAL HOMEOPATHIC NEURO PROGRAM

We went to see a chiropractor that had knowledge of homeopathic programs for rebuilding and restructuring the brain. Many holistic practitioners are familiar with the company Seroyal and their homeopathic Unda products. This particular program is done in four different phases and must be done in order. It is a way to take the system back through the stages of development in the order it developed. Below is a journal of our experience.

Clear emotional triggers first, Tapping or Neuro Emotional Technique (both explained in the Alternative Therapies chapter) are two good ways to do this. Once this has been done, then start this neuro program.

THE SEROYAL HOMEOPATHIC NEURO PROGRAM

You *must* begin with phase one and move through in sequential order. Even if the person is 50 years old, you would begin with phase one. Only go as high as the person's age or "stage". For example: start with one, then do two but if a child is under the age of seven you would not go any further because stage two takes the system through the developmental years up to age seven. Test and see if you need to continue stages one and two for a longer period of time. Once your child has gone through the phases in order one time, you may find that they only need to go through the last phase one more time.

Phase I: Birth to 18 months. This is known as the adrenal phase. It is about survival in the world.

Phase II: Thyroid. 18 months to age 7. When the thymus gland develops.

Phase III: Pituitary, age 7 to puberty. Note: some children seem to go through fears at this age, specifically at night. I've wondered if this is because their pituitary, and therefore, their pineal gland, are developing rapidly and they are more affected by hormonal shifts and melatonin production variations. I hear from parents that their child who has slept through the night in their own bed for years is now coming to them in the night for security with fears and night terrors.

Phase IV: The hormonal phase, puberty onward. This phase is designated as male or female for the individual being treated.

Jacob Seroyal/Unda Neuro Program Journal

Began April 23, 2010

Phase I was done for 7 days, then phase II was done for 7 days, then phase III was done for 7 days, then phase IV was done for 7 days. At this time, we went back to phase I and started the same cycle over again. This was done until all products are gone.

Day 3 of phase I:

Jacob is already showing more initiative, less aggression, and less impulsivity. He is much calmer and more focused.

I came home from taking my daughter to school and he was already up brushing his teeth and was getting himself ready for school—without being asked! I noticed that he was already less hostile and far less aggressive or bothered by the small things that would normally disturb him.

He talked in a more focused and easy-going manner. Eye contact also definitely improved. This process continued to get better every day.

Phase II:

Day 1: Jacob came home from school with a headache that was bad enough that he asked me if I had something to give him for it. I offered him craniosacral work, but he said never mind and left the room.

Day 2: He became very nauseas on the car ride home from karate. He was exceptionally tired today.

Day 3: Still very tired (could be hormones) but overall much more calm and not as easily angered. Far less hostile than usual.

Phase III:

Days 1 and 2: Remained calm.

Day 3: Mother's Day. Carly picked at him relentlessly to get out of bed. He finally blew and chased her through the house until he caught her and became violent with her. Afterward, he felt remorse and even cried. He said he didn't want to go to the beach with us because he didn't want to be around people. Said it was harder to be around people, and he'd rather be alone because it was easier. After coaxing, he finally went to breakfast with us in Cambria and was calm and polite during breakfast and throughout the rest of the day.

Day 4: He seemed to still be thinking about his actions the day before and almost seemed embarrassed. Again, calm and polite.

Phase IV:

First day quickest and most noticeable improvement. After school, he showed extreme kindness toward his sister. He gave her a gift he had received from his teacher as a prize. It was a child's purse he picked out for Carly. He let her hug him and did not resist.

Day3: Jacob has shown tremendous maturity, focus, eye contact, increased social skills and seems more social altogether since on Phase IV. I cannot recall any moments of hostility. If he has an issue he talks about it with me in a calm manner.

I have seen the most drastic improvement from Phase IV!

DEWORMING

Once the body and the brain are balanced, it is a good idea to consider deworming. It is always suggested for those on the autism spectrum or with learning or behavioral issues. Refer back to the chapter on pathogenic microbes for further information.

SUMMARY

Neurons carry messages to and from the brain. They can be damaged by both physical and chemical injury. Luckily, once the toxins are removed and the right nutritional, supplemental, and physical support are offered the brain can heal and rebuild itself.

We have already discussed craniosacral therapy and neurofeedback in the chapter on alternative therapies. They are both very helpful in assisting balance in the brain.

The products found in this chapter can be found at http://naturallyhealingautism.com/a-healthy-home/

CHAPTER 30

THE THREE STAGES QUICK GUIDE SUMMARY

Muscle test prior to any new stage to ask the body if it is ready for what you intend to offer it. Also muscle test for dosages.

Some people will want to test for pathogenic bacteria first; the choice is yours. Candida is likely overgrown, and there may be other pathogens, but the gut-healing process is going to balance a lot of these problems anyway. The easy spit test can be of help with Candida, before and after to test on your own at home. There are tests noted for other microbes in the chapter on different pathogenic microbes.

The issues that are not taken care of are the possibility of Lyme disease and the mold biotoxin illness. If your child has either of these, it is important to know. If the child inherited Lyme from the mother, she will have a history of feeling extreme fatigue and illness. This can be the same for either mom or dad if he has the mold biotoxin illness; it is genetic.

To simplify, look at the history of the parents. Test for microbes via spit test, stool, and urine. Once the diet, cleansing products, and detoxification have been completed, you can see who your child really is. If he still has symptoms of Lyme and the mold biotoxins illness, then a blood test is important to find it or rule it out. You do not want to miss these issues if they exist.

IMPORTANT NOTE: If behaviors or learning are extremely impaired, you may wish to begin some brain support supplements as soon as stage one. As gut pathology heals, there may be less of a need, but sometimes we need help right away. Examples: L-tyrosine for focus, or GABA for anxiety, or 5-HTP and St. Johns Wort for depression. See the chapter on individual brain supplements for more information.

STAGE ONE

SUPPORTING THE LIVER AND THE ADRENALS

WEEK ONE: Begin taking a liver support supplement such as Liver Life by Bioray. For adrenal support Drenamin from Standard Process (small pill form can be crushed up). Sold by many natural health care practitioners and can be found at www.pureformulas.com, OR

Ribes Nigrum Gemmo homeopathic liquid by Seroyal is a good choice. It is available at www.pureformulas.com.

HEALING THE GUT

WEEK TWO: Begin probiotics and enzymes and slowly reducing the bad foods from his diet. Be on probiotics for at least two weeks before getting strict on the diet.

WEEK THREE: Begin taking Glutagenics and chlorella.

WEEK FOUR: Begin a more strict form of the diet.

WEEK SEVEN OR EIGHT: Be on probiotics for at least six weeks or more before beginning Candida cleansing products. Always muscle test to be sure the body is ready to begin this phase and for dosage levels.

STAGE TWO

HEAVY METAL DETOXIFICATION

ABOUT WEEK 10 (or about three weeks after candida cleansing products have begun)

Muscle test to determine if it is time. If you have become comfortable with muscle test assessment then you can do this yourself, otherwise, ask for the help of your trusted practitioner who is versed in muscle testing. Ask the question, "is the body ready for heavy metal detoxification?" If the answer is "no", then continue on the candida cleansing products another week and re-test again with the question.

If the answer is "yes" then proceed to Dr. Andrew Cutler's method of heavy metal detoxification (as noted in the chapter in heavy metals). Get the help of a practitioner who is willing to assist you in following this specific protocol.

Dr. Klinghardt offers an additional example of heavy metal detoxification. This can also be seen at www.klinghardtacademy.com.

STAGE THREE

BRAIN SUPPORT (TIMING BASED ON INDIVIDUAL CHOICE)

Now that your child's body is free of pathogens and toxins, you are able to see his true personality, or who he really is, without all of those issues invading his brain.

If you haven't already done so, this is a good time to do neurofeedback. Homeopathic remedies are also very helpful with this. If you choose homeopathy, seek a professional homeopathic doctor for help.

The brain behaviors still left will be what you will work with per his individuality. For this reason, I refer you back to the chapter on brain support supplements.

There are also homeopathic remedies that are helpful with this.

IMPORTANT NOTE: If behaviors or learning are extremely impaired, you may wish to begin some brain support supplements as soon as stage one. As pathology heals, there may be less of a need, but sometimes we need help right away. Examples: L-tyrosine for focus, or GABA for anxiety, 5-HTP and St. John's Wort for depression.

DEWORMING (optional, but a good idea)

Once things are balanced, it is a good idea to consider deworming. It is always suggested for those on the autism spectrum or with learning or behavioral issues. The product Mimosa Pudica is best.

Unfortunately, it has a very strong, sour taste. I encapsulate it for my children. If your child will not take pills, you can hide the powder it in a smoothie.

See the chapter on pathogenic microbes for more information on deworming.

SUMMARY

Determine your child's baseline for health prior to beginning the program with muscle testing and any tests you feel would be helpful to you. Supplementation to support the brain and varying behavioral needs can be started as soon as you feel necessary.

As a parent who spends the most time with your child you can decide, per symptoms, which healing stage he needs to be on and when it is time to go to the next one. Watch for symptom changes. If you feel you have progressed too quickly then go back to the previous stage for a longer period of time or lower the dosage of supplements. Muscle testing can be helpful in determining your child's needs along the way. Don't be afraid to ask his body what it needs or what dosage is best at this time.

The products found in this chapter can be found at http://naturallyhealingautism.com/a-healthy-home/

CHAPTER 31

PREVENTION

A LOOK AT THE PARENTS TO BE

First, it is critical to identify the underlying issue. A survey of the gut pathology of both mother and father is a good place to start. A simple survey can be conducted prior to pregnancy to establish the health the GI tract of both parents. Candida and other pathogens can be transferred via the placenta to the baby in utero.

Have you or your partner ever experienced physical or emotional symptoms of digestive problems of any kind, trouble with elimination, irritability, anxiety? Do either of you have multiple cavities or problems with the teeth or mouth. Do you still, even intermittently, experience them, and if so, to what degree? If you would like to know specifically what your own flora is doing prior to conception, then you can order the Genova Labs tests for Microbiology analysis. This will tell you about your good bacteria levels, bad bacteria levels, and yeast. If there is concern of parasites, there are also tests for them. All of these tests can be purchased through www.crohns.net, 877-240-7528, and their staff is very helpful if you have questions.

For healthier babies the Candida cleanse should be done six months prior to conception. This would be best if done by both mother and father. If possible, begin the protocol two years prior to conception and continue on a healthy ongoing maintenance program. It is logical to believe that most couples do not have two years time prior to conception to cleanse. Three to six months time is helpful in clearing the gut pathology and heavy metals prior to conception.

SOON AFTER BIRTH

In the first few days after birth, have your child's fecal sample tested for any microforms by a reputable laboratory such as Diagnos-Techs (425)251-0596. A urine test is also a good idea to check for metabolites. Another good laboratory is Genova diagnostics. Their tests can be purchased online, with no doctor's office fee, at www.crohns.net, (877)240 7528. The results are emailed to you and a licensed practitioner is available to go over the results at no additional fee. Do this, especially, prior to any vaccinations. If your child's immune system is suppressed, any vaccines should be postponed until his GI tract is healthy and clear. See the chapter on pathogenic microbes and Candida for more information.

PROTECTING THE BRAIN

Many problems for infants arise in utero. We have talked in detail about the necessity to reduce environmental toxins such as electromagnetic fields, cleaning solutions, and pesticides in your life to assist your child's health and behavior. Proper nutrition is an essential component too.

A good prenatal vitamin contains most of the needed vitamins and minerals, but there are a few nutrients that may not be in sufficient amount or may not be in them at all. The most essential nutrient does not exist in your prenatal vitamin and must be taken during pregnancy, lactation and given to him for the rest of his life. This nutrient is omega-3 fatty acids.

OMEGA-3 FATTY ACIDS

One of the best supplements by far to support the proper health and development of your child's brain are omega-3 fatty acids. We have gone into great detail about them in this book. The importance I stress here is in the mother taking them during pregnancy and lactation for both her needs and the needs of the baby.

Omega-3 fatty acids are needed throughout the entire pregnancy and beyond, but are especially important during the last trimester of pregnancy. This is the period where the unborn child's neurological needs increase greatly. The most important component of omega-3s at this time is DHA. Studies have shown that even small amounts of omega-3s during pregnancy showed benefits. They are important in both fetal brain development and a child's neurodevelopment. A decrease in omega-3 fatty acids during pregnancy has showed both impaired developmental and behavioral scores. Studies have shown that infants and children whose mothers supplemented with only 200 mg of omega-3 fatty acids during pregnancy and lactation had a decreased risk of developing food allergies and IgE-associated eczema. Omega-3s are also neuroprotective.

By supplementing the mother's diet with an adequate amount of omega-3, it can assist both the mother and child with their essential fatty acid needs. DHA facilitates in the health of the reproductive organs for both men and women. They also assist in the production of breast milk. Mothers who take adequate amounts of omega-3 fatty acids have been shown to have reduced postpartum depression and more stable moods. This supplement should continue throughout breastfeeding and his entire life to support the needs of his nervous system.

The following recommendations are the minimal daily dosages established by the International Society for the Study of Fatty Acids and Lipids (ISSFAL).

- Infants (1 to 18 months): 0 to 15 pounds, 32 mg per pound
- Children (1.5 to 15 years): 15 mg per pound
- Adults: 500 mg (With a minimum of 220 mg EPA and 220 mg DHA)
- Pregnant and lactating women: 300 mg DHA per day

Of course, it is best to consult a physician for your personal needs. Children on the autism spectrum or with behavioral or learning disabilities often need more than a child who does not.

PROBIOTICS

All pregnant and lactating women need probiotics. They help to maintain the proper intestinal flora and are not contained in prenatal vitamins. If there are any probiotics in a vitamin, I can assure you it is not enough and the quality is minimal. If you have not taken probiotics previously, be sure to add them in slowly to minimize die-off reactions.

IODINE

More and more research is linking children on the autism spectrum and those with learning disabilities to iodine deficiency. The thyroid gland requires the proper amount of iodine to function normally. Thyroid hormones affect the development and functioning of the kidneys and the liver in utero, two of our key detoxifying organs. Iodine deficiency during pregnancy can cause the baby to have mental disabilities, mental retardation, deafness and an inability to thrive. It is also linked to autoimmune diseases. Discuss your needs with your doctor to be assured of adequate supplementation.

VITAMIN D

If a woman is deficient of vitamin D during her pregnancy, then the deficiency will be passed on to the baby. This can be especially common for babies born in the winter months since we get much of our vitamin D from the sun. Vitamin D helps neurons grow and survive. It is important in brain development and its protection. Vitamin D decreases heavy metal damage to the brain. It is also anti-inflammatory, assists with respiratory infections and asthma.

COMMON BIRTHING PRACTICES

EPIDERALS AND OXYTOCIN

Pitocin affects the levels of oxytocin in an unborn child. Oxytocin assists in the connection between mother and child, especially in the first six days after birth. If pitocin was given to the mother to hasten the birthing process, the level of oxytocin in the child could be altered. If oxytocin is altered it could affect the child's ability to connect emotionally with people. This has been seen in children with autism when they have difficulty with social interaction as well as empathy and showing affection.

CUTTING THE UMBILICAL CORD TOO SOON

The liver can become congested as early as birth. By cutting or clamping the umbilical cord before has completed its pulsing (less than about an hour after birth), it leaves the baby with a reduced volume of nutrient-filled blood, and an increased toxic load that was unable to be filtered out via the placenta. When burdened, the liver cannot filter toxins from food, water, air pollution, pesticides, medications, vaccinations, and more. This sets up the liver for early childhood development of gallstones, and adrenal weakness. See more information in chapter five on supporting the organs of detoxification.

GOOD PREVENTION:

1. Prior to conception I would have my husband's and my own metabolites checked for toxins via the U.S. Biotek's Environmental Pollutants Biomarker urine test from www.labinterpretation.com.
2. Prior to pregnancy, I would take the supplements recommended with the diet in this book. One month into the diet, I would begin the Candida cleansing products listed in the chapter "Candida Cleansing Supplements". If pregnant, I would use the diet to balance my system and slowly add in only probiotic use, unless otherwise advised by my doctor. I would take the ones I had muscle tested positive for at the dosages tested for so that toxic die-off is not too fast for my body to handle.
3. I would be sure that I took proper multivitamin and mineral supplements as well as a proper dosage of probiotics, essential fatty acids, B vitamins including folic acid, vitamin D, and iodine every day. This would be prior to and during pregnancy, during the duration of breastfeeding, and thereafter.

4. I would eat only organic foods and foods without artificial colors, preservatives, or chemicals, especially the excitotoxins MSG and aspartame.
5. See the dentist prior to conception for a check up. If possible, avoid going to the dentist during pregnancy, especially if I have mercury amalgam fillings or any possibility of infection.
6. Prior to conceiving, remove all mercury amalgam fillings. Be sure this is done by a bio-knowledgeable dentist who can remove the fillings without further toxicity to your body. To find a bio-dentist, go www.toxicteeth.org.
7. I would have the father of my child begin on the same detoxifying program at the same time that I began.
8. I would remove any toxic household cleaning or health products from my home and only use non-toxic formulas.
9. I'd do my best to avoid chemical exposure during pregnancy and after. If I lived in a town that had a large usage of pesticides or a mill that excreted toxic substances, I would move to a safer place. Going away to live with my mother in a different town could be an option. If I have to move myself and my child back to that toxic area after my child is born, my child's developing brain will continue to be exposed during development. Many problems can happen after the child's delivery, and I would not return to that environment.
10. I would be sure that my family was somewhat protected from electromagnetic field pollution by attaching GIA brand cell chips to our home phones, all cell phones, and electrical appliances, and in our vehicles. I would also wear a GIAlife pendant for the duration of my pregnancy and thereafter. I offer my website for those who are interested, www.giawellness.com/karenthomas. I would also turn off and unplug any electrical devices in the room I sleep in.
11. I would breastfeed for at least one solid year to two years without using formula to supplement. If this is not possible, I would add omega-3 fatty acids, with high DHA (docosahexanoic acid), to the child's organic formula and avoid soy.

12. When my child reached the age of six or seven months, I might offer small increments of pureed organic fruits or vegetables.
13. I would not introduce cow's milk at all.
14. I would not have my child use fluoride from any source.
15. I would only feed my child pure water from a source I was certain was free of toxins.
16. I would, after breastfeeding was complete and it was age appropriate, offer a multi-vitamin/mineral supplement to my child that was from a respected company known for its quality and high standards. I would be sure the product did not contain artificial ingredients or fillers.
17. I would minimize products with gluten, dairy, corn, and soy.
18. I would not vaccinate my child on the traditional American medical association schedule. If there were a life threatening epidemic I would do my own research and make my own educated decisions, only looking at single vaccines without toxins (if they existed). Homeopathy has many answers for this also.
19. If any vaccines were chosen, I would prefer it to be after my child was at least four to five years of age so I knew his brain was largely developed, and I could estimate that his immune system was strong and he was growing well. I would also never allow any live viruses to be used. I would choose single viruses, if possible, special ordered through my pharmacy. No vaccinations would be given in a period of less than two months apart.
20. I would not raise my child on the standard American diet of junk food such as sugar, high fructose corn syrup, hydrogenated fats, aspartame, monosodium glutamate, food colorings, and other chemical substances.
21. I would feed my child organic, nitrate-free, chemical-free foods.
22. I would show them my love and give them quality time everyday with minimal time in front of electronic equipment such as televisions, computers, or handheld devices.

These are just some of the things that I would do. What will you do?

What if we ate only healthy, whole, natural foods, limited or removed vaccine use, detoxified our bodies before conception, and did the same for our children. How many lives would change for the better?

FOR YOU MOM

We spend so much time taking care of our children that we often neglect ourselves. There is a serious concern in mothers of children with special needs regarding who will take care of their child if something happens to them. This is a very valid concern. Utilize the information in this book for yourself, and utilize local support groups and online supports groups too. Knowing that you are not alone holds more power for you than you can imagine.

It has been shown that the stress hormones of a mother with a child on the autism spectrum are the same as a soldier returning from the Gulf War. The stress is ongoing, so we must find solace. Do something enjoyable for yourself. Go see a funny movie with friends. Read a book that has nothing to do with health, autism, or children. Find books with a happy ending. Get massages and pedicures.

Remembering to watch him when he sleeps can help a lot. It brings back the thoughts and feelings of when he is pleasant, calm and happy. This helps us too.

SUMMARY

It is a good idea to test gut pathology, and neurological weaknesses prior to conception. This can allow you to detoxify or cleanse your system so that the baby has a healthy internal environment to grow in. If there is a family history of candida, gut issues, chemical sensitivities, or emotional instability for either parent, this should be taken into account in the testing and the results. Quality nutrition and necessary supplementation should be taken by mom to protect his gut and his brain prior to, after conception, during breastfeeding, and for the duration of his life.

After birth have the child's fecal sample tested by a reputable laboratory to be sure his gut pathology is healthy and strong. If needed, follow the many choices in this book to bring that back into balance. Never vaccinate if any brain or gut issues show weakness until you are certain your child is in optimum health. Even then, know that you as the parent have many choices to make based on the knowledge you have researched for yourself. Always practice good prevention.

The products found in this chapter can be found at http://naturallyhealingautism.com/a-healthy-home/

APPENDIX: ADDITIONAL RESOURCES

- Testosterone analysis: Dr. Mark Geier, MD, PH.D., mgeier@comcast.net, and ASDCenters.com 301-989-0548.
- Information on autism from, www.TACAnow.org
- www.autismone.org
- The center for autism related disorders (CARD), www.centerforautism.com
- For vision issues, www.autisticvision.com.
- For information on auditory issues and vestibular stimulation via the Tomatis method, www.tomatis.com.
- The autism research institute is the connection for DAN (defeat autism now) doctors, www.autismresearchinstitute.com. Depending on the doctor they may use traditional drug therapies including chelation methods which I do not recommend.
- National autism association, www.nationalautism.org.
- To look up scientific studies, www.pubmed.com
- www.crayhonresearch.com, (877)CRAYHON
- www.mercola.com
- www.futurehorizons-autism.com
- www.feingold.org
- www.noamalgam.com
- www.labinterpretation.com
- www.parentshelpingparents.com

Additional information on vaccines:

- Congressman Calls for Criminal Penalties at Vaccine Mercury Hearings
- http://mercola.com/2002/jul/3/vaccine_mercury.htm
- The Vaccine Guide: Risks and Benefits for Children and Adults by Randall Neustaedter
- Stephanie Cave's book, What your Doctor May Not Tell You About Children's Vaccinations. The issues and vaccinations are broken down and discussed individually, she offers an alternative schedule as well as some suggestions on how to best optimize the child's outcome if vaccination is the choice.
- Vaccination Risk Awareness Network at eddawest@netidea.com They are located in Winlaw, B.C. Tons of up-to-date information.
- VRAN (Vaccine Research Action Network) newsletter 4x/year.
- Email: cddawcst@@netidea.com
- Another good site: www.tinussmits.nl/english/
- Many books on the topic: many can be had from chiropractic association very cheaply. Also see the bibliography and suggested reading for more.

Websites on Fermented Foods

Many commercially made fermented foods lose their cultures due to processing and pasteurization. Below is a list of websites and recipes to help you make them yourself.

- www.gaps.me
- www.scdiet.org
- www.breakingtheviciouscycle.com
- www.pecanbread.com
- www.uclbs.org

LABORATORIES

If you do not have insurance, do not care for the doctors on your insurance plan and their methods, or prefer to start with self-testing without the added expenses, there are many available resources.

DIAGNOS-TECHS

Many other laboratories will not be able to detect the amoebas and parasites we are looking for. Although not all parasites will be detected even from the best lab, your chances for detection are best with this one. Diagnos-tech's laboratories, www.diagnostechs.com, 425-251-0596 has tests for stress/adrenals, malabsorption, gut inflammation, and more. Most natural practitioners carry these in their offices. Diagnos-techs results sheet offers a scale to show the level of what you have from mild to severe.

GENOVA LABS

Genova labs greatest benefit comes from growing out the bacteria. By doing this, they can assess the strength of the strain you carry. When they give you your results, they supply a panel that shows you a number scale to show the strength or weakness of the pathogen. It also shows you which natural products will work best against that strain in you. This specificity is huge when it comes to eradication.

There are several tests available, and they can be purchased online at www.crohns.net or call them at 877-240-7528.

DOCTORS DATA

www.doctorsdata.com

DIRECTLABS.COM (800)908-0000 (recommended by Dr. Shari Tenpenny.

- Heavy metal allergy test
- Hair analysis
- Saliva tests

- Water testing
- Testing for gluten, dairy, soy, and more: www.enterolab.com.

LABCORP, www.labcorp.com, detects the numbers necessary to find the genetic markers for mold biotoxin allergies.

Quest Diagnostics, www.questdiagnostics.com.

Dr. Mark Schauss, DB

Reno, NV 89511
775-851-3337
marks@labinterpretation.com
www.labinterpretation.com
www.labinterpretation.podhoster.com
www.MarkSchauss.com

BIBLIOGRAPHY AND SUGGESTED READING

All books by Angie Voss on sensory processing disorders.

Amen: Change Your Brain, Change Your Life. New York, Crown, 1998.

Amen: Healing ADD. New York, Berkley Books, 1991.

Amen: Magnificent Mind at Any Age. New York, Random House, 2008.

Amen: Unchain Your Brain. California, Mindworks Press, 2010.

Aron: The Highly Sensitive Child. New York, Broadway Books, 2002.

Atwater: Beyond the Indigo Children. Rochester, VT, Bear & Company, 2005.

Attwood: Asperger's Syndrome. London and Philadelphia, Jessica Kingsley Publishers, 2006.

Atwood: Asperger's Syndrome. London, Jessica Kingsley Publishers, 1998.

Bainbridge: Teenagers, A Natural History. Vancouver, BC, Greystone Books, 2009.

Balch: Prescription for Nutritional Healing. New York, Penguin Putnam, 2000.

Bartlett: The Physics of Miracles. Hillsboro, OR, Atria, 2009.

Bayly: Reflexology Today, The Stimulation of the Body's Healing Forces Through Foot Massage. Rochester, VT. Healing Arts Press, 1988.

Black: The Anti-Inflammation Diet and Recipe Book. Berkeley, Publishers Group West, 2006.

Blaylock: Excitotoxins, The Taste That Kills. Albuquerque, Health Press NA, Inc, 1997.

Blaylock: Health and Nutrition Secrets That Can Change Your Life. Albuquerque: Health Press, 2006.

Blaylock: Health and Nutrition Secrets That Can Save Your
Bock: Healing the New Childhood Epidemics. New York, Ballantine Books, 2007.
Brand-Miller: The New Glucose Revolution. Da Capo, 2009.
Braverman: The Edge Effect, Reverse or Prevent Alzheimer's, Aging, Memory Loss, Weight Gain, Sexual Dysfunction, and more. New York, Sterling Publishing, 2005.
Braverman: Younger Brain, Sharper Mind. New York, Rodale, 2007.
Brizendine: The Female Brain. New York, Broadway Books, 2006.
Brizendine: The Male Brain. New York, Broadway Book, 2010.
Brown, Wolf, King, Bork: The Parent's Guide to College for Students on the Autism Spectrum. Shawnee Mission, APC, 2012.
Brownstein: Iodine; Why You Need It, Why you Can't Live Without It. West Bloomfield, Medical Alternatives Press, 2006.
Brownstein: Overcoming Thyroid Disorders. West Boomfield, Medical Alternatives Press, 2008.
Burrows and Wagner: Understanding Asperger's Syndrome, A Guide for Teachers and Educators to Address the Needs of the Student. Arlington, Future Horizons, 2004.
Burton: The Candida Control Cookbook. Fairfield, Aslan, 2002.
Campbell & Campbell: The China Study. Dallas, BenBella Books, 2006.
Campbell-McBride: Gut and Psychology Syndrome. Cambridge, Medinform Publishing, 2010.
Canfield and Hansen: Chicken soup for Every Mom's Soul. Deerfield Beach, Florida, Health Communications, Inc. 2005.
Carrington: Try It On Everything, Discover the Power of EFT. Bethel, CT. try It Productions, 2008.
Carroll and Tober: The Indigo Children. Hay House International, 2008.
Carroll: The Indigo Children. Carlsbad, Hay House, 1999.
Carter: Mapping The Mind. University of California Press, 1998.
Carter: The Human Brain Book. DK Books, International, 2009.
Cave: What Your Doctor May Not Tell You About Children's Vaccinations. New York, Wellness /central, 2001.
Clark: Herbal Healing For Children. Summertown, Healthy Living Publications, 2011.

Converse: When Your Doctor Is Wrong: Hepatitis B Vaccine & Autism. U.S.A. Xlibris Corporation, 2002.

Coulter & Fisher: A Shot In The Dark. New York, Avery.

Cutler: Amalgam Illness, 1999.

Cutler: Hair Test Interpretation; Finding Hidden Toxicities, 2004.

D'Adamo: Eat Right For Your Type. New York, Penguin Group, 1996.

D'Adamo: Live Right For Your Type. New York, G.P. Putnam's Sons, 2001.

Davis & Keyser: Becoming the Parent You Want To Be. New York, Broadway Books, 1997.

DeFelice: Enzymes For Autism and Other Neurological Conditions. Minnesota, ThunderSnow Interactive, 2008.

DesMaisons: Potatoes Not Prozac. New York, Simon and Schuster, 2008.

Doctors' Prescription for healthy Living Magazine: New Hope For Autism. Topanga, Freedom Press, 2008.

Eden: Energy Medicine. New York, Penguin, 2008.

Eden: The Little Book of Energy Medicine. Penguin, 2012.

Essential Science Publishing: Essential Oils Desk Reference. U.S.A, 2007.

Faber & Mazlish: Siblings Without Rivalry. New York, Harper Collins, 2004.

Fallon: Nourishing Traditions Book of Baby and Childcare, 2013.

Gerber: Vibrational Medicine For the 21st Century. New York, Harper Collins, 2000.

Gershon: The Second Brain. New York, Harper and Collins, 1998.

Gittleman: Guess What Came to Dinner? Parasites and Your Health. New York, Penguin, 2001.

Gittleman: Zapped. New York, Harper Collins, 2010.

Gottschall: Breaking the Vicious Cycle. Baltimore Ontario, Kirkton Press, 2007.

Grandin: Thinking in Pictures. New York, Vintage Books, 2006.

Gray: The New Social Story Book. Arlington, TX, Jenison Public Schools, 2000.

Greene: The Explosive Child. New York, Harper Collins, 2001.

Guyton: Basic Neuroscience. Philadelphia, W.B. Saunders Company, 1991.
Hawkins: Power vs. Force, The Hidden Determinants of Human Behavior. Hay House, 2012.
Holland: The Pot Book: A Complete Guide to Cannabis; Its Role in Medicine, Politics, Science and Culture, 2010.
Holzapfel: Apple Cider Vinegar. Summertown, TN. Book Publishing Company, 2002.
Houghton Mifflin Company, 1984.
Huggins: The Nursing Mother's Companion, 2015.
Jonas and Jacobs: Healing With Homeopathy. New York, Warner, 1996.
Kaptchuk: The Web That Has No Weaver. New York, McGraw Hill Books, 2000.
Kaufmann: The Fungus Link. Rockwall, Media Trition, 2008.
Kelly and Ramundo: You Mean I'm Not Lazy, Stupid or Crazy? New York, Scribner, 2006.
Kirby: Evidence of Harm. New York, St. Martin's Griffin, 2005.
Kranowitz: The Out-Of-Sync Child. New York, Penguin Group, 2005.
Kurcinka: Raising Your Spirited Child. New York, Harper Collins, 1998.
Lancaster: Anger and the Indigo Child. Boulder, Wellness Press, 2002.
Lansky: The Impossible Cure. Portola Valley, R.L. Ranch Press, 2003.
Lee and Rosenbaum: Chlorella, The Sun-Powered Supernutrient and Its Beneficial Properties. New Canaan, CT. Kats Publishing, Inc, 1987.
Lieberman: The Gluten Connection. New York, Rodale, 2007.
Life. Albuquerque, Health Press, 2006.
Lipton: The Wisdom of Your Cells. Sounds True compact disc course, 2006.
Lloyd: The Healing Code. New York, Grand Central Life and Style, 2010.
Lynn: The Asperger Plus Child. Shawnee Mission, Kansas, APC, 2007.
Marshalla: Childhood Apraxia, 2001.
Matthews and Foster: Being smart About Gifted Children. Scottsdale, Great Potential Press, 2005.

McCandless: Children with Starving Brains. Bramble Books, 2007.
McCarthy: Louder Than Words. New York, Penguin Group. 2007.
Milne: The Heart of Listening: A Visionary approach to Craniosacral Work. Berkeley, North Atlantic Books, 1995.
Moritz, Andreas: The Liver and Gallbladder Miracle Cleanse. Berkeley: Ulysses Press, 2007.
Murphy: What Every Parent Should Know About Childhood Immunization. Boston, Earth Healing Products, 1994.
Murray: 5HTP, The Natural Way to Overcome Depression, Obesity, and Insomnia. Bantam Books, U.S. and Canada, 1999.
Myles, Cook, Miller, Rinner, Robbins: Asperger's Syndrome and Sensory Issues-Practical Solutions for Making Sense of the World. Shawnee Mission, Kansas, 2000.
Myles: Asperger Syndrome and Difficult Moments. Shawnee Mission, Kansas, APC, 1999.
Nambudripad: Living Pain Free. Buena Park, Delta, 1997.
Nambudripad: Say Goodbye To Allergy Related Autism: Buena Park: Delta, 1999.
Notbohm: Ten Things Every Child With Autism Wishes You Knew. Arlington, TX. Future Horizons, 2005.
Notbohm: Ten Things Your Student With Autism Wishes You Knew, 2006.
O'Shea: The Sanctity of Human Blood, Vaccination is not Immunization. San Jose, CA, Two Trees, 2005.
Ornstein and Thompson: The Amazing Brain. Boston,
Ortner: The Tapping Solution. Hay House, 2013.
Ozonoff, Dawson & McPartland: A Parent's Guide to Asperger Syndrome & High Functioning Autism. New York, Guilford Press, 2002.
Pera: Is It You, Me or Adult ADD? San Francisco, Alarm Press, 2008.
Price: Nutrition and Physical Degeneration. Lemon Grove, CA. price-Pottenger Nutrition Foundation, 2011.
Robbins: A Symphony in the Brain. New York, Jim Robbins, 2000.
Ross: Zang Fu, The Origin Systems of Traditional Chinese Medicine. London, Longman Group, 1990.
Schauss: Achieving Victory Over A Toxic World.bloomington, IN. author House, 2008.

Schwartz: Brain Lock: Free Yourself From Obsessive Compulsive Behavior. New York, Reganbooks, 1996.

Shapiro and Forrest: EMDR, Eye Movement Desensitization and Reprocessing. New York: Perseus Books, 2004.

Shoemaker: Surviving Mold. Baltimore, Otter Bay Books, 2010.

Shomon: The Thyroid Diet. New York, Harper Collins, 2004.

Taylor: Mind Programming. U.S.A. Hay House, 2009.

Tennant: Healing is Voltage. Jerry Tennant, 2011.

The Dana Foundation: Cerebrum. Washington, DC, Dana Press, 2010.

Trudeau: Natural Cures They don't Want you To Know About. Elk Grove Village, Alliance Publishing, 2004.

Truss: The Missing Diagnosis. Birmingham, The Missing diagnosis, Inc, 1985.

Upledger: A Brain Is Born. Berkeley, North Atlantic Books, 2010.

Verspoor & Smith: Autism: The Journey Back-Recovering the Self Through Heilkunst. Verspoor & P. Smith, 2005.

Virtue: The Care and Feeding of Indigo Children. Hay House Publishing, 2001.

Virtue: The Crystal Children-A Guide to the Newest Generation of Psychic and Sensitive Children. Hay House Publishing, 2003.

Weinberger: Candida Albicans: The Quiet Epidemic. San Anselmo, Stanley Weinberger, 2000.

Weinberger: Parasites: An epidemic in disguise. Larkspur, Stanley Weinberger, 1997.

Willey: Pretending to Be Normal. London, Jessica Kingsley Pubishing, 1999.

Wilson: Adrenal Fatigue. Petaluma, Smart Publications, 2006.

Wolcott: The Metabolic Typing Diet. New York, Random House, 2000.

Wurtman: The Serotonin Solution. New York, Ballantine Books, 2006.

www.gapsguide.com: Gaps Guide, Simple Steps To Heal Bowels, Body and Brain. Lashkov, 2009.

Yasko: Autism: Pathways to Recovery, 2009.

Yasko: Feel Good Nutrigenomics, 2014.

Young & Young: The pH Miracle. New York, Werner Books, 2002.

54463826R00317

Made in the USA
San Bernardino, CA
17 October 2017